CANADIAN SPORT SOCIOLOGY

Second Edition

CANADIAN SPORT SOCIOLOGY

Second Edition

Edited by

Jane Crossman

Lakehead University

THOMSON

NELSON

Australia   Canada   Mexico   Singapore   Spain   United Kingdom   United States

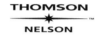

THOMSON

NELSON

Canadian Sport Sociology, Second Edition

Edited by Jane Crossman

**Associate Vice President,
Editorial Director:**
Evelyn Veitch

Publisher:
Veronica Visentin

Senior Acquisitions Editor:
Kevin Smulan

Marketing Manager:
William De Villiers

Senior Developmental Editor:
Katherine Goodes

**Photo Researcher/Permissions
Coordinator:**
Natalie Barrington

Content Production Manager:
Wendy Yano

Copy Editor/Proofreader:
Kelli Howey

Indexer:
Edwin Durbin

Manufacturing Coordinator:
Charmaine Lee-Wah

Design Director:
Ken Phipps

Interior Design:
Katherine Strain

Cover Design:
Dianna Little

Cover Image:
© Randy Faris/Corbis

Compositor:
ICC Macmillan Inc.

Printer:
Webcom

**Library and Archives Canada
Cataloguing in Publication Data**

Canadian sport sociology/edited
by Jane Crossman.—2nd ed.

Includes bibliographical references
and index.
ISBN 978-0-17-610322-4

1. Sports—Social aspects—
Canada—Textbooks. 2. Sports—
Canada—Sociological aspects—
Textbooks. I. Crossman, Jane

GV706.5.C35 2007   306.4'830971
C2007-900236-6

For P.T.
Because the craic with you has always been mighty

TABLE OF CONTENTS

PREFACE

After 25 years of teaching sport sociology, I have noticed that many of my students enter the study of this discipline with their own perceptions of what sport and physical activity are all about. One or two courses later, their perceptions have changed quite remarkably. For example, they learn that the opportunities to participate in sport aren't equitable; that the control of sport is in the hands of a minority, many of whom are Caucasian males of affluence; that racism in sport still exists today even though it may not be readily apparent when watching a contest on television or reading about it in newspapers; that economic and political forces shape what sport is today and what it might look like in the future; and that the mass media act as a filter of what we see and how we see it.

Although this text deliberately has a distinctly Canadian focus, we live in a world of connectedness, largely due to developments in technology. What happens in the world of sport outside our borders influences sport inside our borders. Our American neighbours feed us their sport images via the mass media and, as a result, we cannot help but be influenced by them. Professional teams that comprise the National Hockey League, Major League Baseball, and the National Basketball Association have both American- and Canadian-based teams. For generations, immigrants have been bringing their sports and their ways of doing physical activity to Canada. But we are not simply a carbon copy of another country or an amalgamation of countries. We are uniquely Canadian and, over time, we have shaped our own cultural ideologies and our own ways of interpreting sport.

The second edition of *Canadian Sport Sociology* has been expanded to include three additional chapters: Sociological Theories of Sport, Sport and Social Stratification, and Globalization. Two of the chapters in the first edition pertaining to deviance and violence and aggression have been combined into one chapter entitled Sport and Social Problems.

This book contains 15 chapters. Because the chapter sequence has been purposely coordinated, I recommend that the 15 chapters be read consecutively. However, since their content is so distinctive, it is possible to read the chapters in an altered order.

In the first chapter, I provide a foundation for understanding the study of sport sociology from a Canadian perspective. Following the definition and differentiation of terms relevant to the study of sport sociology, I explore the characteristics of sport and what makes Canadian sport unique. The focus then shifts to how people are socialized into, via, and out of sport.

In the second chapter, Dr. Ian Ritchie presents an overview of sociological theories that are the foundation for understanding the world, and more specifically for our purposes, the world of sport. The author states that since it is not feasible to present a complete inventory of theories, he will focus on four major ones: Durkheim's *functionalism*, Marx's *conflict theory*, Mead's *symbolic interactionism*, and *critical theories* (cultural, feminist, and race studies).

In Chapter 3, Dr. Don Morrow does a masterful job of condensing Canadian sport history from pre-1840 to the present day into one chapter. He highlights the people who influenced sport history as well as the existing social conditions and developments that have had such a profound effect on shaping the development of sport in Canada.

Dr. Rob Beamish, author of Chapter 4, addresses the inequalities of condition and opportunity that exist in sport today. He points out that in Canada we endorse an unequal, performance-based rewards system. Success is linked, for example, to proximity to facilities, gender, social class, and physical ability. He concludes the chapter by discussing the influence that baby boomers (those born between 1945 and 1960) will have on sport.

In Chapter 5, Drs. Victoria Paraschak and Susan Tirone explore discrimination in Canadian sport through race and ethnicity. They point out that sport provides opportunities to feel pride in one's own cultural heritage; unfortunately, the system is structured so that some individuals—that is, those of white, European heritage—feel more pride than others. When this happens, state the authors, those who are discriminated against often form leagues of their own. The sport and leisure preferences of minority ethnic people are described as well as the distinctions between the theories of marginality and ethnicity. How new Canadians pursue sport and leisure is discussed, with specific reference to two studies that examine the meaning of sport and leisure for South Asian women and teenagers. The need to create equal opportunities in sport for all Canadian people is a fundamental message in this chapter.

Gender issues are a topic integral to any comprehensive treatment of social issues pertaining to sport sociology. In Chapter 6, Dr. Helen Jefferson Lenskyj helps us understand the current issues relevant to gender and sport. The differences between sexes with regard to sport-related attitudes are outlined. The author explains that simply "opening the door" to more opportunities won't necessarily solve the problems of marginalization and exclusion. Harassment, violence against women, and sexual abuse are also discussed in this chapter.

Dr. Ralph Wheeler, in Chapter 7, outlines the current sport system in Canada for children and youth, including school, community, and private agencies. Potential reasons for the high rate of sport dropout are outlined. From a balanced perspective, Dr. Wheeler presents some of the problems associated with sport for children and youth, and offers solutions to remedy these problems.

In Chapter 8, Dr. Patricia Lally considers the relationship between sport and educational institutions in Canada, from public school through to university. She describes the existing situation in each of the systems and brings to the fore the difficulties inherent in each. The situation, Dr. Lally points out, is not a particularly encouraging one.

Dr. Kevin Wamsley, author of Chapter 9, addresses the fact that sport is replete with social problems. Topics covered include doping, injuries, and violence, and how they are interconnected. The author also explores how such issues are, in part, a result of the ways that sport is organized and understood not only by participants, but also by sport leaders and sport consumers. Theories of aggression are explained along with a historical overview of how violence in sport has grown in our society.

In Chapter 10, Drs. Steve Jackson, Jay Scherer, and Scott Martyn explain the influence, extent, and power the media has in shaping what we know and how we think. The authors point out that the media operate in a global economy. A section in this chapter is devoted to the historical development of televised sport as well as broadcast rights. Finally, light is shed on the multitude of viewing options that are and will be available to sport consumers.

Chapter 11, written by Dr. Marc Lavoie, is comprised largely of a case study of the 2004–05 NHL lockout to demonstrate how, today, economics is the engine that drives the sport machine. Addressed in this chapter are issues such as collective bargaining agreements, salary inflation, revenues and operating losses, payroll caps, revenue sharing, and the role the public sector plays in the construction of sport venues. Students with a keen interest in the economic side of professional sport will find this chapter a fascinating read.

Dr. Jean Harvey, in Chapter 12, focuses on the marriage between politics and sport. He provides a historical overview of the Canadian government's involvement in sport and the reasons for this involvement. Also included in this chapter is the controversial topic of government subsidy for professional sports franchises. Harvey concludes the chapter by discussing programs developed to assist Canadian athletes and sport organizations as well as the health and fitness of the general population.

With the realization that the process of globalization affects sports both culturally and economically, Dr. David Whitson offers an exciting new chapter to this edition. In Chapter 13, he discusses both the upside and downside to globalization, homing in on transnational corporations and the sports labour market. He points out that, thanks to electronic media, professional sport is now marketed and consumed around the globe.

In the penultimate chapter, Dr. Christopher Stevenson discusses the relationships that exist between sport and religion—more specifically, sport and Christianity. He first questions the modern claim that sport *is* religion by outlining the similarities and differences between the two. He then provides a history of the development of the connection between the two from the late fourth century through to today's "muscular Christianity." Contemporary topics such as superstition and sport, the dilemmas that exist for professing Christians involved in competitive sport, and evangelical Christianity's use of sport are discussed.

In the final chapter, Dr. Dwight Zakus discusses current trends in Canadian sport and also what the future may hold. First, he presents models of change. Then, in order to be able to make predictions, he outlines the current trends with regard to population growth and aging, immigration, urbanization, and sport demographics. In a global context, future directions for sport through culture, government involvement, and new technologies are discussed in depth.

On behalf of all the contributors, I hope you enjoy reading this book—and, furthermore, that it provides you with a sound basis for understanding sport sociology from a uniquely Canadian perspective.

—Jane Crossman
January 2007

ACKNOWLEDGMENTS

The completion of this text would not have been possible had it not been for the willingness of the contributors to share their expertise. To each of them I extend my sincere gratitude and I trust that readers will appreciate their knowledge, insights, and wisdom.

The contributors and I greatly appreciated the advice and guidance of our colleagues in their review of the text and the manuscript:

Robert Argue, Ryerson University
Michael Atkinson, McMaster University
Peggy Gallant, St. Francis Xavier University
Larena Hoeber, University of Western Ontario
Ray Kardas, Grande Prairie Regional College
Klaus Meier, University of Western Ontario
Nicole Neverson, McMaster University
Ian Ritchie, Brock University
Monika E. Schloder, University of Calgary
Geoff Smith, Queen's University

Also, I thank Thomson Nelson for their willingness to run with a second edition. Specific thanks go to Cara Yarzab, who kick-started this project; my marvellous and motivating developmental editor, Katherine Goodes; Kelli Howey, the best copy editor I have ever had the privilege of working with; Natalie Barrington, who skilfully handled the inclusion of photographs, tables, and figures; and Wendy Yano, the production editor who willingly continued to share her expertise from the first edition.

A special thank you to Trish McGowan, who provided constructive comments regarding my chapter, and to Paulene McGowan, who has been my mainstay since the earth's crust hardened.

CONTRIBUTORS

EDITOR

Dr. Jane Crossman is a Professor in the School of Kinesiology at Lakehead University, where she is Graduate Coordinator and also an Adjunct Professor in the Department of Sociology. She received her Ph.D. from Ohio State University in 1979. She teaches undergraduate and graduate sport sociology courses and a graduate course in mental training. Her primary research interest in sport sociology pertains to the newspaper coverage of sporting events, most recently the grand slam events in tennis. Jane also has several publications pertaining to the psychosocial dimensions of sports injuries. In 2001, she edited a book entitled *Coping with Sports Injuries: Psychological Strategies for Rehabilitation*. Jane also contributed a chapter to the book *The Sport Scientist's Research Adventures*, in which she gave insights into the challenges and gratification of being a researcher. Jane is on the editorial board of the *Journal of Sport Behavior* and regularly reviews for a number of journals and texts in the fields of sport sociology and psychology. She has helped numerous elite athletes with their mental preparation and is a Fellow of the Association for the Advancement of Applied Sport Psychology and a member of the North American Society for Sport Sociology. During sabbatical leaves, Jane has been a Visiting Professor at the Universities of Exeter and Brighton (UK) and the University of Otago (New Zealand). When not working, Jane enjoys spending time with her family, which includes exercising a lively border collie and writing fiction.

CONTRIBUTORS

Dr. Rob Beamish, a former Associate Dean (Studies) in the Faculty of Arts and Science at Queen's University, Kingston, Ontario, is currently the Head of the Department of Sociology. Rob received his Ph.D. in sociology at the University of Toronto, and after four years on faculty in the Faculty of Physical Education and Health at U of T he began a joint appointment in the Department of Sociology and the School of Kinesiology and Health at Queen's. Rob was a guest professor at the Free University of Berlin in 1989 and 1991. Rob has taught graduate and undergraduate courses in sociology, sport sociology, and sport policy. His research centres on two distinct, yet interrelated areas: the development and presentation of Marx's theoretical ideas, and the critique of high-performance sport. Rob's work on Marx examines how the publication and posthumous presentations of his literary estate impact upon how Marx was, and is, interpreted and understood. *Marx, Method, and the Division of Labor*, and "The Making of the Manifesto" (*Socialist Register*, 1998), are representative pieces in this area. The recently completed (with Ian Ritchie of Brock University) *Fastest, Highest, Strongest: The Critique of High-Performance Sport*, "Marxism and the Critique of Olympic Sport" (*Marxism and Sport*, Routledge), and *Q: What Do You Do For A Living? A: I'm An Athlete* are representative of Rob's writing in the area of sport and work.

Dr. Jean Harvey is a Professor at the School of Human Kinetics and Director of the Research Centre for Sport in Canadian Society at the University of Ottawa. He received his Doctorat de 3ième cycle in sociology at the Université de Paris VII in 1984. He teaches undergraduate and graduate sport sociology courses. His primary research interests are the political economy of sport, sport policy, sport and globalization, and social inequalities and sport. In 1988 he co-edited with Hart Cantelon a book entitled *Not Just a Game: Essays in Canadian Sport Sociology*. Jean has published extensively on sport and social theory, sport and politics, and sport and globalization. He has been and still is principal investigator and co-applicant on several Social Sciences and Humanities Research Council grants and on research contracts with private foundations. Currently, Jean's major research project touches on a longitudinal evaluation of the impact of sport and physical activity programs for underprivileged kids in Quebec funded by Québec en forme, an initiative of the Fondation Lucie et André Chagnon and of the Government of Québec. At 50, Jean enjoys a new sport career as a soccer player in a plus-35 division six league.

Dr. Steve Jackson is a Professor in the School of Physical Education at the University of Otago, Dunedin, New Zealand, and has served as visiting Professor at the University of Jyvaskyla (Finland), National Taiwan Normal University, and the University of British Columbia. He received his undergraduate degree from the University of Western Ontario and his master's and Ph.D. at the University of Illinois. He teaches in the area of Sociology of Sport and Sport Media. His research interests include media, sport, and culture; globalization and sport; and sporting identities. He is co-editor of three books: *Sport, Culture & Advertising: Identities, Commodities and the Politics of Representation*; *Sport Stars: The Cultural Politics of Sporting Celebrity*; and *Sport in New Zealand Society*. He has published in a wide range of journals, including the *Sociology of Sport Journal*, *International Review for the Sociology of Sport*, *Journal of Sport and Social Issues*, *Culture, Sport & Society*, *Media, Culture and Society*, and the *Journal of Sport Management*. He has served on the editorial boards of the *Sociology of Sport Journal*, the *International Review for the Sociology of Sport*, and the *International Journal of Sport Management and Marketing*. He is currently the General Secretary for the International Sociology of Sport Association (ISSA). Steve enjoys travel and playing ice hockey.

Dr. Patricia Lally is an Associate Professor in the Health and Physical Education Department at Lock Haven University, where she teaches psychological and sociological aspects of sport and physical activity and is coordinator of the minor in Sport and Exercise Psychology. Trish received her undergraduate degree from McGill University, her master's degree from the University of Ottawa, and her doctorate from the University of Toronto, where she also completed a post-doctoral fellowship. Trish's research focuses on the psychosocial development of youth and young adults through sport and physical activity, particularly identity and career development and issues of retirement and transition. Trish has published numerous journal articles on athletic identity and retirement, as well as book chapters on coaching, athletic injury and coping, and initiations in sport. She regularly presents at national conferences and is an active member of the Association for the Advancement of Applied Sport Psychology. She is a regular reviewer for *the Journal of Sport Behavior* and guest reviewer for the *Journal of Applied Sport Psychology* and *The Sport Psychologist*. Trish also works and volunteers as a sport psychology consultant with athletes, coaches, and parents in developmental and elite-level sport. Originally from Ottawa, Trish lives with her husband and daughter in State College, Pennsylvania, is an avid runner, and has run several marathons including the Boston Marathon.

Dr. Marc Lavoie is a Professor in the Department of Economics at the University of Ottawa, where he started teaching in 1979, having obtained a B.A. (1976) at Carleton University and a Ph.D. (1979) at the University of Paris (Panthéon-Sorbonne). He is a member of the

Research Centre on Sport in Canadian Society and a vice-president of the International Association of Sports Economists. He has published two books on the economics of ice hockey: *Avantage numérique, l'argent dans la Ligue nationale de hockey* (1997) and *Désavantage numérique, les francophones dans la LNH* (1998), and nearly 20 articles on the economics of sport or about discrimination in sport. Lavoie is also an expert in heterodox economics, having published *Foundations of Post-Keynesian Economic Analysis* (1992) and *Introduction to Post-Keynesian Economics* (2006). He was the co-editor of a book on the works of Milton Friedman (1993) and on *Central Banking in the Modern World* (2004), and an associate editor of the *Encyclopedia of Political Economy* (1999). Lavoie has been a Visiting Professor at the Universities of Bordeaux, Nice, Rennes, Dijon, Grenoble, Limoges, Lille, Paris 1 and Paris 13, and Curtin University in Perth (Australia). Previously, he was a carded athlete and a member of the fencing squad of the Canadian Olympic Team in 1976 and 1984; he was seven times Canadian senior sabre champion between 1975 and 1986.

Dr. Helen Jefferson Lenskyj is a Professor in the Department of Sociology and Equity Studies in Education, Ontario Institute for Studies in Education, University of Toronto, and has a cross-appointment to the Faculty of Physical Education and Health. A sport sociologist, she has written eight books, her first being *Out of Bounds: Women, Sport and Sexuality* (Women's Press, 1986), as well as more than 60 articles in journals and magazines. Her most recent sport-related books are *Inside the Olympic Industry: Power, Politics and Activism* (SUNY, 2000), *The Best Olympics Ever? Social Impacts of Sydney 2000* (SUNY, 2002), and *Out on the Field: Gender, Sport and Sexualities* (Women's Press, 2003). Her most recent book, *A Lot to Learn: Women and Education in 20th Century Australia and Canada* (Women's Press, 2005), uses family history and her own autobiography to explore girls' and women's education. She is currently working on a sequel titled *Growing Up in the 50s: Places, People and Identities in an Australian Girl's Childhood.* She is a recreational athlete with a particular passion for swimming and canoeing.

Dr. Scott Martyn is an Associate Professor in the Faculty of Human Kinetics at the University of Windsor. As a former Social Sciences and Humanities Research Council of Canada Doctoral Fellow, Scott spends much of his time investigating the historical evolution of the Olympic Games and affiliated insignia as sport marketing properties. He has served on the executive council of the International Centre for Olympic Studies, and continues to serve on executive councils of the North American Society for Sport History and the International Society for Comparative Physical Education and Sport. Along with an ever-increasing number of edited volumes, chapters, articles, and presentations, he has co-authored a book entitled *Selling the Five Rings: The IOC and the Rise of Olympic Commercialism* (University of Utah Press, 2002), with a revised edition released in July 2004. He is the chief editor of *International Sports Studies* and the managing editor of *Olympika: The International Journal of Olympic Studies,* and regularly reviews for a number of other journals and texts in the fields of sport history and commercialism. He is currently the principal investigator in a SSHRC-funded project entitled "Buying the Five Rings: Television Networks, Corporate Sponsors, and Olympic Commercialism" and a co-investigator in two other funded projects. Scott's knowledge in computer web-based design has enabled him to edit for several scholarly websites. His technologically advanced skills and teaching methods allow him to realize the full potential of the multimedia classroom.

Dr. Don Morrow is a Professor in the Faculty of Health Sciences at the University of Western Ontario, London, Ontario, where he is the Director of the Bachelor of Health Sciences Program. He received his Ph.D. from the University of Alberta. He teaches and does research in the academic areas of sport history, primarily Canadian, and sport literature. Don is the recent co-author of *Sport in Canada: A History* (Oxford University Press, 2005), his seventh book. In terms of historical research, his primary areas of research interest include Montreal sport and the organization of sport in the nineteenth century; sport journalism and journalists and the media language of sport; biographies, "heroes," and stars in sport; and festivals and celebrations connected to sporting events. Don has been the editor-in-chief of *Sport History Review* (formerly the *Canadian Journal of History of Sport*) since 1996 and he has served as a president of both the North American Society for Sport History and the Sport Literature Association. An elected International Fellow of the American Academy of Kinesiology and Physical Education, Don also serves as the Chair of the Research and Development Committee of the International Coach Federation (ICF). The ICF is the world's largest organization devoted to the development of life/executive/personal coaching and coaching research.

Dr. Victoria Paraschak is an Associate Professor of Kinesiology at the University of Windsor, where she teaches sociology of sport, government and sport, social construction of leisure, and outdoor recreation. She received a BPE from McMaster University in 1977, an MHK from the University of Windsor in 1978, and a Ph.D. from the University of Alberta in 1983. The primary focus of her research is Aboriginal peoples in sport, and in physical cultural practices more broadly. An integral part of this work is her involvement in government sport and recreation policy in the Northwest Territories. Her work focuses on power relations, social construction, self-determination, and the creation, reproduction, and/or reshaping of cultural practices through the duality of structure. In 1999, she took a year's leave to work with seven different Northwest Territories sport and recreation organizations and establish a direction for the new millennium. This was done through the creation of a joint vision, principles, priorities, and strategic plans for the sport and recreation system. In her 2006–07 sabbatical, she looked at the creation of health services for the Canada Games held in Whitehorse, Yukon, in February 2007. She examined the interface between sport and public health perspectives on such services and the health services legacy for the Yukon from these Games, and created a transfer of knowledge document on healthcare capacity requirements for hosting future Canada Games.

Dr. Ian Ritchie is Associate Professor in the Department of Physical Education and Kinesiology at Brock University, St. Catharines, Ontario. Ian received his Ph.D. in sociology from Bowling Green State University, Ohio, where his studies concentrated on classical and contemporary sociological theory. He teaches courses in sport sociology and sociology of the modern Olympic Games. Ian's research interests include performance-enhancing drug use in sport, media, gender, and the modern Olympic movement; his publications have been included in the *International Review for the Sociology of Sport*, *Sport History Review*, *The International Journal of the History of Sport*, the *International Journal of Sport Management and Marketing*, in addition to other journals and edited volumes; he most recently co-authored (with Rob Beamish) the book *Fastest, Highest, Strongest: A Critique of High-Performance Sport* (Routledge, 2006). Ian is also a member of the International Sociological Association and the International Sociology of Sport Association. A former varsity rower and coach, he now enjoys long-distance trail and marathon running, hiking, golfing, and cycling, along with regular outdoor travel, hiking, and camping, in particular in various mountainous regions of North America including the American southwest and southern Utah, Yukon Territory, Alaska, and Baffin Island.

Dr. Jay Scherer is an Assistant Professor in the Faculty of Physical Education and Recreation at the University of Alberta, Edmonton, Alberta. He received his Ph.D. from the University of Otago (New Zealand) in 2004. Jay teaches undergraduate courses in sport sociology and a graduate course in sport and popular culture. His primary research interests include globalization and sport, the commodification of national sporting mythologies, and sport and popular culture. Jay's research has been published in a number of journals including the *Sociology of Sport Journal*, *Policy Sciences*, *New Media & Society*, *Sport in Society*, *Cultural Studies/Critical Methodologies*, the *International Journal of Sport Management and Marketing*, and the *International Journal of Sports Marketing and Sponsorship*. Jay enjoys reading, playing the guitar, travel, and hiking in Canada's Rocky Mountains.

Dr. Christopher Stevenson is a Professor in the Faculty of Kinesiology at the University of New Brunswick, Fredricton, New Brunswick. He completed his undergraduate degree in England as a double major in zoology and botany. He took a master's degree in exercise physiology at the University of British Columbia in Vancouver, but during that time took a sociology course as an elective and his eyes were opened. He went to Stanford University in California and did an M.A. in sociology and a Ph.D., and soon after came to teach at the University of New Brunswick. His research interests have included examining the careers of athletes; the dilemmas of Christian athletes in attempting to reconcile the values of their faith with the expectations, demands, and values of elite competitive sport; and, most recently, various aspects of masters swimming. Chris is the past-editor of the *Sociology of Sport Journal*, and former Dean of the Faculty of Kinesiology at the University of New Brunswick.

Dr. Susan Tirone is the Associate Director (Graduate Program) and Associate Professor in the School of Health and Human Performance, Dalhousie University, Halifax, Nova Scotia. She completed her Ph.D. at the University of Waterloo in the field of Leisure Studies and teaches undergraduate and graduate courses at Dalhousie. Susan's research focuses on people who live at the margins of Canadian society with an emphasis on their leisure. Her studies have explored how leisure is either enhanced or constrained by various societal factors such as immigration status, poverty, race, and ethnicity. In recent years she has conducted several studies of children and families who are immigrants to Canada from non-Western countries, a study of families and children living in a low-income housing development in Atlantic Canada, and is a member of a national research team that studied the accessibility of municipal recreation services for children and families in low-income communities. She is the principal investigator for a longitudinal study of South Asian Canadians and a member of the Coasts Under Stress research project, which produced several publications including book chapters, journal articles, and a video about the lives of youth in Northern Newfoundland called *It's Who We Are, It's Our Ways*. Susan's recent publications include book chapters and articles appearing in *Canadian Ethnic Studies*, *Leisure/Loisir*, and *Canadian Journal of Community Mental Health*. Susan is a member of a small special-interest choir in Halifax and is a member of the local dory rowing club in the coastal community where she lives.

Dr. Kevin Wamsley is Professor in the School of Kinesiology and Associate Dean of the Faculty of Health Sciences at The University of Western Ontario, London, Ontario. He received his Ph.D. from the University of Alberta in 1992. He has two primary areas of research interest: sport and masculinity in nineteenth-century Canada, and politics and gender in the Olympic Games. In 2005, he co-authored *Sport in Canada: A History*. Between 1999 and 2005, he was Director of the International Centre for Olympic Studies and co-editor of *Olympika: The International Journal for Olympic Studies*. In 2005, he co-edited *Global Olympics: Historical and Sociological Studies of the Modern Games*. Kevin has published numerous articles in international journals and chapters in books related to these areas of research interest.

Dr. Ralph Wheeler is an Associate Professor in the School of Human Kinetics and Recreation at Memorial University, St. John's, Newfoundland. Since 1982, he has played a significant role in the development of a strong physical education preparation program within the faculty. Ralph, who completed his Ph.D. at the University of Alberta, has been instrumental in the review and enhancement of the physical education school program over the years and in providing pre-service teachers with the necessary skills to become successful teachers. He has been active as well in the education of many of the province's coaches, involved for more than 20 years as a course conductor and provincial coordinator (swimming) under the National Coaching Certification Program. Ralph has served on many provincial and national committees promoting physical education and sport and in 1996 served as the general chair for the National CAHPERD Conference. He continues to play a significant role in the development of a strong physical education preparation program within the faculty. In 2006, Ralph was awarded the Certificate of Honor from the Provincial Physical Education Council for his outstanding contribution to the profession.

Dr. David Whitson is a Professor in the Department of Political Science at the University of Alberta, Edmonton, Alberta. He did his Ph.D. at the University of Queensland in Australia, and has taught at Queen's University and in the UK. He is co-author, with Rick Gruneau, of the widely acclaimed *Hockey Night in Canada: Sport, Identities, and Cultural Politics* (Garamond, 1993), and more recently co-editor, also with Rick Gruneau, of *Artificial Ice: Hockey, Culture, and Commerce* (Broadview, 2006). He is an enthusiastic fan of hockey and soccer, and an active cyclist and runner. In addition to his interests in sports, David is also interested in the effects of globalization in rural Canada, and produced a pair of radio shows on this topic, with Roger Epp, for CBC *Ideas* in 2004. He is also co-editor, with Roger Epp, of *Writing Off the Rural West: Globalization, Governments, and the Transformation of Rural Communities* (University of Alberta Press, 2001).

Dr. Dwight Zakus is a Senior Lecturer in the Department of Tourism, Leisure, Hotel and Sport Management at Griffith University on the Gold Coast of Queensland, Australia. His doctorate was earned form the University of Alberta. Dwight teaches human resource management, organizational theory, and sport studies at both the undergraduate and postgraduate levels in the sport management program at the Griffith Business School. His publications include a book on ethical decision-making in sport and recreation, and a wide variety of articles and book chapters in his main research areas of the Olympic movement, social capital, and volunteering, as well as in his general research interests of sport studies and sport philosophy. Dwight is on the editorial board of *Sporting Traditions* and the *Journal of the International Committee for Health, Physical Education, Recreation, Sport and Dance* and completes a wide number of ad hoc reviews. He belongs to an eclectic number of scholarly groups across disciplines (NASSM, IRSS, SMAANZY, EASM, ASSH). Dwight has been a visiting scholar at the Vaxjo University (Sweden), the National University of Education (Singapore), Leicester University (England), and the University of Regina (Canada). When not bogged down in academic work, he attempts to be a golfer, enjoys watching rugby, and spends time with his wife and their dog.

CHAPTER 1

SPORT SOCIOLOGY IN THE CANADIAN CONTEXT: AN INTRODUCTION

Jane Crossman

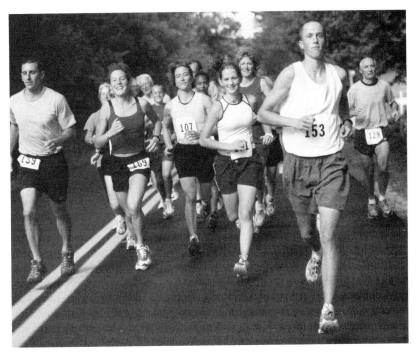

Sport provides people of all ages opportunities for socialization.

Yellow Dog Productions/The Image Bank/Getty Images

We run, not because we think it is doing us good, but because we enjoy it and cannot help ourselves. The more restricted our society and work become, the more necessary it will be to find some outlet for this craving for freedom. No one can say, "You must not run faster than this, or jump higher than that." The human spirit is indomitable.
Sir Roger Bannister (the first sub–four minute miler)

I am a huge believer in giving back and helping out in the community and the world. Think globally, act locally . . . I believe that the measure of a person's life is the effect they have on others.
Steve Nash (National Basketball Association player, who is Canadian)

Students study sport sociology for varied reasons: as a requirement of their course of study; because of a keen or casual interest in sports either as active participants or as spectators; or perhaps simply because the course fits into their timetable! Whatever the reason, one thing is certain: sport is an indelible part of the fabric that makes up Canadian society. In addition to the weather, sport is a common topic of conversation among Canadians of all ages—a kind of social lubricant, so to speak. We discuss the latest scandal that has rocked the sports world, the chances of our favourite National Hockey League (NHL) team making the playoffs, how our curling foursome is playing, or how the local soccer league is progressing.

For better or worse, sport is all around us. Just about every time we turn on the television and flip around the stations, we see sport. The Internet is loaded with sports-specific sites that offer live feeds, recent and past game results and statistics, insider information about teams and players, and even fantasy leagues where participants can control the destiny of their chosen players. Most city newspapers devote an entire section to sports, knowing that approximately 25 percent of readers purchase newspapers for their sports coverage alone. Many of the radio stations we listen to have frequent sports updates.

But we aren't just a nation that follows sports. Some parents devote huge amounts of their time, energy, and money so that their children can participate in organized sport. Provinces, mindful of the declining fitness levels and soaring obesity rates of children and youth, are taking a hard look at extending the number of hours per week devoted to physical education. Colleges and universities offer a wide range of intramural and interschool sports for both women and men. The choice of activities for Canadians to participate in abounds. For example, Canada has approximately 2,200 arenas and 1,300 curling rinks, and more than 2,500 golf courses—650 in Ontario alone, making it one of the most concentrated golf regions in North America. Many of these activities are not just sports; they're social and cultural events played for the fun of friendly competition. Some baby boomers now reaching retirement are spending significant amounts of their leisure time actively involved in their favourite sport and physical activity.

Minority groups, who have traditionally been left out of the sport equation, are now finding more opportunities to compete. For example, the 2006 Winter Paralympic Games in Torino, Italy, had 477 competitors from 39 countries. The North American Indigenous Games held in Denver, Colorado, in 2006 had 8,000 competitors. Sydney, Australia, home of the 2002 Gay Games, saw 11,000 athletes from 70 countries competing. While there is no doubt that the opportunities to "do sport" have increased for minority groups, their participation is still marginalized and trivialized by the media and society at large. While the number of women actively participating in sport has swelled in the past decade, they are still underrepresented in administrative and leadership positions. For example, in 2006 women comprised only 12.2 percent of the 115-member International Olympic Committee (IOC), and of the 434 coaches in the Canadian Interuniversity Sport (CIS) only 20 percent were women.

While a layperson may think that the world of sport is devoid of the problems that plague our society, nothing could be further from the truth. The ability to share in the sport experience is still a struggle for some segments of our Canadian society—segments that will be clearly identified in this text. Sport continues to make the headlines, but all too often for the wrong reasons. Moral reasoning decreases as the seriousness and organizational structure of sport increases. Inequality of opportunity, discriminatory practices, exploitation, strikes, drug use, and illegal gambling have become the unfortunate byproducts of an industry where the focus has shifted away from the process to the product.

My students walk into their first sport sociology class with preconceived ideas about the world of sport and how it works. For example, because of the predominance of African American athletes in certain sports, some of them have the misconception that racism doesn't exist in sport. These ideas have been formed through their own experiences and observations and those of others. It is certain that by studying sport sociology from a scientific and analytical perspective, eyes are opened about what is real and what is true about sport as we know it today.

SO WHERE DOES THE STUDY OF SPORT SOCIOLOGY FIT IN?

Sociology is the study of human social behaviour. Sociologists study social interactions that take place between humans, groups, and societies. They examine the ways in which social structures and institutions (e.g., family, class, and social problems) influence society. They are concerned with the social rules and processes that not only bind people, but also separate them. Because sociology is concerned with our behaviour as social beings, subdisciplines have emerged that are broad in scope and diverse in nature. One of those subdisciplines is called *sport sociology*. Sport sociologists study humans involved in sport (e.g., athletes, coaches, fans, team owners), the institutions and social structures that affect their sport experience (e.g., education, mass media, economics, politics, religion), and the processes that occur in conjunction with sport (e.g., social stratification and mobility, deviance, violence, inequality).

The study of sport and its meaning in Canadian society today is a complex, controversial, critical, and oftentimes disturbing pursuit. It is also fascinating—so much so that it can foster stimulating discussion on a diverse range of topics. Like it or not, sport is an integral component of the fabric of Canadian society.

ORIGINS OF SPORT SOCIOLOGY

The academic study of sport sociology is relatively new. Scientific research in the field didn't exist prior to 1960. From 1965 to 1969, Gerald Kenyon of the University of Wisconsin published a series of articles devoted to the sociology of sport, positioning it "firmly within the positivistic perspective of science" (Sage, 1997, p. 326). In the late 1960s the annual meetings of the American Alliance for Health, Physical Education and Recreation (Dance was added in 1979) included a session devoted to the sociology of sport. In 1976, this same association founded the Sociology of Sport Academy with the purpose of coordinating and promoting the study of sport sociology (Sage, 1997).

The 1960s and 70s constituted an important time for the development of the study of sport sociology. During that time there was much unrest in North America, particularly with regard to the United States' involvement in the war in Vietnam, as well as the civil rights movement. In 1968, during the medal presentation at the Summer Olympics in Mexico City, two African American athletes, John Carlos and Tommie Smith, made a gloved black power salute, thereby using sport as a vehicle to broadcast to the world their despondency with the plight of African Americans. This gesture was symbolic of the imbalance of power that prevailed not only for African Americans, but also for other minority groups, and sport was no exception. Sport sociologists understood that they needed to re-examine sport, and so an organized structure came into being.

A society for the study of sport sociology (which later became the North American Society for Sport Sociology [NASSS]) emerged after a Big Ten Symposium in 1978, thanks largely to the rallying cry of sport sociologist Andrew Yiannakis. The society's first newsletter, known as *The NASSS Newsletter,* was published in that same year; in 1980 the first NASSS conference took place in Denver. Canada has hosted this annual conference six times (Toronto, 1982; Edmonton, 1987; Ottawa, 1993; Toronto, 1997; Montreal, 2003; Vancouver, 2006). (See "Web Links" at the end of this chapter for the NASSS website.)

DEFINITION OF SPORT

Often, laypersons interchange the use of the words *play, games,* and *sport* as if they were the same. Social scientists have determined that they are not, and for this reason it is important to draw clear distinctions.

Play is "a physical or mental leisure activity that is undertaken purely for enjoyment or amusement and has no other objective" (Play therapy, UK, n.d.). Play is more concerned with how we do it, rather than what we do. Therefore, it is self-initiated, free activity with no fixed start or stop times. If there are rules, they are made up as play progresses. Play has no tangible outcomes such as prizes or ribbons, and victory and reward are not features in this form of activity. Five characteristics differentiate play from games and sport (Caillois, 1961): it is free; there are no limitations to space and time; the outcome cannot be determined; the purpose of the activity is intrinsic in nature; and it may contain the element of make-believe. Many people equate play with children because it is a natural activity essential for healthy social development. An example of play occurs when neighbourhood children get together spontaneously after dinner to play a game of tag.

Games involve activities with agreed-upon time, space, and terrain. Rules and game outcomes are introduced at this level. Participants may be involved for both intrinsic reasons (e.g., the feel-good factor) and extrinsic reasons (e.g., prestige, recognition, and status). Playing a game of squash with a roommate or going for a round of golf with a friend are examples of a game.

The word *sport* may have a different meaning for you than it has for others in your class or circle of friends and family. Some people think of sport as a physical activity that, in the extreme, involves only large muscle groups and physical exertion. For others, sport combines both physical and mental components. Some people think that windsurfing, Ultimate Frisbee, rock climbing, cheerleading, billiards, and martial arts are bona fide sports. Others regard them more as recreational pursuits. A critical factor that differentiates sport from games and play is that sport becomes organized at some level. So, does that make chess boxing (an 11-round match consisting of alternate rounds of boxing and "blitz" chess sessions) and rock, paper, scissors events sports in the conventional sense? The World Chess Boxing Organization and the World Rock, Paper, Scissors Society may think so. Others may not.

Also consider the made-for-TV coverage of the World Series of Poker. Mike Dodd, in his article "Sport or Not a Sport? Pot Is Split on Poker" (*USA Today,* Friday, 28 April 2006), considers this question. Is poker a sport just because they show it on ESPN? The ESPN executives might think so, considering that the 2005 World Series of Poker was watched in 1.1 million households compared to other sporting events broadcast on ESPN in 2005: PGA Tour (812,000 households), NCAA women's basketball (218,000 households), major league soccer (203,000 households). ESPN (the E standing for Entertainment) never called poker a sport. Certainly, a mental component is required to play poker. But is there a physical component? Some poker players, such as Doyle Brunson, age 72, argue that there is, because of the length of tournaments: "The last tournament I won, I played 18 hours one day, 16 hours the next day and 16 hours the last day. That's pretty tough" (Dodd, 2006, p. 13C). On the other hand, some athletes might object to the use of the words *poker* and *sport* in the same sentence. Bryan Clay, the 2004 Olympic silver medalist in the decathlon, feels that "the word athlete and the word sport are getting so watered down." Even though the International Olympic Committee (IOC) hasn't recognized poker, it does recognize another card game: bridge. Additionally, federations representing billiards, chess, and ballroom dancing have been granted provisional recognition by the IOC. So that brings us to how, for the purposes of this text, we define sport.

One definition of sport that is commonly used is "an active diversion requiring physical exertion and competition" (WordNet, n.d.). However, the following definition is more comprehensive: "institutionalized competitive activities that involve rigorous physical exertion or the use of relatively complex physical skills by participants motivated by personal enjoyment and external rewards" (Coakley, 2004, p. 20). An examination of the components of this definition is worthwhile.

1. *Competitive activity is institutionalized.* For an activity to be institutionalized, the following four criteria must be in place: (i) rules of the activity must become standardized; (ii) a regulatory body is in place to oversee rule enforcement; (iii) the organizational and technical aspects become important, including equipment and training protocol; and (iv) the learning of the game and the skills therein becomes formalized—for example, in structured coaching situations.
2. *Rigorous physical exertion or the use of relatively complex physical skills is involved.* Many people equate sport with physical exertion. But according to the definition above, this does not necessarily have to be the case as long as there are complex skills involved. Throwing a curling rock would not be considered a rigorous activity for most people, but it does involve fine motor coordination.
3. *Participants are motivated by personal enjoyment and external rewards.* Personal enjoyment may wane as the level of participation increases and external rewards may become increasingly important. The late Willie Stargell, a major league baseball player, dubbed the term "work ball" instead of "play ball," reflecting his perception that the game had become more a means to earn a living than a way of seeking pleasure and fulfillment.

Sport is a social construct—that is, we invent sport for our own purposes and according to what we value in our own culture. Furthermore, a certain activity that is considered to be a sport in one culture or subculture may not be considered a sport in another. For example, in the past the lower class in particular held little reverence toward animals and engaged in such "sports" as dog and cock fighting. Today, most people would be horrified at the prospect of taking part in such activity and would be equally reluctant to consider these activities as sports.

Undeniably, since the advent of television, three unique forms of sport have emerged: corporate sport, pseudosport, and mediasport. *Corporate sport* is aligned to big business and—as in big business—the primary motive is profit. Sports leagues engage in profit sharing; official sponsors of the Olympic Games are given the right to use the Olympic logo alongside their own company's logo; television networks buy the rights to broadcast a series of games and, in turn, sell advertising slots to the highest bidders. Money is the fuel that feeds corporate sport's engine, and the byproduct is sometimes corruption and greed. The loss of the 2005–06 NHL season was an example of corporate greed, where billionaire owners were pitted against millionaire players and the pawns in the melée were the disenchanted and disgruntled fans who were denied the opportunity to watch the Canadian national winter sport. Chapter 11, The Economics of Sport and the NHL Lockout, covers the events and outcomes of the strike in detail.

Pseudosports (sometimes referred to as "trash sports") are events or activities that have been invented largely for the purposes of entertainment. According to the definition of sport that has been provided, pseudosports should not be considered bona fide sports. For the most part, they have been invented for television and often incorporate people and machinery that are big, noisy, and violent. Monster trucks, roller derby, and the World Wrestling Entertainment (WWE) are examples of pseudosports.

Another category of sport that has emerged largely because of people's insatiable need for sport on television is one I refer to as *mediasport*. These are events that restructure the rules of established sports so as to maximize the drama between contestants. Often in these contests either great amounts of money or athletic prestige are on the line—sometimes both. Examples of such sports are skins games in golf or curling, all-star games, or battles of the superstars (whereby athletes from various sports compete against one another in a variety of physical challenges).

Basketball as Play, Game, and Sport

Basketball can be categorized as play, a game, or sport depending on the structure of the activity. Father and son shooting hoops on the driveway after dinner is an example of basketball as a form of *play*. The rules (if there are any) are made up as they go and there is no predetermined start and stop time. University students playing a game of pickup basketball during free gym time is an example of a *game*. What differentiates it from play is that there are now rules in place so that the game has some sort of form and structure. What differentiates it from sport is that it is not institutionalized. In other words, the game evolved because a few people showed up and others joined in, and not because there was an organizing body in place. The men's or women's university intercollegiate basketball team playing a home game against another university squad is an example of *sport*. The team is now part of a league; that is, an organizational structure, under the jurisdiction of the CIS.

CHARACTERISTICS OF SPORT

Now that we have made an attempt to define sport in all its varied forms, it is important to understand what features characterize sport. In other words, what qualities make up sport that differentiate it from anything else?

Involvement

The first characteristic is that a sport is characterized by some form of *involvement* at the behavioural, cognitive, or affective level (Kenyon, 1969).

Involvement at the Behavioural Level

At the *behavioural* level, we actively get involved in sport. For example, children play hockey, pretending to be Eric Staal or Hayley Wickenheiser; adolescents become members of their intercollegiate or intramural volleyball teams; middle-aged adults join a local badminton club; and seniors compete in masters' games in swimming. The most popular participation sports for those over 15 years of age are golf, hockey, baseball, and swimming. Unfortunately, only 34.2 percent of Canadians over the age of 15 (males, 43.1 percent; females, 25.7 percent) report that they regularly participate in sport. The 15- to 18-year-old category is the most active (68 percent); however, the gender gap is pronounced: 80 percent of males regularly participated versus 55 percent of females. Unfortunately, after 20 years of age participation levels continually decrease.

The data for children ages 5 to 14 are far from acceptable, with only 54 percent active in sports (Statistics Canada, 2004a). In this age group, boys (61 percent) tend to be more active than girls (48 percent). For those who participate, soccer is the most popular sport (31 percent), followed by swimming (24 percent) and hockey (24 percent). There is an ever-increasing concern about the inactive lifestyles and obesity rates for children and youth. As electronic entertainment options such as video games, the Internet, and TV become more and more popular, children and youth are becoming increasingly inactive. Televised poker, video games, and online fantasy leagues have taken the place of physical activity. This point was driven home to me this summer when a nephew came to visit and announced that he was going to play baseball. I had in mind what I did when I was his age—and that was to head out to the backyard with a ball and bat, round up a few friends, and have a pickup game. His interpretation, however, was that he was going to pick up his PlayStation game and give his thumbs a workout.

There are regional differences as well with regard to amateur sport participation, with Quebec (38 percent) and Alberta (37 percent) having the highest rates, and Prince Edward Island (25 percent) and Newfoundland and Labrador (27 percent) having the lowest. Furthermore, there appears to be an ethnic difference in involvement in competitive sport between anglophones and francophones. For both sexes, anglophones were found to be more involved in competitive sport when compared to francophones, who were less likely to report that they were involved for reasons of "challenge" and "competition" (White & Curtis, 1990). There are also geographical differences. Curtis and Birch (1987) found that more professional and Olympic hockey players were from small towns than large cities.

Canadians today are interested in sport, but all too frequently are content to let others "do" while they watch (see Table 1.1). Canadians' favourite professional sports to watch are hockey (45.4 percent), baseball (14.6 percent), football (12.3 percent), and basketball (9.3 percent). Furthermore, Canadians prefer their own brand of football to the American version (39.3 versus 22.4 percent, respectively) (Leger Marketing Poll, February 2002), believing that the Canadian rules make for a more exciting game than the American (three downs instead of four and a wider field).

The same survey found that in the last several years 33.8 percent of spectators were less interested in watching professional sport, while 47 percent had the same interest level and 13.5 percent reported that their interest had risen. The primary reason given by the one-third whose interest had waned was as a result of the "ridiculously high" player salaries, followed by the departure of Canadian franchises, weak performances by Canadian teams, and player strikes.

Involvement at the Cognitive Level

Sport also requires involvement at the *cognitive* level. This "refers to a person's knowledge about sport" (Leonard II, 1998, p. 115), whether it is, for example, an athlete's, coach's, or fan's. Examples include learning the rules, skills, and strategy involved in sport; knowing about a favourite player; or following sport via the mass media (television, radio, newspaper, or the Internet). In Canada, the primary organization that has improved the knowledge of coaches is the Coaching Association of Canada. This association launched the National Coaching Certification Program (NCCP), which has been a benchmark program for coaching education in the world, certifying approximately 900,000 coaches since its inception in 1974.

With the marriage of technology and sport, athletes and coaches need to be ever-vigilant of new ways of improving performance, be they new training programs, stronger and more durable equipment, dietary considerations, or mental training strategies. Sport science is changing at such a rapid rate that most national and international teams travel with their own entourage of experts including exercise physiologists, biomechanists, sport psychologists, and massage therapists.

Table 1.1   Participation Rates (%) for the Canadian Population
15 Years and Older

Sport	Total	Male	Female
Golf	7.4	11.1	3.9
Ice hockey	6.2	12.0	0.5
Baseball	5.5	8.0	3.1
Swimming	4.6	3.6	5.6
Basketball	3.2	4.6	1.9
Volleyball	3.1	3.3	2.8
Soccer	3.0	4.6	1.5
Tennis	2.7	3.6	1.8
Alpine skiing	2.7	2.9	2.6
Cycling	2.5	3.0	2.0
Cross-country skiing	2.1	1.7	2.5
Weightlifting	1.8	2.5	1.1
Badminton	1.7	1.7	1.7
Football	1.6	2.9	0.3
Curling	1.3	1.5	1.1
Bowling—10 pin	1.2	1.1	1.2
Softball	0.9	1.0	0.7
Bowling—5 pin	0.8	0.7	1.0
Squash	0.7	*	*
Karate	0.5	0.7	0.4
Figure skating	0.5	0.4	0.6
Rugby	0.4	*	*
Ball hockey	0.4	*	*
Snowboarding	0.3	*	*
In-line skating	0.3	*	*
Racquetball	0.2	*	*

* Data unavailable, not applicable, or confidential

Source: Based on data from the Statistics Canada General Social Survey, 1998.

Involvement at the Affective Level

The third type of involvement in sport is *affective*. The affective domain refers to the feeling or emotive processes that a person experiences as a result of sport involvement. Athletes, from weekend warriors to professionals, experience an array of positive and negative feelings associated with their sport. A tennis enthusiast might feel energized while playing a match and envious of the calibre of play while watching the Wimbledon Championships. An Olympian who has recently retired may feel a mixture of emotions including relief at not having the pressures of training and competition and sadness at being away from teammates and the limelight.

When you think of your favourite sport to participate in, what feelings do you have? Some students might feel exhilarated after playing a game of soccer or elated after snowboarding down a hill of powdered snow on a sunny day. How about the feelings you have when you watch your favourite sport or team? Tense when the contest is close; joyful when the team or player you're rooting for is victorious; or disappointed or frustrated when they lose? Fans feel a sense of vicarious achievement when their team beats a league rival. The feelings one has toward a sport are specific to the person and circumstance. For example, some students may feel excited to go to the Rogers Centre to watch the Toronto Blue Jays play baseball—others may feel bored.

Unpredictability

The second characteristic of sport is the element of *unpredictability*. If we could always predict the outcome of a sport contest, would many people bother watching or participating? Have you ever set your video recorder on your television so that you could catch a sport contest that you were unable to watch live? On the way home to watch the match that had already occurred, did you avoid listening to the radio for fear of hearing the outcome? What if, inadvertently, you found out the final score before viewing the tape? How would you feel? Would you bother watching the game on video once you knew what had already happened? Many people wouldn't bother, because the element of unpredictability has been removed. Another example is the 2000 Summer Olympic Games in Sydney, Australia. Because Australia is about a half-day ahead of North America, live events were held in the middle of our night. So if you watched the Games when you woke up, the outcome was already well known thanks to the mass media. It's no wonder more North Americans followed these Games via the Internet than ever before. "In any sport, the anticipation of what might happen is almost as important as what actually happens" (Costas, 2000, p. 133).

Paradox

Sport can be a *paradox*. The American Broadcasting Corporation (ABC) television network once started its sports broadcasts with the caption: "The thrill of victory and the agony of defeat." Joy and agony are opposites invoked from the same thing—sport. And so a paradox is a statement that seems contradictory, but may actually be true. Sport is rife with paradoxes. For example, sport is something that is supposed to promote health, but athletes sometimes play in pain or when injured. Likewise, athletes take performance-enhancing substances to get the edge on competition knowing full well that their health may be jeopardized. In the first chapter of his book *Sport in Contemporary Society: An Anthology*, Stanley Eitzen (2005) provides in-depth examples of present-day paradoxes in sport.

Drama

The final characteristic of sport is that there is usually a *drama* unfolding. This drama could be a contest between a pitcher and a batter, or the suspense of whether the offence in football will move the ball 10 yards in order to gain a first down. Spectator sports that typically have done well in North America are ones that offer lots of drama. In the past decade, fan support for the National Basketball Association (NBA) and, more recently, the Women's National Basketball Association (WNBA) has increased considerably due in part to the quickly unfolding drama (will the team on offence score a basket or will the defence stop them?). Penalty shootouts in soccer (football, as it is known outside of North America) and ice hockey have certainly added a dramatic way to end a tied game. However, soccer has been a tough sell in North America (even though it is the most popular spectator sport in the world) because of the perceived lack of drama as a result of the low-scoring games. Other strikes against the establishment of soccer as a popular spectator sport in North America are that it hasn't historically been part of our culture and that it must compete with at least four other team sports that are well ingrained into the fabric of our society—baseball, basketball, football, and hockey.

Some sports have changed their rules to make them more dramatic and, hence, more sellable. For example, before the advent of televised golf, golfers played under the rules of match play (head-to-head play). To heighten the drama for television, they moved to stroke play, in which a cumulative score for each golfer is kept throughout the tournament so that winning (or losing) could come down to the last putt in the last round. This produces more drama and excitement, which pays dividends come television ratings time.

IS SPORT JUST A MICROCOSM OF SOCIETY?

For some time, sport sociologists claimed that sport reflects or mirrors society. They then modified their thinking on this matter by suggesting that rather than simply mirroring society, sport is a miniature version of it—or, *sport is a microcosm of society*. That is, the situations and circumstances that occurred in sport also occurred in society. For example, how minorities such as the Aboriginal peoples were treated in sport reflected the way they were treated in society at large. This relationship can also be reciprocal: how society views Aboriginal peoples was reflected in the way they were viewed when, for example, playing lacrosse.

Current thinking is that rather than being a mirror or even a miniature version of society, sport shapes how we think and what we value. Jean Harvey (2000) (author of Chapter 12) summarizes this thought:

> Sport is something more than a mirror of the societies in which it is played. It is not a carbon copy of their inequalities and problems. It is a world in its own right, with its own life and its own contradictions. (p. 19)

Instead of standing on the sidelines waiting for society to dictate the nature of sport, the institution of sport, largely via the mass media, is proactive in shaping what we value; how we think, act, and feel; and what we believe. For example, the small percentage of print and photo space that Canadian newspapers devote to women's sport (as opposed to the large amount of coverage given to white male athletes participating in professional team sports) might influence the importance that people place on women's sport participation and, to a greater extent, women's role within society today. This is one of the ways that sport reflects the inequalities found in society.

CULTURAL CONGRUENCY

To understand the term *cultural congruency* and its relationship to sport, we must first understand the term *culture*. Culture is a set of learned behaviours or activities common to a group of people passed down from generation to generation. From that, a template is formed comprised of how the culture should be organized and what the beliefs, practices, thoughts, actions, attitudes, and values of its members should be. Culture also encompasses a society's customs and habits including language, material goods (e.g., what its members wear, how they are housed), religious beliefs, and how its members govern themselves.

How a culture feels, acts, and thinks is reflected in what is important in that culture. The same can be said for sport. Different cultures approach sport in different ways. What is valued in one culture—competition, perhaps—may not be valued in another. This link between sport and culture is called cultural congruency. For example, North Americans live in a capitalist, market-driven economy in which competition and beating one's opponents is important. That attitude is reflected in the way we play sport. In competitive sport, one of our primary goals is to overcome obstacles in order to triumph over an opponent. This same goal is reflected in many business practices in our Western industrial society. However, when a culture evolves in extreme climates, such as in the northern territories in Canada, then cooperation among people is necessary in order to survive. This, then, plays out in the types of physical activities that are chosen; that is, ones that are predominantly cooperative rather than competitive in nature. Examples of this relationship are shown in Chapter 5, Race and Ethnicity in Canadian Sport, written by Victoria Paraschak and Susan Tirone.

The sports that we participate in are the ones that our parents, siblings, educators, and peers (or other social agents) taught us and the ones that our parents, grandparents, and perhaps great-grandparents brought from their countries of origin. Curling, for example, as Don Morrow points out in Chapter 3, has Scottish roots; the British school system, as Patricia Lally states in Chapter 9, has influenced the importance that the Canadian educational system places on academics versus athletics.

But the sports that are congruent to our culture are not necessarily those that are integral to other cultures. This became all too apparent to me when I was a Visiting Professor in England, New Zealand, and Australia. Our popular spectator sports (hockey, football, baseball, and basketball) are not the ones that fill the stands or get the television sets turned on. Rather, soccer, rugby, cricket, and netball command the most attention. On my last visit to Australia, I was talking to a friend who was an avid sports fan about who the greatest athletes in the world were. I mentioned Wayne Gretzky as a possibility, but my suggestion resulted in a blank look on my friend's face. He had never heard of Wayne Gretzky. Impossible, you might think. He then told me who *he* thought was a great athlete—a storied cricket player whom I had never heard of. The point is that every culture can have a rather myopic view of the world of sport and the players who comprise that world. One of the benefits of travel is that eyes are opened to different cultures and what sports are important to that culture.

SO WHAT MAKES SPORT IN CANADA UNIQUE?

David Whitson in Chapter 13 will make it clear that, as a result of the influence of the mass media, we are made aware of the happenings around the globe on a daily basis. Sport is no exception. In 2006, we watched Italy win the World Cup of Soccer in Germany with 32 nations qualifying; Tiger Woods win the British Open Golf Championships; Maria Sharapova (Russia) and Roger Federer (Switzerland) win the singles events in the US Open Tennis Championships; and the European team win golf's Ryder Cup played in Ireland. So to claim that Canadian sport is a unique entity thriving on its own without any external influences would be naïve and inaccurate. To say that Canada is any more "sports mad" than other countries would be erroneous. As mentioned previously, I have lived in England and New Zealand and have visited Australia and know that some fans love their cricket, football (what we refer to as soccer), and rugby as much as we love our ice hockey. Certainly, we are influenced by our neighbours to the south in many respects—sport is just one example. One only has to turn on the TV on the weekend or on Monday nights from September to January to get examples of this: from NCAA football and basketball to Major League Baseball, the National Football League (NFL), and the NBA. Many of our treasured NHL teams have drifted south to larger market areas. But surely there are some aspects of Canadian sport that set us apart from how other countries do sport. In other words, what makes Canadian sport unique?

One way we differ is in the sports that are prominent in our country, and certainly our climate factors into that. Canada's long winters make winter sports viable options five to six months a year. Golfers go indoors to curl, and many Canadians jump on snowboards and skis (cross-country and alpine) to make the most of living in the northern hemisphere. Boards go up in most neighbourhoods for ice rinks and, when the weather gets cold enough, surfaces are flooded.

In terms of the Olympic Games, Canada has experienced more success at the Winter Olympic Games (WOG) than the Summer Olympic Games (SOG). For example, in the 2006 WOG in Torino, Italy, Canada placed 5th overall among the countries present, with a total of 24 medals. However, at the 2004 SOG in Athens, Greece, Canada placed 21st, with a total of 12 medals. At those games, Canadian athletes won gold in gymnastics, cycling, canoeing, and wheelchair racing. In terms of WOG success, speed skaters have reached the podium on numerous occasions: Gaéton Boucher won two gold medals in 1984; Catriona LeMay Doan won two medals in 1998 and gold in 2002; the men's speed-skating foursome won a gold medal in the 500-metre relay in 2006; and Canada's most decorated Olympian, Cindy Klassen, won one medal in 2002 and five in 2006 (see the photograph below). But speed skating isn't the only WOG sport where Canadians have excelled. For example, in 2002 Becky Scott won gold in cross-country skiing, our curling teams won gold (men's) and bronze (women's), and our men's and women's ice hockey teams experienced gold medal success—with the women repeating in 2006. So in terms of whom our Olympic sport heroes are, the WOG competitors figure largely into the equation. Undoubtedly, with the next WOG in Vancouver, new Canadian sport heroes will emerge.

But let's not forget that we also play and watch numerous sports when snow isn't on the ground. As has already been mentioned, there are more than 2,500 golf courses in Canada, and soccer pitches and baseball diamonds dot green spaces in every town and city. We follow Mike

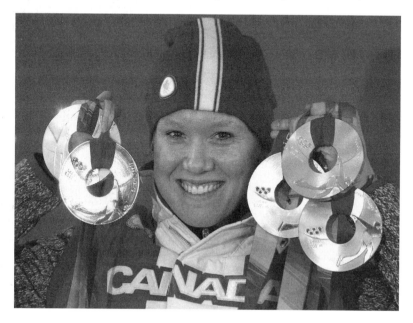

Speed skater Cindy Klassen displays the five Olympic medals (one gold, two silver, and two bronze) she won at the 2006 Winter Olympics in Torino, Italy.
MATT DUNHAM/AP/CP Images

Weir, winner of the 2003 Masters Golf Championship (see the photograph below), and Stephen Ames as they compete on the Professional Golfers Association (PGA) tour, and Lori Kane in the Ladies Professional Golf Association (LPGA) tour.

REASONS WHY CANADIANS FOLLOW SPORT

Canadians follow sport in many different ways and for a variety of reasons. We watch sports live, follow the action via the mass media (television, newsprint, radio, and the Internet), see films with sport themes, and read books about our favourite players and teams. The question posed in this section is, Why do people follow sport in Canada? The reasons can be divided into two categories: personal and social.

Personal Reasons

For many, sport is a primary means of entertainment or pastime. It piques our interest and alleviates the boredom of the everyday routine. Imagine working in a mundane job every day where nothing much changes. Sport provides a stress-seeking opportunity to raise the heart rate and get excited about a team or an athlete. Remember, one characteristic that defines sport is that it is unpredictable. This element of the unpredictable is what attracts some to avidly follow sport.

Some sport enthusiasts possess a strong identity with their favourite team and, in some cases, live vicariously through this identity. If the team wins, they win. If the team loses, this loss rests on their shoulders as well. In the summer and autumn, many Canadians cheer on their favourite Canadian Football League (CFL) team, although many football fans prefer to follow the progress of NFL teams. When major league baseball came to Canada, many Canadians became either Montreal Expos (now the Washington Senators) or Toronto Blue Jays fans. The Toronto Raptors provide us with an NBA team to support. Our sport heroes are those who excel in the sports that are the focus of our sporting traditions.

For some, sport provides an opportunity to view violence and aggression. It also provides some followers with an opportunity to have something to gamble on; one can find everything from *parimutuel* betting on horses to hockey pools at work.

Social Reasons

Watching sport contests is, for many people, a social experience. For example, family and friends gather to watch the Grey Cup, the

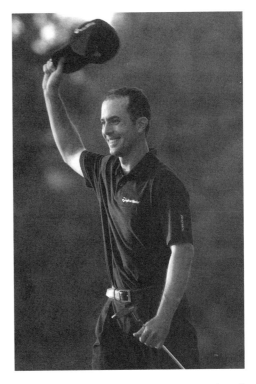

Mike Weir becomes the first Canadian to win a major golf tournament, and the first left-hander to take the Masters.
DAVE MARTIN/AP/CP Images

World Series, or the Stanley Cup finals. For some people, the primary objective is to watch the game. Less enthusiastic sports fans enjoy the company of others and partake in food, fun, and festivities. Whatever the purpose in following sport, it is a popular pastime of Canadians and will likely remain so in the foreseeable future. I grew up watching *Hockey Night in Canada* on television every Saturday night, as many Canadian baby boomers did. We did this because, in part, our parents were interested in doing the same or they felt that it was one way the family could socialize together.

SOCIALIZATION INTO, VIA, AND OUT OF SPORT

Socialization Into Sport

Being involved in sport is not only a physical experience; it also creates opportunities for socialization experiences to occur. Socialization is a "means by which a society preserves its norms and perpetuates itself" (Eitzen & Sage, 2003, p. 61). This process of learning a culture and becoming a contributing member of society is what Leonard II (1998) called a "social metamorphosis" (p. 106). Furthermore, socialization is a reciprocally interactive process whereby one learns attitudes, knowledge, and values and adapts to the society of which he or she is a member. In turn, the person doing the learning (and, hence, being socialized) can exert influence on the social agents doing the teaching. These social agents exert varying degrees of influence (depending on the person and his or her life circumstances) and comprise a combination of family and friends, coaches, and teachers working in institutions such as schools, churches, and the community at large. In the last century, the mass media have also become a socializing agent. Over the years I have heard many explanations from individuals about why they get into sport—from getting involved because an older sibling was involved to avoiding having to do something less desirable. It is worth noting that children are exposed to a variety of social experiences, some of which are sport-related and many of which are not.

Certainly, parents are predominant socializing agents when it comes to sport involvement. If one (or both) parents are actively involved in and enthusiastic about a particular sport or activity, this attitude will usually affect their children in a positive way (Statistics Canada, 1998). Moreover, if the parents include their children in their sporting ventures, they not only learn how to do a particular sport, but also often develop a lifelong appreciation for it at the same time (Welk, 1999). In other words, active children generally come from supportive families. Early experiences in sport are critical in shaping future attitudes and behaviours.

Greendorfer and Lewko (1978) and McElroy (1983) found that within the family structure, fathers were the most significant socializing agents for sport and, furthermore, were the most important predictor of sport participation for both boys and girls. This finding is particularly interesting in today's society, in which a large percentage of children are raised in lone-parent families. More recently, findings from the General Social Survey (Statistics Canada, 1998) showed that being raised in a two-parent versus single-parent family did not significantly affect the children's participation rates (54 percent versus 53 percent, respectively).

Kenyon and McPherson (1973) believe that the process of being socialized into sport is more complicated than just making a positive connection with influential social agents. They contend that personal attributes and socializing situations also play an important role in determining an individual's likelihood of participating in sport.

Personal attributes are the characteristics that make up the individual; they can be either physical (e.g., height, weight, and age), psychological (e.g., mental toughness, determination), or social-psychological (e.g., the ability to work as part of a team). Despite having the physical attributes necessary to play a sport, a child may be hesitant to participate if he or she does not possess the preferred mental requisites, such as aggressiveness or determination. However, if a child possesses all the desired personal attributes and experiences repeated success, he or she will likely be more than willing to continue participating.

Socializing situations consist of "the individual's unique blend of opportunities and life experiences" (Bryant & McElroy, 1997, p. 33). A relationship exists between household income and sport participation: the higher the income, the higher the sport participation. For example, only 25.2 percent of Canadian children from homes with household incomes under $20,000 participated in sport, compared to 34.4 percent with household incomes in the $30,000 to $50,000 range and 50.6 percent of households with an income of more than $80,000 (Statistics Canada, 1998). But financial resources are only one factor that plays into sport participation. Another factor is education, and the higher the education, the higher the probability of sport participation. In 1998, 46 percent of those with a university degree regularly participated compared to 29 percent for those with some secondary schooling or less. Certainly, one's social class and environment influence the opportunity to participate in certain sports. This topic will be dealt with in greater detail by Rob Beamish in Chapter 4, Sport and Social Stratification.

Socialization Via Sport

It has long been the mantra of sport enthusiasts that sport provides a forum through which we learn "life's lessons." Discipline, hard work, dedication to a common cause, and other laudable personal qualities are supposed to be the outcome of having been involved in sport. In some circumstances, this may very well be the case; but in others, regrettably, this is not so. Sport is inherently a teacher neither of what is good nor of what is bad. Rather, it is the nature of the experiences in sport that may provide opportunities for socialization. While one coach may model and expound the virtues of sportsmanship and fair play to his or her athletes, another may be teaching and condoning illegal field tactics and modelling unsportsmanlike conduct.

It is particularly important for children to have positive experiences in sport because these early experiences (both positive and negative) will shape the attitudes they have to sport and physical activity in their later years. It is imperative that coaches of young children make the children's growth and development needs paramount. Children's sports should not be a scaled-down version of how older people play. For example, playing the best players at the expense of the lesser-skilled players should not happen in children's organized sport. Every child should ideally walk away from the experience feeling that he or she had fun and experienced an equal opportunity to play—and wanting to return again. More discussion regarding this issue can be found in Chapter 7, Children, Youth, and Parental Involvement in Organized Sport, by Ralph Wheeler.

Socialization Out of Sport

While some people are socialized into sport, others are socialized out of it. For a variety of reasons, people cease doing a particular sport or all sports for a period of time or permanently. For children it may be the demands of the activity or the feeling that they aren't contributing members of the team that demotivate them; for adolescents it may be the ability to drive a car or an interest in dating and other social activities; for young adults it may be that other roles, for example work or family, demand their time and money; and for adults it may be not being particularly skilled or competent. We might reason that one drops out of sport because something negative has happened to the participant that deterred him or her from continuing—perhaps lack of time, money, or opportunity. This is not necessarily the case. As was pointed out above, sometimes other life choices need to be made at a particular point in a person's life, and for a time sport isn't a primary pursuit.

Research has shown that one does not simply drop out of sport; that is, one day you're in and the next, you're out (Koukouris, 1994). In fact, leaving sport completely or for just a period of time frequently coincides with other life-changing events. A new job or the arrival of a baby may mean other things that were part of a person's life, including sport participation, have to take a back seat for the time being. This does not mean that the person will never return to sport. If a return does occur, it may be to a different sport and perhaps at a different level. When children and adolescents drop out of sport, it is of concern to those who believe that regular sport participation has many benefits. The major reasons Canadians over age 15 give for not participating in sport are lack of time (31.3 percent), lack of interest (26.1 percent), and limitations due to health/injury (12.7 percent) or age (12.6 percent). Reasons for non-participation vary by age. For example, Canadians ages 20 to 54 cite "lack of time" as their primary reason for not participating; those between 15 and 19 cite "lack of interest" as their primary reason; and those over 55 say "age" is the predominant factor.

Gould (1984, p. 87) found that the primary reasons for dropping out included an overemphasis on winning, lack of success, not playing, other conflicting activities, boredom, little improvement, and too much pressure. Furthermore, Anshel (1997) categorized children's reasons for dropping out of sport into three areas: *comparative appraisal* (children are constantly comparing their own motor abilities with the abilities of others their own age, often resulting in a feeling of inferiority); *perceived lack of ability* (how children often attribute a failed performance); *low intrinsic motivation* (instead of wanting to do the sport for its own sake or for the simple joy and fun of participation, which is motivational, children who participate primarily for the tangible rewards and prestige associated with it frequently find themselves demotivated and contemplate quitting).

Numerous strategies exist to combat the dropout phenomenon, and many of them come down to the fact that participants need to feel a sense of accomplishment. Consequently, improvement should be based on self-improvement rather than a comparison to others. Children who drop out of sport will be discussed in greater depth in Chapter 7.

If sport participation is one important way athletes define themselves, then both the integration into and out of sport are pivotal points in an athlete's career. Retirement is one way athletes drop out of sport. The word *retirement* can be a misnomer because, for many athletes, retirement is best described as a transition and a process rather than a single event (Danish, Owens, Green, & Brunelle, 1997; Greendorfer & Blinde, 1985). Athletes don't usually wake up one morning deciding to retire that day from sport. Ideally, they prepare for it by planning how to end that phase of their competitive careers and move on to other activities and life goals. In other words, athletes gradually build an image of retirement from competition during their competitive careers (Torregrosa, Boixadós, Valiente, & Cruz, 2004).

As is the case with others who drop out of sport, this career transitional process often occurs in conjunction with other changes in an athlete's life. Some doors in the person's life are shut, while others are opened. As old sport identities are dropped, new ones are adopted. "The process of leaving a role means that one also is being socialized into a new role" (Tremaine Drahota & Eitzen, 1998, p. 266). For example, one moves from being a competitive swimmer to a competitive rower, or a professional football player to a recreational squash player, or from direct-primary involvement (a participant) to indirect-primary involvement (a coach or administrator).

Athletes make a career transition for a number of reasons, both *voluntary* (conflicting family responsibilities; not enjoying the pressures of competing or travel; lack of commitment or interest; dissatisfaction with the organization, coach, or administrators; not enjoying the self-sacrifice needed to succeed; financial considerations; and frustration with the preoccupation with training and diet) and *involuntary* (injury and selection). The age at which participants retire varies across sports, between sexes, and among able and disabled athletes (North & Lavallee, 2004). Kerr and Dacyshyn (2000) point out that the distinction between voluntary and involuntary retirement is unclear and, furthermore, voluntary retirement does not necessarily mean that the athlete won't experience adjustment difficulties. Ex-athletes making career transitions may face "social, professional and even bodily changes and adjustments" (Stephan, Bilard, Ninot, & Delignières, 2003a, p. 192). The Canadian Olympic Career Centre reports that, on average, ex-Olympians take 18 months to fully adjust to their new identities.

Because athletic careers are relatively short when compared to other professions, athletes in transition often have numerous questions. "What now? How will I make a living?" and, in some cases, "How will I dig myself out of the debt that has mounted up while I was in training?" What is certain is that athletes need to be prepared for this transition and frequently are not (Baillie & Danish, 1992). Retirement is much less problematic when it is planned rather than an event (Torregrosa et al., 2004) and is made easy when athletes develop transferable skills during their sport career (Stephan et al., 2003b). Those who make a reasonably successful transition to life beyond sport do so because they have prepared (Baillie & Danish, 1992; Schlossberg, 1981). They have obtained post-secondary education and obtained qualifications; they have networked with people who can make the right connections for them; they have been exposed to positive role models who have taught them social skills; and, more often than not, they have the support of their family and friends who provide not only monetary assistance but also social support (Grove, Lavallee, & Gordon, 1997; McGowan & Rail, 1996).

Alfermann, Stambulova, and Zemanaityte (2004) found that when European national and international athletes plan their retirement, they have significantly better cognitive, emotional, and behavioural adaptation. Fortunately, professional players' associations have increased their awareness of the importance of assisting athletes in making a successful transition. Some facilitate the process of having their athletes return to formal education, while others provide incentives to branch out into different careers. Lavallee (2005) found that among retired professional soccer players, those who participated in an intervention package to assist them with career transition coped better with this transition when compared to those who did not.

A system to support retired Olympians in making a smooth and successful transition has evolved in Canada. In 1985, the Canadian Olympic Association started the Olympic Career Centre. In 1994, Calgary was the only National Sport Centre; however, in 1998–99 seven more centres, now called Canadian Sport Centres, were added (Victoria, Vancouver, Saskatchewan, Manitoba, Toronto, Montreal, Atlantic Canada). These centres provide career counselling to former Olympians, including training in job-search techniques and assistance in résumé preparation to help athletes (both retired and active) become the best persons they can be. This holistic approach, which is used by both active and ex-Olympians, attempts to help athletes balance all aspects of their lives. Career planning and transition services are expanding across the globe, with Australia and Great Britain taking the lead with their athlete career and education programs. In 2000, 2003, and 2006 international forums were held to discuss best practices with regard to athlete career planning and transition (J. Goss, personal communication, 5 October 2006).

CONCLUSIONS: THE BAD NEWS/THE GOOD NEWS

Some sociologists paint a rather dim picture of the situation in sport today. Certainly, it would be naïve to think sport does not have more than its fair share of issues that need mending at the least and overhauling in some cases. Examples of those issues that will be included in the subsequent chapters in this book include:

- the pressure placed on children by coaches and parents to excel
- children who "do" sport via video games and the Internet rather than actively participating, thereby risking their health
- educational systems that are not providing enough time for physical education
- inequalities that still exist with regard to how minorities, such as women, Aboriginal peoples, and persons with disabilities, are treated
- social problems such as drug use, cheating, violence, and gambling
- the control of sport by the minority elite
- collective bargaining disputes between players' associations and owners
- large, multinational sport equipment manufacturing companies that fail to pay fair wages to third-world employees
- political interference in sport such as boycotts and the use of sport by politicians for political gains
- the influence the mass media can have in shaping our ideals and values, oftentimes giving preferential coverage to Caucasian men playing professional team sports

Sport sociologists need not only to uncover the problems that exist in sport today, but also to offer solutions.

Having mentioned some of the imbalances and injustices, I would rather end this introductory chapter on a positive note. Sport involvement can provide a potentially healthy, invigorating, exhilarating, and rewarding way of spending time. Moments of genuine pleasure and achievement are often realized. And the good news is that some of the problems cited above are being addressed. For example:

- provinces are putting more emphasis on physical education for school children
- the federal government has included in the 2006 budget a $500 children's fitness tax credit to support Canadian parents who enrol children under 16 years old in organized physical sports activities
- the World Anti-Doping Agency (WADA) and professional sports leagues are clamping down on drug use in sport and sanctions for violators are becoming stiffer
- there is a trend in the NHL toward fewer fights (fights per game in the 2003–04 season was 0.64, versus 0.38 in the 2005–06 season)
- there are increased competitive opportunities for minorities in sport such as the North American Indigenous Games, Gay Games, Out Games, Paralympic Games, and Masters Games
- codes of conduct have been instituted in children's organized sport to combat inappropriate behaviour by parents
- provincial and territorial ministers are urging the federal government (as of October 2006) to make a multibillion-dollar investment into Canada's crumbling venues for recreational and amateur sport
- professional women athletes in certain sports such as tennis and golf are getting more media coverage
- some sport equipment companies that employ third-world labour have instituted a fair wage policy.

The sports world today is by no means a perfect one, but steps, some large and some small, are being taken to correct this. The first step in the healing process is an awareness of the issues. It is my wish that this book opens students' eyes and challenges them not only to think about the structure and shortcomings of sport today, but also to envision what it can be in the future.

CRITICAL THINKING QUESTIONS

1. Discuss the reasons why a course in the sociology of sport and physical activity should be part of an undergraduate curriculum in a kinesiology/human kinetics/physical education/sport science program.
2. List and briefly describe who the various agents were that socialized you into sport.
3. Why do you think sport is so popular in Canadian society today?
4. Using baseball as an example, provide an example where it is a) play, b) a game, and c) a sport.
5. Why do you think pseudosports are popular among the working class?
6. Should poker be considered a sport? Does it belong in the Olympics? Justify your response.
7. Provide three examples of cultural congruency in sport today.
8. Think of a country other than Canada that you have visited or lived in. What are the similarities and differences between how the two countries "do" and celebrate sport?
9. Do you feel that a) women, b) ethnic minorities, and c) persons with disabilities are still trivialized and marginalized in sport today? If so, in what ways?
10. Research has shown that those athletes making a career transition who participate in an intervention package coped better. What do you think this package should consist of?

SUGGESTED READINGS

Bergmann-Drewe, S. (2003). *Why sport? An introduction to the philosophy of sport*. Toronto: Thompson.

Blackshaw, T., & Crabbe, T. (2004). *New perspectives on sport and "deviance."* Oxfordshire: Routledge.

Eitzen, D. S. (1996). Classism in sport: The powerless bear the burden. *Journal of Sport & Social Issues, 20*, 95–105.

Eitzen, D. S. (2005). *Sport in contemporary society: An anthology*. Boulder: Paradigm.

Gruneau, R. (1999). *Class, sports, and social development*. Champaign, IL: Human Kinetics.

Houlihan, B. (Ed.). (2003). *Sport & society: A student introduction*. London: Sage.

Jarvie, G. (2006). *Sport, culture and society: An introduction*. Oxfordshire: Routledge.

Malloy, D. C., Ross, S., & Zakus, D. H. (2003). *Sport ethics: Concepts and cases in sport and recreation*. Toronto: Thompson.

WEB LINKS

North American Society for the Sociology of Sport (NASSS)

http://www.nasss.org

NASSS's website, with information on conferences, members, the history of the organization, and so on.

North American Sport Library Network (NASLIN)

http://www.naslin.org

Communication and resource sharing.

Sport Canada

http://www.pch.gc.ca/sportcanada/

Home page of Sport Canada.

SPORTDiscus

http://www.sirc.ca/products/sportdiscus.cfm

Sports, fitness, and sports medicine database.

Canadian Olympic Association

http://www.olympic.ca/

News and events from Canada's Olympic Committee.

CHAPTER 2

SOCIOLOGICAL THEORIES OF SPORT

Ian Ritchie

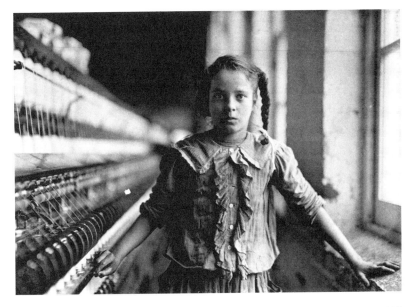

A young girl working in a cotton mill in the early twentieth century in the United States. Child labour was one of many hardships the first sociologists attempted to understand during the early days of the industrial revolution.

© CORBIS

Common sense is the collection of prejudices acquired by age eighteen.

Albert Einstein

Sociological theory is the foundation of the discipline of sociology in general, and its particular understanding of sport and physical activity in sport sociology. This chapter introduces four major theoretical perspectives: structural functionalism, conflict theory, symbolic interactionism, and critical social theories. The theories offer competing perspectives but at the same time occasionally complement one another in their attempts to answer questions about the nature of social and cultural life. Examples from the study of sport and physical activity demonstrate that the perspectives often raise serious challenges to many common assumptions about sport.

SOCIOLOGICAL THEORY: GENERAL THEMES AND HISTORICAL CONTEXTS

Lying at the foundation of sociology—as is the case with any discipline, whether in the physical sciences, social sciences, or humanities—is theory. Theory is the central tool that sociologists use to understand the human world around us in general, and more specifically the role that sport and physical culture play within that world. In simple terms, sociological theory is a proposition or set of propositions about the nature of the social world and people's roles or active engagement in that world.

People "theorize" about the world around them all the time, in the sense that they ponder various aspects of social, cultural, or political life, or perhaps just about the conduct of other people around them in their everyday lives. However, what sets serious theory apart from common, everyday ideas about the world is the fact that sociological theories must ultimately be accountable, in the sense that they must prove themselves through a process of verification with the facts of the social world. In other words, they must withstand the test of systematic verification, whether in the form of facts and statistics or simply careful and systematic observations about certain aspects of social life.

Despite this fundamental difference between sociological theory and everyday observations, it is still useful to think of what sociologists attempt to do in understanding the social world through theory as really not too different from what people in human societies have always done since time immemorial. People have always created accounts or stories about the nature of the social world around them in order to understand it better and, in turn, understand themselves. For example, anthropologists have identified the important role *myths* play in human cultures, in that they explain to people the nature of the world around them and their role in the greater scheme of things. Myths, it should be pointed out, and contrary to the literal meaning of the term itself, are really stories that are based not only on fictionalized or exaggerated accounts, but also at the same time on factual ones. Canadians, for example, have mythologized or told stories about their country through the sport of hockey, and those stories are based on fictionalized or exaggerated accounts of the country and its history as much as they are on the bare "facts" of the game or its history (Gruneau & Whitson, 1993, pp. 131–52).

But again, sound sociological theory must withstand the test of time through constant refinement and rigorous debate, and it must be provable through careful observation and systematic verification. Sometimes the results are contrary to common perceptions or "common sense." When the terms common sense are used they typically mean that someone is using sound and practical judgment. However, here the terms are meant in the more literal meaning; that is, that there are often ideas that people—perhaps many people—have in common. Einstein's statement at the beginning of this chapter, however, points to the problem with this kind of sense—it is quite often wrong. We accumulate ideas through various sources as we grow, Einstein suggests, but that does not mean those accumulated sets of ideas are accurate or a true reflection of the world around us.

So, one of the first points about sociological theory to keep in mind is that it does not always support common-sense notions about the nature of the social world. The use of performance-enhancing substances in high-performance sport provides an example. Few would question or think twice about the legitimacy of rules against the use of drugs in sport, because it is taken for granted that the use of certain banned substances is inherently unethical. Indeed, the World Anti-Doping Agency (WADA), which oversees anti-doping efforts in the Olympic Games and is the largest and most important drug detection organization in the world of sport, reflects this common-sense view that the use of drugs is inherently unethical. The central justification for banning drugs—and for using urine and, more recently, blood detection and screening procedures—as WADA's *World Anti-Doping Code* states quite clearly is, "to preserve what is intrinsically valuable about sport . . . [t]he intrinsic value is often referred to as 'the spirit of sport'; it is the essence of Olympism" (World Anti-Doping Agency, 2003, p. 3).

But what exactly does the "spirit of sport" mean? The terms suggest that sport has a certain "essence" and, by implication, has been the same throughout history, which has given sport its "spirit." Sound historical research, however, informed in turn by equally sound theory, does not support the idea that sport has been the same throughout history, making the "spirit" to which the *Code* refers vague at best and very likely inaccurate. In one of the best historical accounts of drug use in sport, Yesalis and Bahrke (2002) demonstrate that there was very little if any moral condemnation of drug use until almost midway into the twentieth century. In fact, the authors point out, in many competitions "there was no attempt to conceal drug use with the possible exception of some trainers who guarded against the proprietary interest in their own special 'doping recipes' " (p. 46).

Other historical accounts support Yesalis's and Bahrke's claims. There is little evidence, for example, that the ancient Greeks, in their version of the Olympic Games, condemned athletes for the use of any substances that might enhance their performances in any way. Part of the reason for this is the fact that the ancients adopted a "winner take all" approach that far outweighed our own today. So serious was the attempt to win at all costs in ancient Greece that extremely violent acts in wrestling were commonplace and victorious athletes were held up as almost the equivalent to the gods themselves (Public Broadcasting Service, 2004). As Kidd (1984) says, "[t]he modern handshake would have seemed an act of cowardice" because of the dramatically different approach the ancients took to their sport (p. 76). In short, while it just seems to make common sense that drugs are incompatible with some natural, timeless, or perhaps "spiritual" aspect of sport, real history demonstrates that this is not the case; the moral condemnation of drug use in sport is a reflection of only very recent, modern sensibilities—there is little evidence of such condemnations in the history of sport otherwise.

Besides the challenges that sociological theories and the discipline of sociology as a whole often bring to some common understandings of sport, there are a few other important points to keep in mind before considering the theories themselves. The first point flows from the example of historical differences in attitudes regarding the use of performance-enhancing substances. The theoretical perspectives offer not only an interpretation of social conditions at present; they also offer interpretations of history. They do this in two senses. First, events in history are interpreted according to the tenets of the particular theory, or in other words theory will guide the manner in which events of the past are viewed. History is not thought of as a *static* accumulation of facts but rather a *dynamic* set of events, and which interpretations of events or what "facts" are considered important is guided by theory. Second, each of the theoretical perspectives encourages us to think about and evaluate social conditions as they currently are by putting those conditions into historical context. In other words, we can learn a lot about the way things are today by looking back and placing events in their proper historical context. You will find that many of the authors of chapters in this text remind us of important elements of Canadian sport history so that we might in turn better understand current issues.

The discipline of sociology itself should be thought of in this historical context. While the events that lay the foundation of sociology are many and complex, two stand out. The first event is a series of *democratic revolutions* that led to the emergence of democratic institutions and forms of government. The democratic revolutions in France and the United States in the late-eighteenth century are the most obvious examples, although equally important over time was the gradual *evolution* into democratic traditions in many countries, including Canada. These changes brought about the idea that governments are responsible to people, and that people as citizens can actively and rationally play a role in the affairs of the state. Sociology emerged, in part, to consider these changes and to contemplate the newly envisioned role of democratic institutions and people's relationship to those institutions. Today, the fundamental rights and freedoms of Canadians, as they are spelled out in the Canadian Charter of Rights and Freedoms, ratified as part of the Constitution Act of 1982, is but one important example in a long history of democratic development in Canada.

The second—and likely more important—event is the *industrial revolution*. In fact, so important was the development of industrial society to the emergence of sociology that the discipline in its earliest days during the late-nineteenth and early-twentieth centuries was more or less defined as the study of the causes and consequences of the industrial revolution. The industrial revolution dramatically changed the way in which goods were produced and the way in which people laboured. But for the vast majority of people it also brought new social problems: mass exoduses of people from rural settings to urban cities, miserable and often dangerous working and living conditions, new forms of crime, vast inequalities between the rich and the poor, and a general sense of alienation or disaffection caused by the dramatic changes in people's lives.

Out of these two historical contexts, sociology emerged to consider two main questions or issues. The first was the *issue of social problems*. In light of the hardships wrought by the industrial revolution, the earliest sociologists were concerned with how to create a social order that could resolve some of the fundamental problems: food production and distribution in growing cities, the availability of clean water, poor hygienic living conditions, the physical hardships from long hours of strenuous work in factories, child labour, vast inequalities between the rich and poor, and so forth. The issue of social problems continues to play an important role in sociology, and Kevin Wamsley's discussion in Chapter 8 is a reflection of this continued role.

The second was the *question of community, authority, and tradition*. As peasants were lifted—often forced—from their land to work in cities as labourers, as small manufacturers were replaced by big companies, as urban living quickly replaced rural life, questions arose as to how to maintain and develop authority structures in the new social order, how to provide people with a sense of community in light of rapid changes, and how to answer questions regarding loss of rural and religious traditions as society became more secularized. How should the new social order be organized and established? What was the role of individual citizens in relation to newly emerging state-run institutions and forms of government? What social bonds would unite people in newly emerging urban communities? These were some of the important questions the first sociologists attempted to answer.

There are two additional points about these historical contexts that are important. First, while sociology has become much more diverse since these events began in the eighteenth and nineteenth centuries, the same fundamental problems persist and continue to be considered, even if their form has changed somewhat: *stratification* or inequalities between classes of people (discussed by Rob Beamish in Chapter 4); crime and deviance; poverty and access to the fundamentals of life, including food, clean water, clothing, and shelter; and debates and conflicts over the social and political order and people's role in it continue to be issues and questions that remain with us today.

Second, the dominant social practices of sport as we know them today emerged out of the same time period, the same conditions, and the same problems. For example, in Canada the first major sports organizations emerged during the early years of the country's industrial and social development. The first sports organizations appeared in Canada during the mid-to-late 1800s, and by the early-to-mid twentieth century Canada had a very developed—albeit loosely organized—system of sport organizations and competitions that was quickly becoming part of an international sporting scene (Kidd, 1996b).

Another important point to keep in mind before considering the theories is that sociology is a discipline that encourages a personal relationship to the topic matter. This idea is perhaps most clearly expressed by American sociologist C. Wright Mills (1959). In his book by the same title, Mills describes *the sociological imagination* as the ability to link general social issues with everyday life and personal problems. Mills uses the example of unemployment, a problem that, if experienced directly, people typically treat in only personal ways with individual solutions. However, Mills points out that the problem must also be approached as a problem of social structure, especially when unemployment rates are quite high, or when "[t]he very structure of opportunities has collapsed." Then, Mills explains, "the correct statement of the problem and the range of possible solutions require us to consider the economic and political institutions of the society, and not merely the personal situation and character of a scatter of individuals" (p. 9). Sociological theory, in short, encourages us to evaluate our own lives in different ways, and our roles in the greater social and cultural world around us.

Also, the theories we are about to consider should not be thought of as static, but instead in a constant *dynamic* state in which debate and refinement have led and will continue to lead to their change and evolution. The temptation at first in reading accounts of theories is to look for the one that is "right"; however, that search will likely be futile. Instead, each theory should be thought of as having certain strengths that help to ascertain certain elements of the social world, but also weaknesses or areas it does not consider. Indeed, theories that have attempted to make all-encompassing universal claims about the nature of the social world as a whole have ultimately failed because they have attempted to do too much.

Importantly, sociological theories all have in common a political motivation to understand the nature of the social world around us in order to make it a better one for everyone. This motivation dates back to the historical foundations of the discipline itself and the first questions and issues it addressed, as discussed earlier. One of the natural consequences of this is that the theories often point to the many problems that exist in the social world. This *critical* element of the theories should in no way overshadow sociology's recognition of the many ways in which sport and physical culture more generally can play an active and very positive role in human social life. Identifying problems, however, is a necessary step in making the very positive aspects of physical activity and sport available for as many people as possible.

Finally, the theories discussed here do not by any means represent a complete inventory of theories in sociology. The discipline offers a dizzying array of perspectives, and they continue to grow. However, what follows provides a concise summary of major perspectives that have guided thinking in sociology's past and continue to guide thinking currently, have laid the foundation of sociological inquiries in sport and physical activity, and will put into context the various topics in the chapters that follow. The theories presented here are also very general and in most cases there is a diversity of more specific perspectives that fall within each. As such, they should be thought of as general guidelines, as opposed to theoretical "formulae" into which sport can simply be plugged. Having said that, all sections will include, quite naturally, a discussion of the application of theories to sport using both general examples but also ones specific to Canada.

ÉMILE DURKHEIM AND STRUCTURAL FUNCTIONALISM

The foundations of *structural functionalism*—often referred to synonymously as *functionalism*—are very old and can be traced to elements of ancient Greek thought and, much more recently, British social philosophy (McQuarie, 1995, pp. 1–2). In terms of the latter, an important early expression of structural functionalist ideas came from Herbert Spencer (1802–1903). Influenced by Charles Darwin's theory of evolution, Spencer equated social processes with biological or organic ones, claiming that society operates according to principles similar to that of animal life and the manner in which that life develops and evolves. "It is also a character of social bodies, as of living bodies, that while they increase in size they increase in structure" Spencer (1961, p. 140) wrote in *The Principles of Sociology* in 1898. Here, Spencer expresses in naturalistic and evolutionary terms two ideas that would eventually become staples of structural functionalist thought: that social systems can be thought of as real entities operating according to scientific laws, and that society has a "structure."

The most important and influential figure to develop and more fully express these basic functionalist tenets was Émile Durkheim (1858–1917). While active in French politics and social life generally, Durkheim's most noted accomplishments were realized in his active reforms of French education, and he is generally recognized as the "father" of French sociology. During his lifetime, the new discipline of sociology was not generally respected in higher academics and Durkheim should be credited with working to gain its respect. Many identify Durkheim as being the single most important early founder of the discipline (see Loy and Booth, 2002, pp. 41–3).

The essential elements of Durkheim's theories on social life can be seen in what many consider to be his most important work, *Suicide: A Study in Sociology*, published in 1897. *Suicide*, a classic in the history of social science research, gives us not only Durkheim's sociological view of the act of suicide itself, but by expanding upon its central themes an indication of the more general elements of structural functionalism as a whole. Indeed, the subtitle of the book informs us that the study is about both the specific act of suicide, but at the same time a guide to Durkheim's view of what the emerging discipline of sociology might look like and what his general theory of society is all about.

Durkheim makes what appears to be the counterintuitive claim that the act of suicide is much more than just a personal act by an individual. It is, instead, a social act and in fact operates according to social laws. Durkheim referred to any human activities of this sort as *social facts*, by which he meant any phenomena that operated according to social rules or laws independent of any one individual. His notion of social facts was the basis for Durkheim's more general vision of how human social life should be studied. As he clearly states, "[s]ociological method as we practice it rests wholly on the basic principle that social facts must be studied as things, that is, as realities external to the individual" (Durkheim, 1951, pp. 37–8).

Claiming that suicide is a social act independent of the particular motivation of any one individual who commits that act sets Durkheim's view dramatically apart from common ideas about suicide, particularly in his own day. He challenged two major ways of thinking about the act of suicide in the late nineteenth century: individual notions of the act, and in particular an emerging body of work in psychology that explained suicide according the inner laws of the mind; and Christian religious thinking that thought of the act as a sin against God.

Durkheim met one of the litmus tests of sound theory mentioned earlier—that it must be verified through systematic accumulation and observation of facts or statistics—by first of all collecting a remarkable inventory of statistics on suicide rates across Europe. This in and of itself was no small feat given the very limited technology and media of communication available to him in the late nineteenth century. After collecting his data, Durkheim observed that suicide rates follow identifiable social patterns. For example, men committed suicide at significantly higher rates than women, Protestants committed suicide more than Catholics, unmarried people more than married people, and wealthy people, interestingly, more than poorer people. Durkheim identified other categories, but a common theme emerged, one that is crucial to understanding his theory of society more generally: that levels of *social integration* across categories of people significantly impact the chances of a particular individual committing suicide or not.

By *social integration*, Durkheim meant common ties or bonds that hold people together and give them a common outlook and a feeling of solidarity with the social world around them. As stated clearly in his own terms: "suicide varies inversely with the degree of integration of the social groups of which the individual forms a part" (Durkheim, 1951, p. 209). So, while for example men and those who are wealthy might achieve greater autonomy and independence, it comes at a cost of reduced integration and social bonds, and thus a greater chance of suicide.

Durkheim and then other functionalist theorists who followed him in the twentieth century expanded upon this essential notion of the role of social integration to develop a much more general and complex theory of society. The theory became particularly strong by the middle of the twentieth century, especially in the United States under the direction and influence of Harvard professor Talcott Parsons, whose dominance in American sociology was so great that sociology at one point was almost synonymous with "Parsonian structural functionalism" (McQuarie, 1995, pp. 4–5).

In general, structural functionalism views society as a *complex system in which all of the different elements of its structure work to promote stability and solidarity within that system*. The essential elements of the theory's view of society can be seen in the two terms in the name of the theory. First, society has a *structure*, which means it has a stable and persistent pattern of elements, including institutions, patterns of interpersonal behaviour, and values and norms. In terms of *function*, all elements function or contribute to the overall stability of the structure of society (Parsons, 1961).

While at times somewhat difficult to comprehend when expressed in theoretical terms, the example of education might help explain the theory. The institution of education, according to structural functionalism, will take on a particular form only if it functions to reinforce the overall structure of the social system as a whole and reinforce its dominant values and norms. So, in simple terms, by far the most common reason university students cite for attending university and potentially receiving a degree of higher learning is to get a better job than they would otherwise. Here, education is both reinforcing and reflecting the economy, and the values and norms of students are in turn a reflection of, or function to reinforce the values important to, the work world.

For understanding sport, functionalism has been important in terms of considering several important vital functions sport serves to wider society. Also, the theory was dominant in the discipline of sociology when the specific subdiscipline of sport sociology was first developing in the 1960s and 1970s.

Sport, according to the structural functionalist analysis, functions to develop group bonds, to encourage a sense of community, and to integrate people into society's dominant values. Sport also acts as a significant agent of socialization and helps children, in particular, develop solid social skills. In addition, sport functions as positive entertainment and as an "escape valve" from some of the more laborious aspects of everyday life. Finally, it is often argued that sport functions to deter youth and others from deviant and antisocial behaviour (Loy & Booth, 2000, 2002).

In Canada, we can think of the many ways in which sport plays a crucial role in the construction of a common sense of nationhood. Athletes supported under Sport Canada and its system of funding and development for elite national and international competition serve as both a means to enhance nationalism and a common identity domestically, while simultaneously acting as international ambassadors. Following Ben Johnson's world-record medal performance at the World Track and Field Championships in Rome in 1987—and before the infamous scandal that resulted from his positive drug test one year later—Minister of State for Fitness and Amateur Sport Otto Jelinek said that "Ben Johnson, doing what he's doing for Canadians in Rome, is probably worth more than a dozen delegations of high-powered diplomats" (Beamish & Borowy, 1988, p. 11).

While it dominated sociology by the mid-twentieth century and influenced the first research on sport in the 1960s and 1970s, structural functionalism then declined in influence because of two major criticisms. The first was a criticism of the internal logic of the theory. There is an inherent logical *tautology*—a circular argument that does not have any real meaning—in the theory in the sense that the elements of social systems are assumed to be functional by the very fact that they exist, but at the same time they exist because they are functional. The circular argument turns on itself, and becomes meaningless as a result, critics argued.

But this internal criticism is less important than the criticism of the social and political conservatism inherent in the theory. All elements of society are viewed as necessary and good for the simple fact that they exist to reinforce the overall structure of the system as a whole. But surely not all elements of social systems are justified? In its insistence on the importance of social order and the functional utility of the various elements of that order, functionalism overstates the positive components of society. It is questionable how poverty, violence, crime, institutionalized racism or sexism, and many other social problems can be thought to be positive elements of a social system, especially, of course, for those on the receiving end of those problems. But ironically this is an implication of functionalist theory. Functionalism reached its lowest point in this regard when it was suggested by two theorists of social stratification, Kingsley Davis and Wilbert Moore (1945), that class inequalities are inevitable components of social systems and play important functional roles. Their proof was based on their observation that class stratification has existed in all social systems and, they argued, it is necessary to reward those who spend time and effort training and working in jobs that are more important for society as a whole with greater compensation in the form of status or wealth. While at one level the Davis–Moore thesis may make sense because some jobs do in fact require greater training, skill, and knowledge, critics pointed out that this by no means justified the often huge inequalities or discrepancies in terms of status or pay. The most successful and highly paid professional athletes come to mind right away, in that, while they may provide great entertainment, it is difficult to justify their multimillion-dollar salaries given their questionable utility or usefulness to society otherwise.

In some senses the Davis–Moore thesis drew the proverbial line in the sand in debates about sociological theory. Statements such as theirs eventually led to the downfall of functionalist theory and the rise of a competing perspective that attempted to account in a much more realistic fashion for the existence of social problems and inequalities.

KARL MARX AND CONFLICT THEORY

Like structural functionalism, some of the central tenets of modern conflict sociology are very old and can be traced back to ancient times. However, the theory's more modern form owes itself to one individual in particular: Karl Marx (1818–83) (McQuarie, 1995, pp. 63–5). Marx was born in Trier, in the Rhineland (in what is now Germany), and in his earliest years as a student he became interested in the study of law and philosophy before turning his attention later to journalism, political activism, and writing in social and political critique. His radical politics and involvement in workers' organizations were partly the cause for his migration—sometimes forced—from Germany to France and eventually England (Beamish, 2002, pp. 25–39).

Marx sought to develop a social theory that understood the world around him and at the same time actively help create social conditions that would be more egalitarian and democratic. Marx's political commitment was due to a large degree to the harsh conditions of life, discussed earlier, encountered by a majority of people in the emerging industrial revolution. His famous words "[t]he philosophers have only *interpreted* the world, in various ways; the point, however, is to *change* it" (Marx, 1972, p. 109) are a clear reflection of his political commitment. Indeed, that same political commitment would have a lasting legacy on the conflict tradition in sociology years after Marx was gone, as it would on various social movements throughout the twentieth century and now into the twenty-first.

What was unique about Marx's analysis of society and what lay at the foundation of his ideas was, first, his recognition that the *economic* conditions of social life formed the base or foundation of social life more generally; second, his ability to synthesize and expand his observations regarding the basic economic conditions of social life into a more general theory regarding the nature of social, cultural, and individual life; and third, his observations regarding the important role *social conflict* played in social and cultural life and the history of societies.

The idea that economic conditions lay the foundation for social life is really at the core of Marx's theory. Marx observed that throughout history different economic forms shaped social systems and, in turn, people's lives within those systems. He referred to these forms as the *mode of production*. Within each mode of production—and Marx studied many in human history, including ancient society, feudalism, and capitalism—Marx also observed that classes emerged

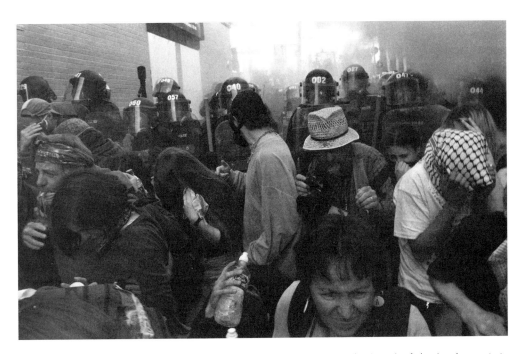

Modern-day protests over free trade liberalization and globalization—such as the Summit of the Americas protests in Quebec City in April 2001—reflect some of the same free-market tensions that Marx was concerned with in the nineteenth century.

KEVIN FRAYER/CP Images

based on their ability to wrest control over economic resources and the means of producing goods. This, Marx observed, had led to a state of *conflict* between the respective groups in each case. The opening lines of *The Communist Manifesto*, one of the most important political documents in modern history, state this clearly:

> The history of all hitherto existing society is the history of class struggles. Freeman and slave, patrician and plebeian, lord and serf, guildmaster and journeyman, in a word, oppressor and oppressed, stood in constant opposition to one another, carried on an uninterrupted, now hidden, now open fight, a fight that each time ended, either in a revolutionary reconstitution of society at large, or in the common ruin of the contending classes. (Marx & Engels, 1948, p. 9)

While Marx was interested in various modes of production throughout history and the conflicts that emerged from them, the *capitalist* mode of production drew the lion's share of his attention and work. In his most important work, *Capital*, published in 1867, Marx attempted to explain in scientific terms the manner in which the capitalist mode of production worked (Marx, 1977). His central insight is that capitalism, in its unyielding drive to create profit, produces two separate classes—capitalists who realize the profits and surpluses from the system, and workers who do not. The strength of the capitalist mode of production, however—one unlike other modes of production—is that workers *appear* to be acting freely and of their own choice. However, workers do not realize their full potential because their labour is *alienated* labour; that is, labour that ultimately benefits those who profit from it. As Marx states clearly: "work is *external* to the worker . . . consequently, he does not fulfil himself in his work but denies himself. . . . His work is not voluntary but imposed, *forced labour*. It is not the satisfaction of a need, but only a *means* for satisfying other needs" (Marx, 1963, pp. 124–5). Marx's dual insights regarding the production of the class system within the capitalist mode of production and the alienation of the worker would many years later be central to both Marxist and conflict-based analyses of sport.

Marx's insights into the role of class conflict formed the base of *conflict theory* more generally. The central difference between Marx's analysis and the one of conflict theory is that the latter developed a much broader and encompassing definition of conflict, especially as the theory was adopted in U.S. sociology in the post-WWII era (McQuarie, 1995). Conflict was recognized to be much more ubiquitous in society, beyond the conflicts between the capitalists and working classes as Marx saw them. Examples include conflicts between workers and middle-managers in industrial settings; between authority figures and subordinates in many different bureaucratic organizational contexts; or between political elites and citizens or secondary-level government members in totalitarian political regimes, under socialist–communism, or, for that matter, in liberal–democratic societies.

Conflict theorist Ralf Dahrendorf expresses the essential elements of conflict theory as a series of four postulates:

(a) Every society is subjected at every moment to change: change is ubiquitous.
(b) Every society experiences at every moment social conflict: social conflict is ubiquitous.
(c) Every element in a society contributes to its change.
(d) Every society rests on constraint of some of its members by others. (Dahrendorf, 1995, p. 78)

It should be obvious from Dahrendorf's summary just how dramatically different the conflict model is from the vision of society proposed by structural functionalism. Whereas structural functionalism sees a smoothly operating, coordinated, and stable system, conflict sees constant power, inequality, and change.

In terms of the analysis of sport, three overarching questions or issues flow from Marx's central insights and the more general conflict model that followed from them. First, how does sport contribute to or reinforce class and other power structures in society? While we may not tend to think of sport as reinforcing class inequalities or other forms of power, sport has in fact played a very important role in Canada's history in this regard (Gruneau, 1983). In his landmark book *The Struggle for Canadian Sport*, author Bruce Kidd (1996b) demonstrates that the active political power struggles between various groups during the period between the two World Wars created the foundation for some of the most important elements of the Canadian sport landscape. One for-profit business cartel, the National Hockey League, was particularly successful in setting the agenda for Canadian sport; however, Kidd demonstrates that this did not come without a cost: the handful of owners—all men—were successful but were so at the expense of other vibrant sporting traditions, including a very successful women's organization under the direction of the Women's Amateur Athletic Federation. Also, amateur leaders, who in general supported middle- to upper-class sporting clubs and the elite men—again, all men—that made up their membership, came into conflict with a vibrant workers' sport movement—one that has been largely erased from Canada's sporting history—which attempted to use sport as a means to fight for workers' rights. Conflict based on class differences, various political objectives, and the attempt to define the *meaning* of sport was common in early Canadian sport and significantly shaped the country's early cultural landscape.

A second issue that arises from conflict theory is the manner in which conflict and change occur within sporting organizations and practices. Donald MacIntosh's and David Whitson's (author of Chapter 13, Globalization) *The Game Planners: Transforming Canada's Sport System* (1990) is a classic example of this. The authors demonstrate that during the development of the government-run and -funded sport system from the 1960s to the late 1980s, particular political objectives combined with an emerging cadre of sport "professionals" determined the direction of the sport system to meet their own interests and agendas. As a result, despite the fact that the first legislation supporting government involvement in sport in 1961 called for support for sport at both the high-performance level and the everyday grassroots level, the former has completely overshadowed the latter because high-performance sport satisfies the political and professional objectives of those within the system. One major and, as the authors argue, unfortunate consequence is there has been very little support, other than lip service, for grassroots efforts to support mass recreation and sport at the local or everyday level. A second consequence is one that has influenced physical education and allied disciplines. MacIntosh and Whitson point out that as the federal sport system developed, physical education programs changed to reflect the need to produce performances at the national and international levels:

> In the model of "professionality" that now dominates Canadian physical education, the young sport scientist or sport manager is encouraged to see his or her job as the production of performance . . . and is seldom seriously introduced to the social and political questions that surround the concentration of resources on elite sport. (MacIntosh & Whitson, 1990, p. 120)

University physical education, in other words, has been directly implicated in the power struggles to define what is important for the sport "system" at the federal level. MacIntosh's and Whitson's analysis continues to have direct relevance today. Interestingly, as there has been increased support for the federal high-performance sport system over time, participation rates and activity levels of Canadian youth have shrunk.

The third issue stems directly from Marx's idea about the alienation of the worker in the capitalist mode of production. Some conflict theorists have claimed that sport, as a reflection of that system, has produced an alienated experience. In *Sport: A Prison of Measured Time*, French social and political theorist Jean-Marie Brohm (1978) gives a classic Marxist-inspired condemnation of sport and, in particular, the Olympic Games. Sport, Brohm claims, is an institutional form through which capitalist class inequalities are reproduced and excessive attention to work has become an unquestioned ideal. Athletes, Brohm claims, pay excessive attention to the details of time (thus the subtitle of the book) and the command of space at the exclusion of other forms of physical activity that might be more liberating and fulfilling. Expressed in his own no uncertain terms, Brohm claims that "sport is the *ideology of the body/machine*—the body turned into a robot, alienated by capitalist labour" (p. 77).

Rob Beamish (author of Chapter 4) has also expressed the dynamic of sport's potential combined with the problem of limiting that potential under alienating conditions:

> If sporting activity is so rich with creative potential—so robust with opportunities for indi-
> viduals to explore their own limits and the limitations of human physical performance—the
> loss of control of the product can have devastating consequences for the creative potential of
> physical activity. . . . rather than realising the full productive potential of the athlete, sport
> stands against the athlete and builds the power of the market's influence over sport while
> restricting the expressive potential of the athletes themselves. (Beamish, 2002, p. 37)

It was mentioned at the beginning of this chapter that all sociological theories used to study sport have a political motivation. The legacy of Marx's ideas and conflict theory as a whole is the identification of inequalities and the manner in which they influence the experience of sport, and the promise of an unalienated full expression of physical movement for as many people as possible.

GEORGE HERBERT MEAD AND SYMBOLIC INTERACTIONISM

Symbolic interactionism is part of a much bigger tradition in sociology called *microsociology*, which in general studies and attempts to understand the real-life behaviours of people in society. Microsociological approaches are generally critical of *macrosociology* or "grand theories"—such as structural functionalism and conflict theories—because of their overemphasis on sweeping structural processes at the expense of understanding how *people* actually understand the world around them and interact. In 1964, when microsociological perspectives were first coming into their own, George Homans' scathing critique of macrosociology's overemphasis on social structure at the expense of understanding people's real-life experiences was expressed clearly: "What I ask is that we bring what we say about theory into line with what we actually do, and so put an end to out intellectual hypocrisy" (Homans, 1964, p. 818).

The most important individual in terms of the development of symbolic interactionism was George Herbert Mead (1863–1931). Mead taught at the University of Chicago from 1894 until he died in 1931. During his years at Chicago the university had an influential department of sociology, although Mead taught social psychology courses in the philosophy department. His teaching history is important because, despite the fact that he did not publish a single book during his lifetime, his teaching would influence generations of students and help form an entire subdiscipline in sociology, one that influenced other academic areas as well. He was known to be a powerful orator and lecturer; students were so enthralled with his teaching that a group of them collaborated to publish his work posthumously based on their notes from his lectures. The result was *Mind, Self, and Society*, first published in 1934 and considered a classic in sociology (Mead, 1962; see also Donnelly, 2002, pp. 83–5; McQuarie, 1995, pp. 188–90).

Mead's theoretical insights were a reaction against, first, the structural or macrosociological theories and, second, a tradition in psychology called *behaviourism*, which held that human behaviour could be equated with animal behaviour and explained according to natural and automatic responses to stimuli in the environment. This, Mead believed, grossly underestimated the role of human thought and volitional action. In particular, behaviourism did not account for the *symbolic* nature of human thought and the ability of humans to interpret and give meaning to the world around them through language. It also did no justice to the *social context* or role of *social interaction* in determining human behaviour. These two fundamental insights are the foundation of Mead's thinking and, combined, the source of the perspective that would eventually become known as *symbolic interactionism*.

At the heart of Mead's theory is the manner in which humans develop a sense of *self*. When the term is used in everyday language it usually is meant in a purely individual sense, as in my*self*. However, Mead pointed out that the self is a dynamic, not a static thing. In other words, we do not simply *have* a self; rather, we continually *develop* a sense of self over time—it is an ongoing process. Mead spent much time explaining the development of the self in children as they grew, pointing out that children grow through a series of stages, each of which gives them a greater sense of themselves as individuals and at the same time a greater sense of others' images of them and how they *think* others view them (Mead, 1962, pp. 144–64).

The latter point regarding the image others have of a person gets to the core of a second important point Mead made about the self. Mead described two components of the self, which he called the *I* and the *Me*. While the terms are very simple, the ideas they represent are much more profound. The I for Mead is the internal component of our self—the part of the self that is subjectively experienced and initiates a person's actions in the world. This is the part of the self we associate with our internal feelings, motivations, and general purpose in life. The Me, however, is the image humans have of themselves that comes from outside of ourselves—how others view us and how we believe or think others view us. While the I is the subjective experience of the self, then, the Me is the objective experience. In Mead's own words:

> The "I" is the response of the organism to the attitudes of the others; the "me" is the organized set of attitudes of others which one himself assumes. The attitudes of the others constitutes the organized "me," and then one reacts toward that as an "I." (Mead, 1962, p. 175)

For Mead, the two parts can be separated at the conceptual level, but not at the real-life level as they are actually experienced; we constantly live through, and with, both the I and the Me at the same time. But what is important in making the conceptual break for Mead lies at the heart of his theory and its impact on sociology: the Me component of the self is created from the wider social world, meaning our very sense of our*selves* is, in essence, and at one and the same time, part of a social identity.

Intuitively, we can think of what Mead is trying to suggest by thinking about our own day-to-day experiences. For example, we have all seen people who are self-conscious about the way they are dressed, to the extent that they frequently look at themselves to make sure whatever pieces of clothing they are wearing on a given day are appropriate. They may also fix their hair, or perhaps carry their bodies in particular ways to appear a certain way. The feeling that people have when they go through this process represents perfectly Mead's notions of the self as it is comprised of the I and the Me. The person's identity and sense of him or herself is "wrapped up," so to speak, in the presentation of self through physical appearance. But who is doing the "looking" here? Certainly, it's an internal process, in the sense that the person asks "How do I look?" But of course the second part of the process—perhaps the more important one—is external. The imaginary mirror that the person is holding up, which generates the external image the person has of him or herself, is the social world itself. The social world is looking in and has become a part of the person's personality or sense of self as he/she learns how to dress and look a certain way, and carry or "comport" him or herself in a certain way. This, in essence, is the Me component of the self Mead is describing. The important part of Mead's analysis is that the self, human identity, and even the very act of being conscious of oneself, is *social*.

After Mead, a number of theorists debated the role of the self in relation to wider social structure, but it was one of Mead's students, Herbert Blumer, who coined the term *symbolic interactionism*. The foundation of social life, Blumer said, is implied by the two terms in the theory's name. Blumer (1995) makes this clear when he says that "symbolic interaction" refers to the

> fact that human beings interpret or "define" each other's actions instead of merely reacting to each others actions. Their "response" is not made directly to the actions of one another but instead is based on the meaning which they attach to such actions. Thus, human interaction is mediated by symbols, by interpretation, or by ascertaining the meaning of one another's action. (p. 206)

Here Blumer, following Mead, makes it clear that understanding human interaction is much more complex than behavioural psychology or structural functionalism in sociology would have it. Meaning is created by humans and not through social structure "from above." Blumer purposely puts "response" in quotation marks to point out that the stimulus–response theory of the behaviourists is clearly a simplistic view of how human beings understand the world and interact with others.

The fundamental insights in symbolic interactionism have formed the basis of various methods for studying everyday life, loosely summarized under the terms *interpretive sociology*. Interpretive sociology refers to a collection of methods for understanding the meaning that people bring to their own lives and actions, the lives and actions of others around them, and the complex interaction between people's everyday lives and the wider social structure (Beal, 2002). The theories and methods have grown and become much more complex since Mead's day; however, in general his foundational observations regarding the manner in which the self is developed within a social context form the central motivation for interpretive sociology (Donnelly, 2002).

For sports studies, two major themes have emerged. The first is the study of *socialization* and the processes through which people are both socialized into sport, and socialized through sport. Socialization *into* sport means the active process of learning sport's rules, codes, values, and norms. Socialization *through* sport, on the other hand, refers to the lessons that are learned from sport that have some application to wider society. While much of the research in socialization has concentrated, not surprisingly, on children's sport, it should be pointed out that socialization is a life-long process. One example of this is the development of mid-life sports identities, such as is gained through any one of the many adult Masters sport organizations and competitions. Also, sociologists are only just beginning to understand the experience of sport and physical movement for older adults.

The second major theme in interpretive sociology of sport is sport *subcultures*. Here, research has attempted to understand the process through which subcultural groups form their own unique language, belief system, normative structure, and general inner-group identity. Some so-called alternative sports, such as surfing, rock climbing, extreme sports, skateboarding, Ultimate Frisbee, and others provide interesting and accessible contexts to understand the process through which members develop subcultural identities; however, members of all long-standing traditional sports develop their own unique language, belief system, and identity as well.

One of the ways in which the study of socialization and subcultures intersect is in the career paths of athletes. Here, the process of becoming an athlete, maintaining an athlete identity, and retiring or disengaging from a sport is studied. Christopher Stevenson, author of Chapter 14, has studied the process of becoming a high-performance athlete. Stevenson interviewed several Canadian and British high-performance athletes in an attempt to understand the process through which a serious athlete identity is formed. Among his findings was the fact that the process of developing and maintaining an identity is very complex and goes far beyond just knowing the particulars of the sport itself and performing well in it. The process also involved an important social and interactive element, in which athletes formed bonds that themselves determined whether an athlete would stick with the sport or not (Stevenson, 1999).

Interpretive sociology has a bright future because research has only just scratched the surface in terms of understanding people's experiences in sport and in the development of sporting identities.

CRITICAL SOCIAL THEORIES

Critical social theories are first of all, as the name suggests, a number of theories, not just one. They are also a more recent development in the sociology of sport and so should be thought of as a "work in progress." If any generalization about critical social theories can be made, it is that they are a combination, reflection, and development of two of the theories mentioned to this point: conflict theory and symbolic interactionism. Power and inequality tends to be a continuing concern in critical theories, but generally they differ from conflict theory in two major respects. First, it is not assumed that people are simply subservient, passive "dupes." People and groups in critical theories have *agency*, meaning they can control, at least to some degree, the conditions of the world around them, even in the face of power relations that might try to limit them. Humans actively and often imaginatively interpret and give meaning to the world and in doing so challenge dominant ways of seeing things. People can challenge power relations in order to evoke change, and to make sense of their lives while they are doing so. Second, critical theories tend to expand notions of power and authority beyond that of conflict theory, in particular to an understanding of gender and sexual relations on the one hand and race relations on the other. These two strands within critical social theories are outlined below. Jay Coakley and Peter Donnelly (2004a) explain the combination of these two differences. Critical social theories, they point out, explain:

> how power is produced and reproduced [and] how people struggle over the ideas and meanings they use to make sense out of the world, form identities, interact with others, and transform the conditions of their lives. (p. 42)

Three major strands can be identified within critical social theories. The first strand is *cultural studies*. While cultural studies itself encompasses a growing and diverse body of work, certain historical predecessors denote common elements. One important inspiration for the development of cultural studies was Antonio Gramsci (1891–1937), an Italian social and political theorist and activist who was arrested in 1926 because of his involvement in the Central Committee of the Italian Communist Party in Italy. Gramsci was particularly interested in the manner in which power and control are maintained in capitalist economies under liberal–democratic forms of government, both of which were still in relatively early phases and under contestation from alternate forms of economic planning and political structures in Gramsci's day. Gramsci used the term *hegemony* to describe how this process happens. Instead of direct physical control, Gramsci believed that the power of dominant classes is maintained through a process of developing consent among the populace. This can occur, first, in a structural sense in that groups at different levels of social organization make compromises with ruling classes, such as is the case when labour organizations concede to wage or salary increases, or when volunteer organizations compensate for social inequalities by fundraising.

But consent also occurs through a second manner, when the ideas that benefit the ruling classes are accepted and become "common sense" in the minds of people. For Gramsci, the process is an ongoing one in which consensus of the people always has to be won over. As cultural studies theorists Jennifer Hargreaves and Ian McDonald (2000) explain:

> In Gramsci's formula, it is not simply a matter of class control, but an unstable process which requires the winning of consent from subordinate groups. It is, then, never "complete" or fixed, but rather diverse and always changing. (p. 50)

While rarely do people think of sport playing a "hegemonic" role in reinforcing social power relations, there is no question that it has done so in Canada's history. Interestingly, this was more fully recognized years ago when social and political organizations used sport much more directly for ideological purposes than they typically do today. In the 1920s and 1930s, the Workers' Sports Association of Canada fully realized that amateur organizers would happily use sport as a means to appease the working classes (Kidd, 1996b). Indeed, amateur leader Henry Roxborough's comment in *Maclean's* magazine in 1926 that "A nation that loves sport cannot revolt" could not have been more politically opposite to that from a workers' rights paper the following year:

> The whole capitalist class profits by a system that keeps workers excitedly interested in trivial matters remote from true concerns . . . The brain-numbing narcotic of the sporting page is perhaps more deadly to the average worker than the more active poison of the editorial page. (cited in Kidd, 1996b, pp. 50, 167)

In these words we see the dual parts of power at play as cultural theorists see it; sport is used both as a means of social control but at the same time the workers' rights paper demonstrates that a certain degree of agency or, in this case, resistance is possible.

A second influence on cultural studies was the creation of the Centre for Contemporary Cultural Studies in Birmingham, England in 1964. While the Centre started as a means to study the history of the English working class, cultural studies as it became defined at the Centre developed over time and spread internationally to include both the culture and structure of class in many other countries, and the influence of people's experiences with popular forms of culture, including sport, and how those experiences intersect with power and class (Hargreaves & McDonald, 2000).

A second strand within critical social theories is *feminist studies*. Shona Thompson has expressed feminism's main social and political objectives in clear terms:

> Fundamentally, feminism champions the belief that women have rights to all the benefits and privileges of social life equally with men. For the purposes of those concerned with sport, this means that girls and women have the right to choose to participate in sport and physical activity without constraint, prejudice or coercion, to expect their participation to be respected and taken seriously, and to be as equally valued and rewarded as sportsmen. (Thompson, 2002, p. 106)

Feminist-inspired histories of sport in Canada have identified the very important role that gender relations and ideas about both women and men have played in the country's sporting traditions. A landmark book is Helen Lenskyj's *Out of Bounds: Women, Sport & Sexuality*, published in 1986. The year is important because Lenskyj's book was published at a time when there were very few published works on the history of, or social issues related to, women's sport, a reflection of the fact that the disciplines of sociology and history were dominated by men who as a rule pushed women's issues to the side. Lenskyj (author of Chapter 6, on gender issues in sport) is especially strong in analyzing some of the sources of cultural beliefs that for years justified limiting women's participation. Medical science was particularly important. The scientific doctrine of the "conservation of energy" was used—and abused—to argue that women had a limited amount of "vital energy" and any effort put into vigorous physical activity would come into direct conflict with women's ability to bear and rear children. The "frailty myth" that resulted was so strong that for years to come many people believed that it was simply "unnatural" for women to engage in any sort of vigorous activity (Lenskyj, 1986).

A more recent example in feminist-inspired studies is Ann Hall's (2002) *The Girl and the Game: A History of Women's Sport in Canada*, likely the most complete historical account of women's sport in Canada ever written. Interestingly, Hall's opening line of the book, "The history of modern sport is a history of cultural struggle" (p. 1) replicates, but with significant differences, the opening sentence of *The Communist Manifesto*: "The history of all hitherto existing society is the history of class struggle" (Marx & Engels, 1948, p. 9). Hall's opening line reflects, first, the central difference between feminism and conflict theories—the recognition by the former that power operates at levels conflict theory in its classical theoretical form had not envisioned; second, the "struggle" in Hall's sentence reflects a position common in critical social theories in general—that resistance is possible and power is never complete. While male power and privilege certainly played an important role in women's sport historically, Hall recounts in her text the various ways in which women—and sometimes men—resisted that power and privilege to create opportunities. As Hall says:

> Women's long history of confronting a male preserve like sport illustrates the "double movement of containment and resistance" that characterizes cultural struggles among dominant and subordinate groups. (p. 2)

Feminist theory continues to inspire studies of the various ways in which sex, gender, and sexuality influence sporting experiences; these are discussed in more detail in Chapter 6.

A final strand within critical social theories is *critical race studies*. The discipline of sociology of sport has been largely negligent in understanding the important role of ethnicity, ideas about race, and racism in sport. Critical race studies have emerged in the attempt to overcome this gap by pointing out the important role race relations and racism have played in shaping sporting traditions in Canadian history and how they continue to shape it today.

Generally, critical theories of race are interested in, first, the manner in which sport and physical movement play important roles in the development of ethnic cultural beliefs and heritage; second, the manner in which certain ethnic traditions in Canada have been privileged at the expense of others; and, finally, the manner in which ideas about "race" have been naturalized or reinforced through sport. All of these themes are discussed in more detail in Chapter 5 by authors Victoria Paraschak and Susan Tirone.

One of the important themes taken up by critical race theory—one that has only just begun to be analyzed in relation to sport—is the manner in which ideas about what "Canada" is and what constitutes a "true Canadian" are themselves imbued with assumptions about race. Sociologist Himani Bannerji (2000) has challenged the notion of "Canadianness" by suggesting that this notion has contained within it assumptions about race. The country's colonial history has led to a certain dominant image of Canadianness, but these dominant notions have been based on very specific historical conditions and cultural traditions in which certain groups have been privileged in the development of the image while others have been erased from the picture. In Bannerji's words:

> Official multiculturalism, mainstream political thought and the news media in Canada all rely comfortably on the notion of a nation and its state both called Canada, with legitimate

subjects called Canadians. . . . There is an assumption that this Canada is a singular entity, a moral, cultural and political essence. . . . And yet, when we scrutinize this Canada, what do we see? The answer to this question depends on which side of the nation we inhabit. For those who see it as a homogenous cultural/political entity . . . Canada is unproblematic. For others . . . who have been dispossessed in one sense or another, the answer is quite different. (pp. 104–5)

An example in Canada's history is the "two solitudes" account of the English and French in Canada which, while certainly an important and real part of Canada's history and one that continues to influence the country's social and political life, is also an account of Canada's history that has effectively erased Canada's Aboriginal peoples from the historical picture. Interestingly, in justifying funding for a new federal sport system in a campaign speech he made in 1968, Pierre Trudeau claimed that sport could be used effectively to promote nationalism and ease tensions between the French and the English (MacIntosh & Whitson, 1990; MacIntosh, Bedecki, & Franks, 1987). The sport "system" that developed, however, effectively ignored the many and varied sporting traditions of people who were dispossessed, including Aboriginal sport.

And what type of sport was privileged? International Olympic sport has played a hegemonic role internationally and directly influenced what the government has considered to be "real" sport in justifying its federally run sport system. But consider the comments of the founder of the modern Olympic Games, Pierre de Coubertin, in an article entitled "Why I Revived the Olympic Games" published in 1908:

[t]he work must be lasting, to exercise over the sports of the future that necessary and beneficent influence for which I look—an influence which shall make them the means of bringing to perfection the strong and hopeful youth of our white race, thus again helping towards the perfection of all human society. (de Coubertin, 2000, p. 546)

Pierre de Coubertin's comment regarding the "white race" is in one sense shocking, although it is not clear that he meant literally for Olympic sport to "perfect the white race." Nevertheless, his comments point to the fact that, while the Olympic Games tends to be regarded by many as the world's main representative of "sport," the movement was in fact founded on very particular traditions in Western Europe during a very specific point in time; the sport of France, England, and a few—very few—other nations played the dominant role and dictated in turn the dominant form of sport internationally for the remainder of the twentieth century. Critical race studies are only just beginning to unpack some of the central assumptions about race and ethnicity in sport. Indeed, de Coubertin's comments suggest race and ethnic heritage are woven right into the very fabric of "sport."

CONCLUSIONS

It should be kept in mind that sociological theory is an ongoing and developing process. Part of the purpose of this chapter has been to demonstrate that sociological theories themselves have long heritages and in many cases intersect in terms of perspectives on the social and cultural world. Perhaps the most important thing to keep in mind as you read the chapters that follow, and as you consider the myriad perspectives on the themes presented, is the ultimate political goals of sociological theory and, in turn, the developing discipline of sociology of sport: to make the world the best one possible, one in which sport and physical activity can play important and significant roles in the enrichment of people's lives.

CRITICAL THINKING QUESTIONS

1. This chapter demonstrated that sociology views history itself as a *dynamic* process. What examples can you think of in which having knowledge about some aspect of Canadian sport history has enabled you to understand an issue or controversy in the present?

2. The discipline of sociology emerged out of the problems and issues generated by the emergence of democratic institutions and the industrial revolution. What problems or issues still exist today, similar to the ones the first sociologists were concerned with?

3. C. Wright Mills' use of the "sociological imagination" was discussed in this chapter. What other examples can you think of (besides Mills' example of unemployment) in which what appear to be personal problems should also be thought of as public issues?

4. Put yourself in the shoes of a Marxist thinker. How would you consider the following topics: the Canadian federal government's funding of elite athletes; Nike Corporation's third-world labour practices; public access to facilities and resources for sport and recreation?

5. What examples can you think of in which the "Me" part of the individual character (as defined by George Herbert Mead) is reinforced in sport? In other words, think of examples in which the external social environment leads to individuals taking on a certain sports character or identity.

6. In what ways do gender and sexuality (discussed in the final section of the chapter) continue to play an important role in Canadian sport today in terms of both empowering but also limiting experiences in sport?

SUGGESTED READINGS

Coakley, J., & Donnelly, P. (Eds.). (1999). *Inside sports*. London and New York: Routledge.

Coakley, J., & Dunning, E. (Eds.). (2000). *Handbook of sports studies*. London/Thousand Oaks/New Delhi: Sage Publications. Especially Chapters 1–5.

Gruneau, R. (1999). *Class, sports, and social development*. Champaign, IL: Human Kinetics.

Hall, M. A. (1996). *Feminism and sporting bodies*. Champaign, IL: Human Kinetics.

Maguire, J., & Young, K. (Eds.). (2002). *Theory, sport & society*. Amsterdam: JAI.

WEB LINKS

ISSA International Sociology of Sport Association
http://www.issa.otago.ac.nz/index.html
The International Sociology of Sport Association provides a good general description of the discipline's purpose and links to related websites such as journals, conferences, and related information.

McMaster University, Department of Sociology Virtual Library
http://www.mcmaster.ca/socscidocs/w3virtsoclib/theories.htm
McMaster's Department of Sociology website provides good information and links to sociology in general and sociological theory. It is not specific to sport but is a good general resource.

Feminist Majority Foundation
http://www.feminist.org/sports/
The sports link on the Feminist Majority Foundation website provides information on women's sport history, equity issues, and empowerment through sport.

CHAPTER 3

CANADIAN SPORT IN HISTORICAL PERSPECTIVE

Don Morrow

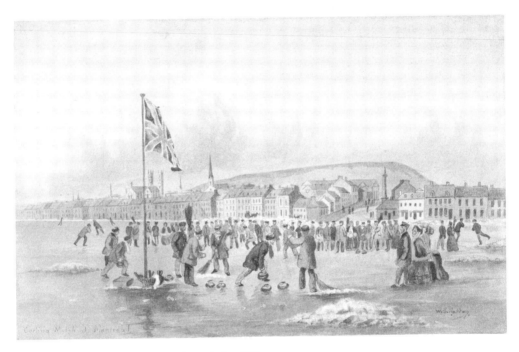

Curling on the St. Lawrence River near Montreal, circa 1850.

Library and Archives Canada/W. H. Coverdale collection of Canadiana/Accession no. 1970-188-2096/C-040148

I know history isn't true Hinnessy, cause it ain't like what I see every day in Halstead Street. If a man comes along with a history for Greece or Rome that'll show me the people fightin', gettin' drunk, makin' love, gettin' married, owin' the grocery man, and bein' without hard coal, I'll believe there was a Greece or Rome but not before.... History is a post mortem examination. It tells you what a country died for. But I'd like to know what a country lived for!
Adapted from Caroline Ware, The Cultural Approach to History

It is the intention of this chapter to provide a historical or cultural–historical context that is fundamental to understanding and analyzing the social constructs/issues in contemporary Canadian sport from a more sociological perspective. Human behaviour has continuity to it; traditions, customs, norms, and cultural and personal values combine to impact behavioural choices and actions over time. Past, present, and future are all connected in important and inextricable ways. Thus, it is exceedingly difficult to comprehend, for example, contemporary gender issues in sport (see Chapter 6) without historical context and perspective.

DOING HISTORY

The term and connotations of the word *history* merit discussion because there is considerable difference between the past and history. In everyday terminology, the word history is used to convey the sense of anything that happened in the past. For example, with regard to a known sporting championship that was won ten years ago, we might say, "that's history." To the contrary, it's not history; that championship is a fact. Is it merely a matter of semantics? Facts (and dates) are important tools in the historian's repertoire but they are not to be equated with history. A list of facts or dates of events is just a list, it's not history. In one sense, history might be perceived as everything that happened in the past. Unequivocally, that's true; equally true is the fact that we can never know everything that happened in the past. Consider your own life. If you were to sit down and make a list of everything, every single event that has happened to you since the day you were born, would it be complete? Would it be accurate? Upon whose memory would you rely? When you finished, would you have anything more than a compilation of dates and facts more akin to a grocery list than to something meaningful and revealing about your life? And whatever list of events (no matter how complete) you compiled, would it by itself convey who you are, how you feel, what is important to you? Not likely. By extension, then, history can never be *the* record of human events, simply because we have only a fragment of records and facts about past events. Events in the past must be interpreted to be made meaningful. That interpretation is the work of the historian.

In reality, history is a method of inquiry about the past. In other words, history is what historians *do*, or, history is what a historian articulates about her subject matter. Famed French philosopher Voltaire satirically claimed, "History is after all nothing but a pack of tricks which we play upon the dead" (Durant, 1926, p. 241). In the same vein, we might say that while some historians might feel they are re-constructing the past when they write history, often they are creating a representation of that past just because of the difficulties of knowing everything that happened concerning an event or a situation or group of people. Historians ask questions about the past in order to *do* history. Inquiry is the basis of all science and social science. Historians often have the advantage of knowing past people's futures; their disadvantage is that they cannot ask questions directly to those people. Instead, historians rely on extant evidence, especially *primary* evidence—diaries, records, newspapers, census data, photographs, drawings—as the basis for formulating questions about events that happened in the past. We might ask, What were the formative factors leading up to the 1972 Canada versus the USSR hockey series? Or, we might ask, What was the nature of Canadian press coverage of the games during that series? Both are valid questions derived from the historian; neither question will reveal everything that happened during that hockey series. Even though it is often the case that historians wish for more data, more abundant evidence, it is really the clear articulation of historical questions that determines the nature and the quality of history that historians do.

Finally, it is important to consider objectivity and perspective in doing history. There are historians and traditional schools of thought that claim historians can be completely objective and reveal events exactly as those events happened without any intervention of the historians' values, biases, and/or beliefs. In basic science, researchers try to eliminate bias through such processes as manipulating a single variable for examination, by structuring control groups in experiments, and by introducing randomization in subject selection and so forth. It is difficult to imagine that one historian can eliminate all his biases. What might be more important is for historians to acknowledge their assumptions and biases and perspectives. In the latter regard, as you learned in Chapter 2, researchers use theoretical frameworks in order to explain human behaviour—theory informs their perspective. For example, Marxist historians often use the concepts inherent in class reproduction to analyze historical events. Our past in Canadian sport abounds with examples of social-class privilege and exclusion (Metcalfe, 1987). Thus, certain rules in sport might have served to preserve social-class distinctions; using a Marxist framework for analysis allows the historian to explain behaviour from that perspective. Other historians take a more narrative approach to doing history; the very word *hi-story* does contain the notion of story. This is not to suggest that history is fiction; rather, it underscores that one historian's version or interpretation of a series of events might be different than any other historian's analysis of the same events. It depends on the questions the historian asks of the data and the perspective used by the historian.

This chapter will provide a perspective on some of the trends in the development of Canadian sport over time, mostly prior to 1960, the point in time when federal government involvement in sport became paramount and pervasive (Chapters 8, 11, 12, and 13 deal with some of the resultant social, economic, political, and international issues). In considerable measure, this analysis will follow the framework and perspective inherent in the author's recent, larger work *Sport in Canada: A History* (Morrow & Wamsley, 2005). Readers might wish to refer to that book along with others listed in the Suggested Readings located at the end of this chapter. More importantly, you are encouraged to read critically; to look for my biases as a historian; and to ask questions about what you read, since reading any text meaningfully involves engaging with the material. In essence, the analysis used in this chapter will be more issue-oriented and thematic; instead of tracing events linearly, certain issues, especially as they relate to social constructs such as race, gender, and social class, will be amplified or explained in different contexts; that is, more a spiralling of events and issues. Any historical discussion of Canadian sport must be preceded by a very brief examination of significant historical antecedents and precedents in sporting evolution from ancient to modern times in Western society.

ANTECEDENTS TO CANADIAN SPORT

Greek Sporting Culture

While many ancient societies show strong evidence of the integration of various forms of physical activity—play, games, sport, dance, recreational activities—into their cultures, it is generally accepted that the roots of modern sport emanate from ancient Greece, the "birthplace" of Western civilization. We have evidence from the earliest works of Western literature, *The Iliad* and *The Odyssey*, in which their author, Homer, interprets Greek sporting events that took place sometime between the twelfth and the ninth centuries BCE. Both narratives describe heroic deeds performed against or within the backdrop of large-scale wars. The form of sport mirrored skills needed for warfare—running various distances, jumping, boxing, wrestling, chariot-racing, and throwing implements that were precursors to javelins and discus. Herein, we can trace the rudiments of track and field activities and horseracing that have been so much a part of Western societies for centuries. Instructive in these contests is the fact that only men participated and that these men wanted to win to honour their gods as well as to be the best warriors. Homer offers us even deeper insights into the value structures that became part of these events. For example, in *The Iliad* the writer describes the funeral games held in tribute to the fallen warrior Patroclus. The events were the same war-like events listed above; however, it is important to note that such games were held in celebration of Patroclus's life. Moreover, in describing those events, Homer is not content merely to tell what happened; instead, he stresses such elements associated with the events as moral virtues, character development, luck, and even cheating. Why and how people participated in sport is often at least as instructive as who played and the list of victors.

The period most associated with the forms and functions of modern sport was the Classical Greek era. It spanned the eighth through to the fifth centuries BCE, approximately. City-states like Athens and Sparta, perhaps the two most renowned among hundreds, developed cultural values that both shaped and were shaped by forms of physical activity and sport.

Athenian society during the Classical Greek era ennobled its citizenry via fostering progressive thought, democracy, and a liberal approach to life. The city itself was a vital commercial and industrial hub of the Western world. Moderation in all things characterized Athenian society. The dictum "a sound mind in a sound body" is a product of this belief system. And yet, Athenian society was very much an elitist society, one that was predicated for its glory of slavery. Similarly, the educational system catered to the all-around training of boys in music, the arts, the sciences, and training of the body. Young Athenian boys attended the *palaestra*, or "wrestling school," as the venue for their education. If an outdoor track was attached to the *palaestra*, the structure was known as a *gymnasium*—the forerunner of our modern concept of an area dedicated to the pursuit of various physical activities. Gymnasia contained all manner of running and exercise areas and were as much meeting areas for philosophical discussion as they were locales for physical endeavours. In the same vein, the most well known contribution to sport by the Greeks, the ancient Olympic Games, were physical, cultural (with music, literature, and artistic events), and religious celebrations.

The Ancient Olympic Games

The ancient Olympic Games originated during the eighth century BCE and were the most prominent of some 1,300 national athletic festivals. Track and field, combative, and horseracing events varied little at the great quadrennial Games and their almost 12 centuries of continuous existence is testament to the significance of sport in Greek culture. Socially, the games were the preserve of the male elite—women could not participate in the Olympic Games, although there are records of female Olympic victories accorded to those women who owned some of the horses used in the equestrian events. In addition, the values of fair play, equality, and amateurism emanate from these Games. Amateurism is virtually a policy of exclusion—who shall compete and under what set of rules and restrictions—and in this era, a slave culture, the Olympic Games were reserved for the male aristocrats. Fair play was certainly part of this amateur code, and the quest for equality/fairness is also revealed in the sophisticated nature of some of the ancient Greek sporting equipment. For example, for the highly prized foot races, the Greeks tried every conceivable form of fair start—the blare of a trumpet was one—until the invention of the *husplex*, or starting gate. It was not until 1956 that researchers were able to identify and explain the use of this ingenious device. Racers stood upright on stone sills; beside each runner was a vertical, wooden post and a horizontal arm (like a modern railway gate) behind which the runner stood. A cord ran from the arm, down the post, under a bronze bracket or two, and back to a starter who held the ropes for all the participants. When the starter dropped the ropes all the railway gate–like arms dropped at the same time, thereby facilitating a fair start (Harris, 1972). It is clear, then, that the Greeks developed sophisticated measures and restrictions to promote their Games. It is intriguing how much modern horse-race starting devices resemble the *husplex,* and equally fascinating that in foot races longer than one lap of the stadium runners ran counterclockwise, a tradition that defies logic and remains as the uncontested way of running multiple-lap events in track competitions today.

Traditions, conventions, rules, and value systems attached to ancient Greek sporting customs have become part of our Canadian sporting inheritance. Values attached to fair play and character development, the discipline of training for competition, the quest for excellence, the joy of the struggle (the Greek *agonistic* ideal), the notion of celebration through sport, and amateurism are all clearly established parameters of sport within ancient Greek culture and are all ones that remain in contemporary sport in a variety of ways. As the Roman Empire became the dominant society in the Western world during the six centuries surrounding the early Christian era (second century BCE to fourth century After the Christian Era, ACE), new value systems were brought to sport and indeed new forms of and forums for sport were developed.

The Roman *Ludi*

Owing in large measure to Roman influence, the national athletic festivals became increasingly professionalized and commercialized by the third and fourth centuries ACE. The Romans greatly transformed existing institutions like sport. Rome itself was an urban marvel, with its aqueducts, paved roads, parks, libraries, and 1.5-million population crammed into an area 17 kilometres in circumference. Imperial domination and commercial successes meant that most Roman citizens enjoyed some 150 holidays per year. In order to appease its population of 100 million at the height of the Empire, prominent Romans or emperors hosted, often at public expense, popular games or *ludi* (from whence we derive our word *ludicrous*). The *ludi* were gargantuan in scope, nature, and impact. Elaborate chariot races were held in the colossal Circus Maximus; wild beast fights with animals versus animals and/or animals versus gladiators (so accurately depicted in the contemporary movie *The Gladiator*) were held in the Roman Colosseum and in amphitheatres all over the Empire (Mannix, 1958). Whereas the Greeks valued participation by their elite, the Roman *ludi* were vast spectacles where spectatorship and entertainment, not participation, were the predominant values. Moreover, professionals—paid performers—were the norm in Roman games and sports, as was gambling on outcomes. Thus, by the end of the Roman era, there is almost a repertoire of forms of sport and values attached to sport from these two ancient cultures. Significantly, modern sport in Canada (and elsewhere) has duplicated, at various points in time, these forms and values attached to sport.

The Chivalric Code

By the end of the fourth century ACE, a number of factors combined to diminish Roman dominance and their games. Economic decline, famine, plagues, earthquakes, and a growing Christian fanaticism that reviled the physical excesses of the *ludi* were all factors that ushered in the Middle Ages, that period of about one millennia that stretched into the fifteenth and sixteenth centuries. Warring elites and poverty of the masses were the norm as *feudal* societies were dominated by the strict *ascetic* doctrines of the Christian church that advocated self-denial and strong anti-physicalism. Physical activity during this era was very much confined among the masses to the hard work of living and serving one's feudal lord. Among the upper classes, the most prevalent competitive activities were the *tournaments* and *jousts* (the latter so vividly portrayed in the modern movie *A Knight's Tale*). Tournaments featured groups of equestrians in combat, while jousting was an individual competition. While these events were lavish displays of medieval pageantry, what was significant about the contests was the code of conduct attached to them, that of *chivalry*. It encompassed ideals or values associated with an amalgam of honour, virtue, knighthood, bravery, loyalty, and sacrifice. Legends and myths related to King Arthur and his knights of the round table together with the Christian Crusades are probably the most well known representation of the *chivalric code* today. The masses or peasants engaged, sporadically at best, in village games and country festivals, but not likely in any sporting activities akin to the tournaments.

FIRST NATIONS GAMES AND CONTESTS

By the fifteenth century, when European conquests of North America took place, sport was clearly an activity that carried great value systems, traditions, and customs. Significantly, the impulse to play games and sports seems timeless. The form and functions of sport before the fifteenth century seem consistent in that sport was a male preserve—women were virtually excluded from games and sporting contests in Western civilization; the forms of sport were mostly related to war-like activities; upper classes dictated the forms and functions of sport; codes of behaviour were endemic and varied from amateurism to professionalism to chivalry; festivals and spectacles and celebrations were often key motivators for sport; beauty, excellence, discipline, and victory were widely evidenced; and finally, it is clear that organization is a key variable in competitive sport, from funeral games to Olympic Games to Roman spectacles to medieval tournaments and jousts. Prior to European contact, the First Nations were the earliest players of games and contests in early Canada.

Aboriginal culture for some 10,000 years before European contact was a nomadic one. Groups such as the Algonquians or the Iroquois and subgroups such as the Mohawk, Neutral, Cree, and Ojibwa travelled to be home, not to get home, and they relied on the resources the land provided and demanded of them. That lifestyle required certain skills and attributes such as strength, endurance, and resistance to pain; these, in turn, were values that were reflected in Aboriginal cultural practices like wrestling, physical contests (arm pull, finger pull, even testicle pull), and greeting games that required little equipment. When subgroups gathered it was always occasion for games and contests wherein gambling of material goods added both excitement and a means to redistribute tools, food, and other elements. Blanket toss, mooseskin ball, pole push, running contests, and early forms of lacrosse called, depending upon the particular group, *baggataway* or *tewaarathon*, were all events that were connected to the land, ways of life, and the skills of survival. Celebration was a paramount virtue in these contests, as was the notion of spiritual significance attached, for example, to a game of *tewaarathon* conducted to commemorate harvest bounty. These were the physical contests, games, and traditions that existed as Europeans infiltrated the area now known as Canada beginning in the late sixteenth and early seventeenth centuries.

FRENCH CONQUESTS

Multiple agendas brought Europeans to this continent. The quest for colonization, presumed riches of gold and other precious metals, a missionary zeal to instil Christianity in every corner of the earth, the allure of a northwest passage to the East, and the discovery of an abundance of fish (the Grand Banks, for example) and animal fur (primarily the beaver) all served as magnetic attractions to the New World. The darkness of the Middle Ages gave way to the progressiveness and idealism of the European Renaissance, an era characterized as the "re-birth" of civilization reminiscent of Classical Greece. Such scientific discoveries as the printing press and medical innovations went part and parcel with a literary renaissance most notably embodied by Shakespeare. Artists such as Leonardo da Vinci and Michelangelo revolutionized notions about the beauty and science of the body. And it was this set of ideals and idealism that permeated the minds of those who set out in conquest of new lands such as Canada.

The areas of Canada to be inhabited first by Europeans were the extreme Maritime coasts closest to the Grand Banks, the vast fur trading lands of central and northern Canada, and a major cluster of settlements that became known as New France (later Lower Canada, subsequently Quebec). New France was founded by French explorer Samuel de Champlain in the early seventeenth century. Early towns established at what became Quebec City and Montreal were vibrant communities for the seigneurial or feudal land development/settlement system that was created to foster economic growth along the St. Lawrence River. Over the course of most of the seventeenth and the first half of the eighteenth centuries, the *habitants* or French peasantry—men and women—worked the long, narrow strips of land and raised families while the fur traders, voyageurs, and the Jesuit missionaries fostered the fur trade and the predominantly Catholic religious institutions. Indeed, it is from the *Jesuit Relations*, a set of documents written by the Jesuit missionaries and sent back to France as propaganda to induce emigration to New France, that we are able to discern the rich social fabric of this era. Comparable to the pastimes of ancient and medieval cultures, the form and function of physical activities were those related to survival (Metcalfe, 1970). Thus, the *habitants* engaged in games and contests of running, wrestling, horseracing, snowshoeing, sleighing, and canoeing together with the clerically despised (for their presumed sinful nature) balls and dances. And the physical prowess of the *coureurs de bois* (runners of the woods) came to be feared and revered and developed into "masculine identities closely linked to the physical demands of their labour: strong, swift, and enduring, combined with fierce independence and a lack of deference to the authority of French administrators" (Morrow & Wamsley, 2005, p. 17).

BRITISH TRADITIONS

At the end of the Seven Years War between the British and the French in 1763, the British assumed control of what we now call Canada and was then termed British North America (BNA). While the French were allowed to retain their culture, religion, customs, and ways of life, Aboriginal groups lost control and ownership of massive tracts of land. The British poured troops and resources into BNA and brought their institutions of justice, religion (primarily Anglican), and social-class structures and governance to the maritime areas of Nova Scotia and New Brunswick and primarily to Upper Canada (now Ontario). The "British" were a composite of English, Irish, and Scottish descent reinforced later in the eighteenth century by United Empire Loyalists or British sympathizers living in the United States who came back to live in British-Canada following the defeat of the British in the American War of Independence. We know from various acts of legislation against gambling, liquor production and consumption, Sabbath-day activity restrictions, and hunting or gaming laws, along with the necessity to license billiards tables, that these activities and practices formed an important part of the lifestyles of early British North Americans.

A great deal more is known about the classic "pioneer" period of BNA, the years between the Rebellions of the Canadas (Upper and Lower) in the 1840s and the time of Confederation in 1867. Relatively massive immigration—from a population of three-quarters of a million in 1821 to more than two million at mid century—reflected an economic prosperity that, in turn, was accompanied by a social stability conducive to games and recreations. For example, circuses literally brought amusement to small towns; weddings and their accompanying *chivarees* or mock serenades were occasions for physical contests and games. So too were *work bees* in rural BNA, when neighbours gathered to raise a barn, make quilts, or harvest crops all followed by dancing, contests like wrestling and games of chance, and, of course, drinking (liquor sold for 25 cents per gallon). Taverns were ubiquitous along the highways and bi-ways of early Canada. By their very presence and fostered atmosphere of conviviality, the taverns served as social and activity centres for the citizenry. In point of fact, the very first sporting club for which we have a written record, the Montreal Curling Club, was formed at Gillis's tavern in 1807 (Lindsay, 1969). Travellers' accounts inform us that hunting and fishing were popular pastimes (obviously derived from subsistence needs) among both upper and lower social classes even though the forms of these activities varied by social class (Gillespie, 2001). By contrast, the 1845 Statutes of Upper Canada list a host of activities that legislators sought to prohibit among the lower classes on Sunday:

> And be it enacted, That if any such Merchant, Tradesman, Artificer, Mechanic, Workman, Labourer, or other person whatsoever, shall . . . purchase any wares, merchandizes, goods, chattels, or personal property, or any real estate whatsoever, on the Lord's Day, commonly called Sunday . . . or shall play at skittles, ball, foot-ball, racket, or any other noisy game, or shall gamble with dice or otherwise, or shall run races on foot, or on horseback, or in carriages, or vehicles of any sort on that day, or if any person or persons shall go out fishing, or hunting or shooting, or in quest of, or shall take, kill, or destroy any deer or other game, or any wild animal, bird, or wild fowl, or fish, except as next hereinafter mentioned, or shall use any dog, fishing rod, gun, rifle, or other machine, or shall set any net or trap for the above mentioned purposes on that day . . . shall pay a fine or penalty not exceeding ten pounds, nor less than five shillings, current money of this Province, for each offence, together with the costs and charges attending the proceedings and conviction. (Lindsay, 1969, p. 353)

What is interesting is that such enactments very likely reveal the prevalence of exact practices of these amusements and games rather than any termination of such activities. In essence, Sabbath restrictions were measures implemented by the governing classes to control what were deemed to be unruly activities of the lower classes.

HORSERACING AND THE GARRISONS

Prior to Confederation, the single sporting activity that crossed all social classes in interest and in direct or vicarious participation was horseracing. Some background information is necessary to understand the prevalence of this activity. The military presence in North America was continuous and widespread; every town was a "garrison" or military post where troops were stationed. Since military engagements were infrequent, officers and non-officers had considerable time at their disposal. Commissioned officers for the most part were members of the upper and middle class—gentlemen from Britain who had received their early education at such British public schools (the Canadian equivalent are private schools) as Eton, Chester, Harrow, and Rugby. Major pedagogical reforms wrought by such educators as Dr. Thomas Arnold, headmaster at Rugby School, advocated school systems of self-governance, hierarchal organization from senior to junior years, prefects, and "houses" or residences that became the social units of the schools. Boys organized themselves into teams for games and activities like hare-and-hounds (cross-country running), rugby, cricket, football (soccer), and boxing, all amidst the prevailing Anglican religion fostered within the schools. By the time of Dr. Arnold's tenure at Rugby, all boys were expected to be both good students and active participants in games and sport. Moreover, the schools and their gaming activities carried a value system, a code of sporting honour that extolled the virtues of team play, loyalty to one's house, fair play—in short, a set of values that came to be recognized as *muscular Christianity*. Nowhere is this value system better portrayed or dispersed than in one of the most popular novels of the nineteenth century, *Tom Brown's School-days* by Thomas Hughes (1857), a tale of Rugby boys and their sporting exploits and attendant values during Arnold's administration at that school. Graduates from the British public schools often became government, civic, and military leaders. Many of the latter served as officers in British North America and carried with them the sporting practices and values promoted in the British public schools. So significant was their impact on early Canadian sport that one researcher stated unequivocally:

> The paramount influence [on the development of sport] for more than a century after the Conquest was derived from the sporting examples set by the British army garrison [officers]. (Lindsay, 1970, p. 33)

Imbued with this British public school sporting tradition, these officers brought their administrative training and expertise, the opportunity afforded by very little active conflict, and their inclinations toward a variety of sports and games—not the least of which was horseracing. The officers supplied the horses, built the racing tracks and venues, purchased the prizes, and provided officials for equestrian events. To all social classes, horserace meetings were spectacles for amusement, competition, and gambling. For example, an 1843 equestrian steeplechase competition in London, Ontario, attracted some ten thousand people. Royal patronage was granted to many of the equestrian events. However, the social and economic impact of the equine contests was dramatic. Tent cities were spawned for the races—town commercial and farming activities halted for the events, where gambling, brawls, and crime were common. In response, the garrison officers tried moving the events further into the country to discourage the "great unwashed" from attending the events; they still came. One prominent Canadian city, Halifax, was such a magnet for horserace competitions and their attendant social consequences that city officials cancelled and disallowed all horseracing competitions for more than a decade around mid-century.

While horseracing was the most universally popular of the garrison officers' leadership initiatives in sport, there were other activities promoted by these men. Fox-hunting, cricket challenge-matches, tandem and sleighing clubs, skating events, and track and field competitions were among the sports and activities fostered by the garrison officers. Evidence for the dependency on the military for the conduct and participation in these pastimes and sports is highlighted by their great decline when British troops were withdrawn during the Crimean War in Europe during the 1850s. With the perceived and real threats of the American Civil War during the 1860s British militia poured back into BNA, and the newspaper evidence for sporting contests shows dramatic increases, especially in cricket and horseracing. In spite of the initiatives of the British garrison officers, it must be pointed out that by Confederation there was a distinct social class and a gendered order to sport. For example, within the military, regular militia men were court-martialed for habitual drunkenness; that is, it was the officers who enjoyed sport participation, not the lower ranks. Similarly, while women worked extremely hard in the home and on the land and demonstrated tremendous physical prowess, "increasingly, social institutions including government, church, school, and private organizations such as men's clubs promoted idealized femininities tied to notions of dependency, domesticity, chastity, and relative weakness—in contradistinction to the daily experiences of most women" (Morrow & Wamsley, 2005, p. 34). It is abundantly clear from this examination of sporting evolution from ancient cultures through to the mid-nineteenth century that, in Western societies, sport was largely the preserve of the male elite citizenry. Quite simply, the roots of sporting practices seem to be tied indivisibly, timelessly, and universally to men and to notions of manliness.

INDUSTRIALIZATION AND TECHNOLOGICAL CHANGES

Within BNA or Canada, up until the middle of the nineteenth century sporting practices were dependent on individual initiatives and upon existing social institutions such as the bee, the tavern, and the managerial resourcefulness of the garrison officers. The transition to modern, "organized" sport was very much a product of the industrial revolution and the concomitant technological changes that characterized the second half of the nineteenth century. Coalitions of interests such as those of the Scots and the Montreal middle class developed strong sporting organizations just as the process of industrialization altered society in general. Sweeping changes in methods of transportation and communication combined with advances in sporting equipment and facilities catalyzed this process of organizational sophistication in sport, sporting practices, and the availability of sport to wider segments of society. By examining these innovations using a cross-section of sports during the nineteenth century, the rate, direction, and magnitude of sporting change can be explained and understood.

Transportation modes up to the early nineteenth century were often cumbersome and relatively slow. One could walk, snowshoe, canoe, ride on horseback, carriage, or sleigh—all methods of conveyance that required time to travel. For sport, this dependency on time of necessity limited most sport participation to the elite. Furthermore, it reflected and contributed to the social nature of early sporting clubs. Instead of a primary, athletic motive, clubs like the Montreal Curling Club were formed and developed mainly for social interests, not athletic. It was the introduction of steam to water craft that led directly to changes in sporting foci and practices. Steamers and steamboats in the second half of the nineteenth century were a form of recreation in themselves; often, bands were on board, steamship companies offered excursions, and rival company boats even raced each other to get to destinations. More specifically, these companies offered prizes for sporting competitions, gave reduced rates to attend cycling and baseball events, and often allowed ferryboats and other steamers to serve as grandstands for rowing events. Certainly, these changes had an accelerative and promotional effect on a variety of sports. When steam was applied to the tracked vehicles used in mining, railway companies quickly developed that form of transportation.

In 1850, there existed some 160 kilometres of track in Canada. Government grants induced railway companies to connect towns and cities that were within 100 kilometres of each other. Thus, areas such as southern Ontario, parts of Quebec, and the Maritimes were served very rapidly by these transit links. By 1900, some 30,000 kilometres of railway linked Canada coast to coast. One of the railway's primary impacts on society was a dramatic reduction in time to travel. Whereas it took some three days to travel by stagecoach from Toronto to Montreal early in the nineteenth century, travel from that Ontario city to Port Moody, British Columbia took only five days at the end of the century. So great was the time reduction factor that a Canadian, Sir Sandford Fleming, invented the concept of creating time zones for different areas of the world. For sport, the impact of the railway was almost immediate and widespread. Primarily, railway transportation permitted more people to engage in sport just because of the time and convenience factors. More profoundly, a universal impact on sport was the potential crystallization of a fundamental concept in organized sport—regularity. Baseball, lacrosse, rowing, and track and field competitions actually could be scheduled well in advance of the events, to the extent that a whole new concept—leagues—could be structured prior to a sporting season. Multi-club events were possible; for example, 32 teams used rail connections to attend a curling bonspiel during the 1860s. International sporting tours, such as the visit of a British cricket team during the 1870s, were enjoyed because of railway passage. Spur lines could be built to serve as grandstands, as they often were, especially in winter for events such as the very popular snowshoe races of the 1870s and 1880s.

Methods and means of communication paralleled methods of transport. Mail delivery, for example, took days and weeks; until mid century, the receiver paid the postage and the bulk of BNA mail went through England. Sports and games could be arranged by letter, or by word of mouth, or by setting out a challenge from one club to another in the press. In the latter regard, the number of newspapers in the country increased from 200 to 1,200 from 1840 to 1900. Sport was irregularly covered for most of this period; the sport pages were more a product of the twentieth century. And there was a time lag in reporting if a sporting contest was covered such that news of an event in Nova Scotia might take some time to appear in the Ontario press, and vice-versa. When the telegraph was invented in the 1850s, communication was revolutionized. Since the Atlantic telegraph cable was completed in 1866, it meant that news in 1867 of the Saint John, New Brunswick four-oared rowing crew's success at the World Championships in Paris, France (that team is known as the "Paris Crew") was instantly transmitted to Canadians. A byproduct of such accelerated coverage of sporting events combined with league schedules very likely meant reciprocal effects in creating and sustaining fan interest in a variety of sports at the local, provincial, national, and international levels.

SPORTING EQUIPMENT EVOLUTION

Socially and economically, the 1850s were prosperous and growth years for Canada. Events such as the Crimean War in Europe meant great demand for wheat and timber; British capital for the development of more railway lines to facilitate exports of these vital products accelerated during this time. In addition, Canada experienced a 37-percent increase in population between 1851 and 1861, a clear reflection of the country's affluence and its allure to immigrants. Prosperity and population increases usually mean positive effects on and with sport, and they certainly did in this case. One of the mass trends in sport and recreation, a virtual skating mania "from Gaspé to Sarnia," was reflected in the media across Canada during the 1860s. A symbiotic part of the zeal for skating was the impact of technology on sporting equipment, in this case skates. For example, interest and demand meant increased production of skates. More patents were taken out regarding improvements in blades and boots, accessibility increased, and costs quickly were reduced. Another direct impact of technology on equipment manufacture, production, and distribution was uniformity or standardization. As lacrosse sticks, baseball bats, rowing shells, and track and field and other implements were mass produced, participants benefited by better quality and more standard equipment. Whereas early competitors in, say, the hammer throwing event at a Caledonian track and field competition in Cape Breton might have had to create and sign an "article of agreement" about the size and weight of the hammers to be thrown, standardization meant that all competitors could use the same equipment. The implications for the sophistication of sporting organization are obvious.

There are myriad transitions in specific sports brought about by technological changes that are too numerous to describe in this chapter. Cost reduction is one general change with wide-reaching repercussions for sport diffusion to the middle and lower classes. Cricket, a very popular sport among the British elite, remained a relatively expensive sport for most of the nineteenth century; often, bats, balls, and pads were sold in jewellery stores. One cricket bat cost anywhere from 6 to 9 dollars, whereas by 1900 one could purchase a lacrosse stick for less than 50 cents. Similarly, facilities for sport were crucial to sport dispersion and interest. Baseball and lacrosse fields demanded relatively little cost, whereas golf courses—the latter were not in evidence until the mid 1870s—were expensive propositions that kept golf an upper-class sport. Skating rinks and curling areas could be cleared on local rivers—or, within cities, fire departments often built outdoor rinks and toboggan runs. Very few indoor facilities for sport existed during the late nineteenth century, but those that did for hockey, skating, and curling increased their respective sport participation and interest when gas lighting permitted an extension of time to play into the evenings, thereby permitting broader working-class interest and opportunity (Jobling, 1970).

Perhaps one of the most intriguing, socially impacting, and recreationally fascinating pieces of equipment in this century was the bicycle. Its derivation stems from France and England, where hobby-horse precursors were used by gardeners to traverse their estate grounds. By mid century bicycles were of the penny-farthing variety, with a 120-centimetre-diameter front wheel over which the rider perched on a spring-less seat and a diminutive back wheel of some 30 centimetres. The first of these machines to reach Canada was likely sometime in the early 1870s. In spite of their height, discomfort to ride, poor roads for riding, and their expense (at least 100 dollars), the public fascination for bicycles was remarkable. Over the next 30 years, mass marketing and innovations in design led to pneumatic tires, equal-sized wheels (dubbed "safeties" by the mid 1880s), all manner of accoutrements like lights, horns, and spring seats, and greatly reduced costs. Riders, often representing bicycle clubs, raced on the penny farthings and on the safeties. However, much like skating, the real impact of the bicycle was in its widespread use for transportation and recreation across social classes and across gender lines and social conventions. Many historians credit the bicycle for offering one of the first means of recreational pastimes and for catalyzing dress reform for women (Hall, 2002). (Specific repercussions on women's sporting development are discussed later in the chapter.)

MONTREAL: THE CRADLE OF ORGANIZED SPORT

Another component of industrialization was the whole phenomenon of urbanization—the tendency for people to settle in clusters of towns and cities. Organized sport is very much an urban-related and urban-facilitated social behaviour. In many respects, as a result of the twin processes of industrialization and urbanization more people had more money and more time to compete in sport. Leaders and leadership in Canadian sport development came from the largest cities, in particular the city of Montreal. Without question, Montreal was the commercial hub of Canada; it was the nexus for timber, fur trading, shipping, and railway companies, and fostered such giants of national industry as the Molson, Redpath, and McGill tycoons. This centrality of economic and industrial prowess was mirrored in sport such that Montreal is often hailed as the "cradle" of organized sport in Canada. Just in terms of fostering certain sports, entrepreneurs in this city were responsible for founding, defining, and developing such sports as snowshoeing, ice hockey, figure skating, speed skating, lacrosse (the non-Native version), cycling, and football. Each of these sports carries its own unique story of evolution. However, for the purposes of this chapter, what is central to comprehend about Montreal's vanguard role in organizing Canadian sport is the formation of the Montreal Amateur Athletic Association (MAAA) in 1881.

A trio of clubs with strong membership and established practices—the Montreal Snowshoe Club (MSSC), the Montreal Lacrosse Club (MLC), and the Montreal Bicycle Club (MBC)—bought the Montreal Gymnasium in the core downtown area as a home for the conglomeration of clubs called the MAAA. The oldest of these three clubs, the MSSC (formed in 1843), played an instrumental role in fostering snowshoe events, races, long-distance tramps or outings, charity events, drama productions, and social events of dinners and dancing (men with men), and generally championed the manly virtues of being a snowshoe participant (Becket, 1882); that is, club members and executives brought a wealth of managerial experience to the MAAA. Its sister organization, with a lot of crossover members, the MLC was regarded as one of the premier competitive lacrosse clubs in Canada. And, of course, the MBC was symbolic of escalating social interests in the bicycle. The MAAA's original stated purpose was practical and unambitious: "The promotion of physical and mental culture among, and the providing of rational amusements and recreation for, its members" (Morrow, 1981, p. 26). However, the MAAA assumed a position of national sport leadership out of all proportion to its stated purpose.

By the 1890s the MAAA membership numbered some 2,500 men, with the three founding clubs plus football, toboggan, and skating clubs, with departments in billiards, shooting, gymnastics, and bowling, and connected clubs in drama, chess, hockey, fencing, and boxing. What was uniquely important about the MAAA was that for the most part its members—if not certainly its club executives—were middle-class businessmen with considerable professional and managerial skills. With the financial and membership stability of the Association itself, these businessmen used their administrative acumen to foster excellence in sport—the MAAA hockey team, to provide only one example, won the first two Stanley Cup championships in the early 1890s—and to found and promote no fewer than 11 national sport-governing bodies such as the Canadian Wheelmen's Association (for cycling), the National Lacrosse Association, and the Canadian Amateur Hockey Federation. In short, executives within the MAAA wielded tremendous power in the development of organized sport in Canada. Nowhere was this more pronounced or more profoundly felt than in fostering the code of amateurism as the guiding principle for Canadian sporting development until late in the twentieth century.

AMATEUR IDEALISM

Earlier in this chapter, the notion of amateurism in ancient Greek sport was discussed along with the more commercial, professional aspects of sport during Roman times. It is quite clear that organized sport, historically, has been the preserve of elite males and that sporting practice usually carried a gentlemanly code of conduct, as it did with the chivalric code and with the British public school notion of muscular Christianity. In Canada, as we have noted, the earliest organized sporting clubs were social first, athletic second in their *raison d'être* and it was the upper class, like the garrison officers, who were the main participants. With the stark and rapid changes accompanying industrialization, sport had the potential of becoming more democratized, by opportunity, to women and to more social classes. Timelessly, amateurism has to be one of the most unique tenets in governing any human behaviour; as a principle, it is a concept cemented to exclusion—who will *not* be allowed to compete in what sports. For example, in the mid 1830s in Canada, a thriving horseracing club in Newark, Ontario, published a "rule" that "no black man shall be allowed to compete under any pretext whatsoever" (Cosentino, 1975). We can only speculate the reasons for this stricture; however, in another sport, snowshoeing, there were standardized lists of race cards enumerating the events from short to longer distances. For these prestigious races in Montreal, it was common to include an event for Natives. The prestige event was the "open" two-mile race, which was understood to be closed to "Indians." In the early 1870s, two Natives lined up for the start of an open event. Considerable controversy ensued, the result of which was to list thereafter the open events as "Open (Indians barred)." Clearly, there was a racial tinge just as there had been in the late 1860s when a Black rower, William Berry, was excluded from the Toronto Bay Rowing Regatta. The real issue was control—or control over the perceived "proper" sporting participants. Canada's first amateur definition, established by the Montreal Pedestrian Club, 1873, encapsulates this issue:

> An amateur is one who has never competed in any open competition or for public money, or for admission money, or with professionals for a prize, public money or admission money, nor has ever, at any period of his life taught or assisted in the pursuit of Athletic exercises as a means of livelihood *or is a labourer or an Indian*. (Morrow, 1986, p. 174)

Part of the issue of amateurism is discrimination; not just negatively, in the sense of racial discrimination, but also in the notion of equality of competition. In some sports, such as rowing, lacrosse, and track and field, the quality of the sport was so high and the emphasis on winning so dominant that some competitors did compete for money or under aliases to get a valuable prize. Some athletes were able to acquire fame and monetary gain and then spend more time training in the quest for victory, prestige, and material reward. For those competitors unable or unwilling to follow suit, it meant inequality of competition, somewhat akin to the whole issue of steroid use in contemporary sport, if steroids are examined just from the issue of equality of competition. Until well into the twentieth century, for the most part, to be labelled a "professional" in sport was to be tarnished as someone who would lie, cheat, fix outcomes—in short, do anything for victory. Thus it was that sport-governing bodies like the Canadian *Amateur* Association of Oarsmen and the Montreal *Amateur* Athletic Association took it upon themselves to use the notion of amateurism as a method to police their perceptions of inequality, be they social, racial, or pecuniary. For the middle-class businessmen of the esteemed and influential MAAA, amateurism became and was promoted as *the* guiding value system in competitive organized sport. So adamant were these men about the significance of this principle that they created the Canadian Amateur Athletic Association (CAAA) in 1884 to be the national custodian of the amateur code. In some iteration or another, the CAAA stayed in continuous existence until the mid 1970s, heavily bolstered by the international prestige attached to the modern Olympic Games, whose administrators revered the same amateur ideal.

TRANSITIONS TO MASS SPORT

In almost every respect, the whole concept of amateurism is very much an elitist, social exclusionary mechanism instituted to preserve the status quo in sport of the male upper and upper-middle classes. Policing the ideal was like trying to herd cats or grasp mercury in one's hand. Nevertheless, this fossil-like principle became the prevailing ethos of sport in Canada. By the turn of the twentieth century, in popular team sports alone, multiple levels of sporting competition existed in baseball, lacrosse, and ice hockey. Winning major trophies in these sports became the central focus of sport; larger and more spectator-enhanced facilities were built; the athletic quality of competition improved, and so forth. At the same time, the Canadian economy and landscape were changing. Federal government initiatives translated into 2.5 million new immigrants coming into Canada between 1900 and 1920, many of them to the newly opened and established provinces in the West. Wheat became one of our central exports; the softwood forests of northern Ontario supplied major European markets; and mining of precious minerals in that same region meant boom times for small communities in the north. In the latter regard, it was the smaller communities of Kirkland Lake, Timmins, Renfrew, Sault Ste. Marie, and so on that first promoted a commercial, professional basis for ice hockey by using mining money to pay the best players to live in these communities and play hockey for the local teams. Newspapers catered to and promoted the proliferation of and interest in sports with the creation of sport pages. Railway connections expanded to cater to the wheat, wood, and mineral markets. Movie houses opened, women's suffrage was granted (1918), and labour unions were formed out of the impetus of the 1919 Winnipeg General Strike. World War I was a key variable in solidifying British loyalties, in creating an even deeper rift between French and English Canadians with the issue of military conscription, and in stimulating the economy. The central point in relating these changes is to underline the prevailing current of commercial growth and prosperity in Canadian society. The same was true in sport; however, the iron-clad rule of amateurism reigned supreme among sport-governing bodies.

ENTREPRENEURIAL INTERESTS

High-level team sports received the most notoriety in the press and in public perception. Concomitant with the commercial trends in society, so too in lacrosse, ice hockey, track and field, and football there was an "outbreak" of professionals (paid and/or non-amateur abiding practitioners) and professional behaviours by 1905. So great was the professional paranoia that even to play against a professional athlete on another team could result in the amateur athlete's suspension from competitive sport. For so-called major sports such as lacrosse and hockey, whole teams were often suspended. At the same time, in order to win league championships, teams and clubs proclaiming their amateur affiliation used job offers and secret payments to recruit the best players. Ironically, it was the MAAA organization that made a bold suggestion to permit amateurs to play with and against professionals as long as everyone knew who the actual professional players were. The upshot was an almost-three-year protracted war among those factions that wanted to remain purely amateur and the MAAA-induced group that wanted more open competition (Morrow, 1986). The pawn in the middle of this conflict was Onandaga Native runner Tom Longboat. Longboat was a phenomenal long-distance runner who was accustomed to all manner of discriminatory behaviours and accusations very similar to those in evidence in the early non-amateur discriminatory practices. As winner of the 1907 Boston marathon, Longboat was the odds-on favourite to win the marathon gold medal at the 1908 London Olympic Games. He had always abided by amateur regulations, and yet during the athletic war the MAAA organization conspired with the American Amateur Athletic Union to accuse Longboat of professional practices in an effort to eliminate him as a marathon competitor. The charges did not stand; however, Longboat was given an overdose of strychnine, a commonly used central nervous system stimulant that resulted in his collapse at the 19-mile mark during the marathon (Kidd, 1983). The attempt to discredit Longboat failed. In the end, amateurism as an ideal prevailed. Growing interests and parallel value systems embedded in the 1908 London Olympic Games aided this resolution of the conflict in Canada.

And yet, the preservation of the ideal often was nominal even by amateur moguls. For example, consider the case of one consummate amateur athlete, race-walker George Goulding. His racing career spanned some ten years beginning in 1906. By the time he retired from racing, he held world records at almost every distance from 1 to 10 miles. His technique was flawless; not once was he even accused of "lifting" in a sport where judges went prostrate to inspect race-walkers who technically might be running, not walking. While Goulding never accepted anything more than travel expenses for his events, his magnetic attraction for spectators was such that holding matched races featuring his name would attract thousands of paying fans, even to the point of filling Madison Square Gardens in New York City. Clearly, sport venue operators made money from his prowess, and amateur officials often went to great lengths to equalize the competition by handicapping Goulding's starting time to let his competitors gain an advantage, or by holding races that had only Goulding and one other major rival. The latter was contrary to the rules and ideals of amateurism since it clearly isolated the top athletes only for a competition (Morrow & Leyshon, 1987).

What the Goulding case and many other examples from individual and team sports show is that the quest for excellence in organized sport almost demanded some method of promotion other than the restrictive blanket of amateurism. What transpired was that entrepreneurs envisioned a commercial basis for high-quality sport, especially for team sports. Thus, hockey, for example, was developed at every level of amateur play in strictly amateur leagues. At the same time, openly professional hockey leagues developed in southern and northern Ontario such that by 1910 the National Hockey Association (the forerunner to the NHL) was formed with contractual obligations that carried rules about how long a player was bound by the contract to play with one team. Lacrosse and baseball did the same thing, although the permanency of the success of these two professional sports in Canada was not the same as hockey. Whereas an athlete like George Goulding had no choice or opportunity to make money from his talent, some ten years later Lionel Conacher, a Toronto-born athlete voted Canada's best all-round athlete of the first half-century, literally was able to capitalize on his athletic abilities. Conacher excelled in baseball, lacrosse, football, wrestling, boxing, and hockey. It was the professional opportunity in hockey that enabled him to "turn pro" and make his livelihood from earning money in sport. In fact, up until 1937 when he retired from pro hockey he was a semi-professional or professional in all six of his chosen sports (Morrow, 1979).

THE HERO/STAR IN SPORT

One of the important byproducts of the burgeoning development of and interest in high-level sporting competition is the notion of stars or heroes in sport. Both Goulding and Conacher were extremely well known in their sporting times. Sport heroes provide windows or texts through which we can see how communities eulogize and celebrate their stars. Individual sport stories, like myths, provide basic images and metaphors that inform the perceptions, memories, and even aspirations of society. And we can never minimize the impact one individual can have on the rate, magnitude, and direction of change in sport. A case in point is Dr. George W. Beers, the Montreal dentist and "flaming lacrosse evangelist." Beers codified the first set of rules for his sport and set up a convention to establish its national sport governing body, both in Confederation year. He also showcased lacrosse to England, the birthplace of modern, organized sport, by leading two very successful international tours in 1876 and 1883—the latter sponsored in part by the federal Department of Agriculture as an immigration-promoting initiative. Because of Beers' incredible lacrosse salesmanship, for more than a century lacrosse was thought to have been formally declared our national sport (it never was during his lifetime, but both hockey and lacrosse were given that sanction in the mid 1990s). Certainly there were other factors in the development and dispersion of lacrosse, but Beers is a striking example of a visionary, single leadership in sport (Lindsay, 1972).

Although Beers played lacrosse as a goaltender, he was not the kind of classic sport hero who dominated his sport as an athlete. It is interesting that perhaps the first such hero in Canadian sport was working class, of Irish descent, and an avowed professional oarsman, Ned Hanlan. World champion from 1880–84, Hanlan absolutely captivated the sporting public during his era. Although smaller in stature than many of his competitors, Hanlan mastered the use of the sliding seat in rowing to the extent that he virtually controlled the pace of his events. His exploits are too numerous to mention here. What is important is that it was Hanlan's skill combined with his business acumen that worked to solidify his heroic status in a public that clearly was awed by him. Even in the United States, for one single event on the Potomac River both Houses of Congress adjourned to join some 100,000 spectators for just one of his races—and that was prior to his world champion achievement. He was an anomaly in terms of his professional status; however, his skill and domination of the sport, abetted by the proclivity toward gambling on his events, elevated him above normal standards and conventions (Cosentino, 1974). Moreover, even when he went to tour and compete in Australia after losing his world title, he was still so widely acclaimed that on two separate trips he was the major drawing card (Brown, 1980, p. 1–44). Hanlan was the consummate hero—male, highly skilled, charismatic, and unabashedly adored internationally.

Culturally, sport stars are very much products of their times and environments. In French Canada, Louis Cyr, hailed during the period from the 1880s to the early twentieth century as "the world's strongest man," embodied the revered physical prowess ennobled by French

Canadians (Weider, 1976). What also intersects heroic status is gender. We have learned how much sport is a male preserve. Socially, for most of the period under historical examination herein, women were marginalized socially, politically, and physically. To a considerable extent, women's bodies were under the rule of medical men who somehow understood the "apparent" fragility of the female body and the attendant tendencies toward "hysteria" of the mind. It was indeed the adoption and adaptation of the bicycle during the 1890s that almost literally emancipated women to become more active physically. Drop-frame safety bicycles led to the invention of bloomers and split skirts, thereby greatly facilitating mere movement for women. There are sporadic records of women participating in all manner of sports from pedestrianism to ice hockey by the start of World War I. Perhaps the most famous and most lasting influence on Canadian women's participation in sport was a group of stars—shooting stars. From 1915 to 1940, the Edmonton Commercial Graduates' basketball team, dubbed simply the Edmonton Grads, absolutely excelled at their sport. Coached the entire time by high school teacher—and, eventually, Alberta Lieutenant Governor—J. Percy Page, the Grads won some 93 percent of more than 400 highly competitive games against local, provincial, national, international, and Olympic (exhibition) teams. With a farm team feeder system, tremendous civic boosterism, and Page's managerial skills, the team was amateur in practice but with all the hallmarks of a skilled, professional team. However, the gendered order of society dictated that they had to be ladies first, athletes second. For example, Page insisted that all players had to remain single; no smoking or drinking was permitted; chaperones were required for all team events; they had to dress off the court as "proper" young women; and fair play was both valued and mandated (Macdonald, 1976). In short, women athletes, if judged by this remarkably successful team, had to live into a gendered standard of behaviour not expected of men in sport.

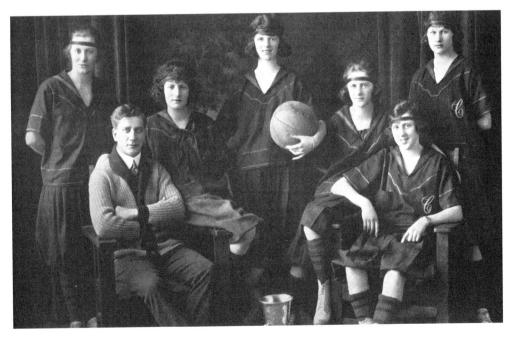

The Edmonton Grads, 1922.

Courtesy of Dr. Don Morrow

Individual women athletes had similar expectations and assumptions placed upon them by society. When Ethel Catherwood, a member of Canada's track and field team in the 1928 Olympic Games, competed in and won a gold medal in the high jump, it was her beauty that captured media attention, not her athletic prowess. Catherwood, a native of Saskatchewan, was proclaimed the "Saskatoon Lily" owing to her perceived good looks. Similarly, Barbara Ann Scott, world and Olympic champion figure skater of the late 1940s, was revered for her good looks, her athletic talent a distant second. Scott, although in three separate years voted Canada's best athlete and therefore winner of our prestigious Lou Marsh award, received the greatest share of her media coverage in Canada in the women's section of the press, not on the sport pages. Instead of her athletic skill, reporters focused on her skating outfits. In many ways, Barbara Ann Scott was created by the media to be petite, feminine, blonde, pretty, a darling on skates, the valentine of Canada (she won one world championship in February near Valentine's Day), Canada's fairy princess (Morrow, 1987). And yet, perhaps owing to the post-war conservatism of her era, it was an image that worked. Handcrafted Barbara Ann Scott dolls were treasured by girls and women during the 1950s.

STATE SPORT

If one were to choose a symbol to represent the dominant trend in Canadian sport between 1900 and 1960, it would likely be the dollar sign. Entrepreneurial, commercial, and professional interests and opportunities in sport were rampant. The other important thread in Canadian sport development during the twentieth century was government involvement in sport, recreation, or fitness. Understandably, the 1867 British North America Act was silent on sport. The federal government's earliest involvement in sport was its immigration-directed investment in the 1883 lacrosse tour to Great Britain (mentioned above) and its sponsorship of Canadian involvement in international rifle competitions such as The Bisley, also in Great Britain. Direct federal intervention came first in the form of the 1911 Strathcona Trust, an act to encourage physical and military training in the Canadian public education system. The Trust was operated by the Department of Militia in the schools and had the decided effect of embedding military drill and physical training in the curriculum, thereby leaving sport as an extracurricular event for more than half a century.

During the Depression, provincial governments in the western provinces reached a cost-sharing agreement with the federal government to support recreation and sport programs for the public. This important dual-funding precedent (known as the Sport-Rec Movement) led to a similar arrangement for the passage of the National Physical Fitness Act (NPFA) in 1943. The NPFA was the direct result of war rejection figures due to the lack of physical fitness. In objectives, the Act was ambitious in that one of its four goals was to encourage physical activity among all Canadians via a $250,000 per capita cost-sharing scheme with the provincial governments. The most significant results of the NPFA were the establishment of physical education degree-training programs in three different provinces and the establishment of a National Advisory Council on Physical Fitness. In 1954, the NPFA was repealed without one dissenting vote in the House of Commons. However, the die of state intervention was cast by these early acts.

During the Cold War of the 1950s, sporting success, particularly in the modern Olympic Games, became a mechanism and a symbol for national political prowess among world super powers. Canadian Olympic achievements were relatively abundant during the first half-century of the Games. For example, the Canadian women's track and field team outperformed all other women's teams in the 1928 Amsterdam Games. At the same Olympiad, Vancouver's Percy

Williams won the coveted 100- and 200-metre sprinting events. However, it was Canada's sheer dominance in Winter Olympic ice hockey from 1920 to 1948 that was our country's trademark. In the three quadrennial festivals beginning in 1952, Canada "failed" to win its coveted first place in the international arena. These events and others inspired the Diefenbaker-led federal government to pass the 1961 Fitness and Amateur Sports Act (FASA).

This significant piece of legislation cemented state supported and administered elite-level sport through to the end of the twentieth century. Managed within the Ministry of National Health and Welfare, the FASA was aimed directly at improvements and victories in national and international sporting competitions. Experts from diverse fields advised the government through a National Advisory Council. The FASA had considerable impact. Its agents established the Canada Games; set up coaching leadership and training programs; initiated provincial cost-sharing programs to set up elite sporting facilities; founded bursary programs for athletes; and set the course for money to be poured into world hockey team developments and competitions. Clearly, the state's target was gold medal production in important international competitions such as the Olympic Games and the various Canada versus the USSR hockey series of the 1970s. The "fitness" component of the FASA seemed hollow by comparison. However, in 1971, after an intensive study of Canadian fitness levels, the federal government created ParticipAction, a not-for-profit, national-level fitness campaign aimed at the personal fitness levels of every Canadian. Still, world-class sport prestige was the vision that propelled massive government support for the 1976 Montreal Olympic Games and the 1988 Calgary Olympic Games. The much-touted 1998 federal Mills Report underscored the economic, social, and cultural impact that international sporting prowess brings to our nation (Morrow & Wamsley, 2005).

CONCLUSIONS

There have been whole histories done on the evolution of single sports, individual athletes, teams, particular events, sporting clubs, and so forth. In this chapter, we have merely touched on some of the stories, events, trends, issues, themes, and processes of sport's development. The connections among values held in the context of sport from ancient to modern times are quite stark. Fair play, male dominance, social class control, amateurism, professionalism, policies of social exclusion, spectatorship, technology, urbanization, and gender orders have all shaped the form and function of sport over time. By the 1950s and the Cold War era, elite sport in Canada had moved more and more toward state intervention and control, resulting in the implementation of the Fitness and Amateur Sport Act that governed elite, non-professional sport in Canada throughout the remainder of the twentieth century.

CRITICAL THINKING QUESTIONS

1. What are some of the important considerations for researchers of sport history?
2. What other policies of exclusion, other than amateurism, are there in sport?
3. How did social class and social stratification influence sport in Canada over time?
4. How did technological changes transform sport in Canada?
5. How and why did Montreal become such a pervasive force in organized sport?
6. How do heroes influence sport and sport behaviours?
7. What examples do we have of a gender order in Canadian sport, and in what ways did that order manifest itself?

SUGGESTED READINGS

Hall, A. M. (2002). *The girl and the game: A history of women's sport in Canada*. Peterborough, ON: Broadview Press.

Howell, C. (2001). *Blood, sweat, and cheers: Sport and the making of modern Canada*. Toronto: University of Toronto Press.

Kidd, B. (1996). *The struggle for Canadian sport*. Toronto: University of Toronto Press.

Morrow, D., & Wamsley, K. B. (2005). *Sport in Canada: A history*. Toronto: Oxford University Press.

WEB LINKS

Note: See also the web links listed at the end of each chapter in Morrow and Wamsley, 2005.

North American Indigenous Games
http://www.virtualmuseum.ca/Exhibitions/Traditions/
Seven museums honour and explain North American indigenous games.

Curling History
http://icing.org/game/history/historya.htm
A brief and general history of curling.

Multiple Links for Snowshoeing in Canada
http://www.out-there.com/htl_ssh.htm
Snowshoeing facts and events, historical and contemporary, with a multitude of links to related websites.

McCord Museum of Canadian History
http://www.mccord-museum.qc.ca/en/
Access through the Museum to some 125,000 images/pictures relevant to Canadian history.

Amateur Athletic Union of Canada—Alberta Branch Files
http://www.glenbow.org/collections/search/findingAids/archhtm/aauc.cfm
Glenbow Museum archival site, accessing primary sources regarding the Amateur Athletic Union of Canada.

Baseball's Invention in Canada, Adam Ford's Letter and Supporting Article
http://www.aafla.org
From the above link, click on Search and search for "Adam Ford" to find his letter on the "invention" of baseball together with a supporting, detailed research article.

1972 Summit Series
http://www.1972summitseries.com/
Information and video clips on the acclaimed 1972 hockey "summit" series.

Canadian Olympians
http://www.collectionscanada.ca/olympians/index-e.html
Searchable database of Canadian Olympic athletes from 1900 to 2004.

CHAPTER 4

SPORT AND SOCIAL STRATIFICATION

Rob Beamish

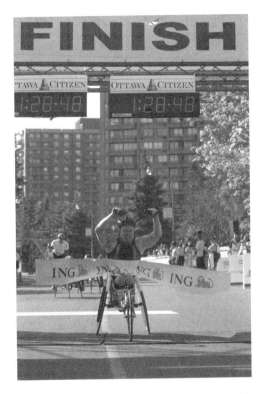

Competitive opportunities are increasing for persons with disabilities.

Photograph by Action Sports International, www.asiphoto.com

The major inequalities in society are in the main social products, created and maintained by the institutions of property and inheritance, of political and military power, and supported by particular beliefs and doctrines, even though they are never entirely resistant to the ambitions of outstanding individuals.

Tom Bottomore, *Elites and Society*, 1964, p. 123

With 24 seconds left to play in the 1972 Canada–Soviet hockey series, Paul Henderson scored a goal that stands out as one of Canada's greatest moments in sport. As important as that goal was, it is rivalled by numerous other significant victories.

The 1978 Commonwealth Games, held in Edmonton, showed that Canada not only could win, but also could decisively outperform its rivals in one of the world's major sporting events. In addition to amassing the largest medal total among the participating nations, Canada had more gold, more silver, and more bronze medals than any other nation.

Just a decade later, Canadian emotions shot to rarefied heights of jubilation when Ben Johnson crushed Carl Lewis in one of the globe's most prestigious sporting events—the 100-metre dash in the Olympic Games. Those emotions plummeted when Johnson tested positive for the banned substance stanozolol, but Canadian pride was restored with Donovan Bailey's 1996 world-record performance in the Games' premier event in Atlanta. The Canadian men's 4x100-metre relay team cemented the nation's prowess by defeating the highly favoured American men right in their own backyard.

Between 1915 and 1940, the Edmonton Grads dominated women's basketball internationally. In a sporting dynasty without equal, the Grads won 502 of 522 games they played during that 25-year reign; they won 17 consecutive world championships and four Olympic gold medals. Now the Canadian women's hockey team has begun to reassert a similar dominance, winning eight consecutive world championships (losing to the USA only in 2005) and both gold medals awarded in Olympic competition. Like the Grads, the women's national hockey team serves as an inspiration to millions of young girls across the nation.

Placing first, despite what people often say, matters to a lot of Canadians—young and old, male and female, people of all abilities. But success in sport, like reaching the upper ranks in other areas of social life, involves far more complex issues than simply placing ahead of the competition—and that is why the world of formal, organized sport provides an ideal opportunity for one to study the most important issues related to social stratification and social inequality in contemporary, market-oriented societies.

The primary outcome of formalized, competitive sport is differentiation and stratification. Sport ranks and unequally rewards all those competing for first place—or the top spot—whether one focuses on the material rewards of victory (for example medals, trophies, money) or the more intangible rewards of personal accomplishment. In sport, someone, or some team, is first—wins gold—leaving the others in second, third, and so on down the ranking to the very bottom: last place. Competitive sport creates a vertical ranking, or hierarchical stratification, of participants based on performance.

Since victory and the unequal distribution of rewards are based on performance—or one's "merit"—competitive sport is often regarded as a genuine meritocracy. A *meritocracy* is a hierarchical ranking and reward system in which merit—one's demonstrated performance—determines where one will end up in the hierarchy. Sport, its supporters argue, rewards those who make the most of their ability through their personal dedication to long-term preparation, sacrifice, and concerted, concentrated effort during competition. When John Munro, then the Federal Minister for Health and Welfare, initiated the steps to what would become Canada's high-performance sport system, he emphasized the social importance of the hierarchical, pyramid structure of sport (Canada, 1970). Those at the top, Munro argued, would act like magnets and draw people into the sport system while its merit-based hierarchy ensured that those who worked hard and produced winning performances would rise to the elite levels of the system.

The acceptance of a hierarchal system of unequal rewards based on performance extends beyond sport. In schools, for example, students are taught a variety of subjects and academic skills and then tested. Students' performances are evaluated and the results produce an overall ranking for each student's performance. A student's overall performance determines whether she or he will be allowed or denied the opportunity to advance further in the education system.

Educational performance—demonstrated, academic merit—is a decisive criterion for certain opportunities of considerable consequence. Educational performance is part of a sorting process that most Canadians not only accept but also believe is the best way to allocate people to different advanced educational opportunities. Admission to university, for example, often depends on not simply meeting the minimum entrance requirements; in certain select, highly sought-after programs or universities one must perform well above the minimal requirement.

The paid labour force into which young Canadians move is also stratified; the specific type and level of qualification are important factors in determining where one might enter into the hierarchy and the financial rewards she or he will receive for acceptable performance in a particular job. The occupational structure in Canada offers different financial rewards depending on one's location in the hierarchy. The stratified income structure in Canada's hierarchically arranged labour force not only is accepted by most Canadians, but also is deemed by many business and government leaders as the best and fairest way to allocate financial rewards and incentives in the paid labour force.

Four points about social stratification stem from the above discussion. First, most Canadians accept a stratified system of rewards based on performance. Whether it is in sport, education, the workplace, or other aspects of our lives, Canadians believe it is appropriate to differentially reward and rank people on the basis of their achievements. As a result, most Canadians accept what many sociologists term "the achievement principle" in determining one's share of the nation's wealth, power, and prestige. This point requires special emphasis because, as this chapter will demonstrate, a genuine, wholehearted commitment to the achievement principle—a full commitment to the unequal allocation of rewards on the basis of merit alone—involves some very unexpected commitments to key questions and issues in social stratification. A commitment to the achievement principle involves the acceptance of some principles and social practices that seem, on the surface at least, to contradict the original commitment to an achievement-based meritocracy.

Because Canadians tend to endorse the achievement principle, they dislike and tend to oppose people receiving high rewards just because of "who they are." In sociological terms, they oppose unequal reward based on *ascribed status*—one's place of birth, sex, race, ethnicity, "station in life," and so on. This is the second point of importance: those who study social stratification draw an important distinction between ascribed (based on birth) and *achievement-based stratification*. In contemporary, market-based societies, inequality based on ascribed characteristics is far less accepted than inequality based on achievement-based characteristics.

Third, while Canadians accept and often endorse inequality in the reward structures that exist in sport, education, income, and some other dimensions of their lives, they do not accept inequality in *all* aspects of their lives. On the contrary, there are many issues and social situations where Canadians firmly oppose inequality. For example, Canadians feel very strongly that everyone deserves equal treatment before the law; they believe that all Canadians should be treated with equal fairness and equal impartiality and not on the basis of their race, sex, or disability, for example, when competing for positions in sport, education, or the paid labour force. As a result, the federal government has enshrined in the Charter of Rights and Freedoms a number of basic rights and freedoms that must apply equally to all Canadians.

Although it might seem inconsistent for Canadians to accept and endorse inequality in some aspects of their lives while making it illegal in others, this is not necessarily the case. It may be perfectly legitimate and logically consistent to affirm inequality in one area of life while supporting equality in another. In any discussion of social stratification, one must clearly identify the "object of inequality." One can discuss, debate, and sort through issues in social stratification only if she or he is clear about what must be, or what may legitimately be allocated unequally (or equally). Only once the object of inequality has been explicitly identified—the ranking that results from sporting competitions, for example, or the unequal allocation of financial rewards to highly successful as opposed to less successful athletes—can one then determine the consistency or inconsistency of apparently contradictory views on other types of inequality, such as the inequality of resources going to support potential podium athletes rather than sharing the resources more equally among all of Canada's high-performance athletes. The acceptance of inequality in one aspect of social life, it is important to emphasize, does not necessarily commit one to accepting inequality in all other aspects of social life. Determining a consistent position begins by identifying the object or outcome under consideration.

Finally, because few Canadians take the time to clearly identify the "object of inequality" when thinking about issues of social stratification and tend to rely upon common-sense notions of stratification, rights, freedoms, and equality, they often hold positions on different issues of stratification and inequality that actually contradict one another. Most Canadians do not always recognize that the acceptance of inequality in one sphere of social life has a direct impact on other areas of social life. For example, can one support the unequal reward structures in sport or education, while arguing that there must be equality of opportunity to take part in sport or education? Can one advocate for inequality in one sphere while advocating for equality in another—or is one committed to supporting inequality in all aspects of social life?

Questions of equality and inequality in social stratification are very complex; it is only through careful reflection and analysis that people can begin to develop positions on stratification, equality, and inequality that are internally consistent and would lead to actions that would enable them to reach the larger goals they feel are important. Fortunately, sport is an ideal vehicle for sorting through and clarifying some of the complexities that exist in the study of social stratification, and this chapter will explore several of the key issues that affect Canadians today.

OPPORTUNITY AND SOCIAL STRATIFICATION

At the 2006 Winter Olympic Games in Torino, Italy, Canada won 24 medals—more than the nation had ever won at the Winter Games. The federal government, which provides vital funding for the Canadian Olympic team's development; the Canadian Olympic Committee (COC), which plays a central role in the organization and operation of Canada's Olympic Games efforts; the Canadian media; and Canadians in general were overjoyed with Canada's success. Prior to the Games, the COC had announced that its performance objectives were simple—to rank third overall in the medal totals and to win 25 medals. Some thought the objectives were unrealistic, but Canadian athletes met the standard—and with 18 fourth-place finishes, they proved that Canada clearly does rank among the top Winter Games nations in the world. So, on the one hand, there was absolutely nothing wrong with Canada's performance—it met national expectations and perhaps surpassed them. Canada's best athletes, on the basis of their own performances—on the basis of their own demonstrated merit—ranked third in the world and held out the tantalizing possibility that they might rank higher at the 2010 Games in Vancouver. But a closer look at Canada's performance shows some interesting trends and raises some important questions about stratification in Canadian sport in particular and social stratification in Canada more generally.

Of Canada's 24 medals, athletes born, living, or training in Alberta won 14. Canada's greatest success came in long-track speed skating, with eight medals (five of these involved Cindy Klassen, though two were team competitions). Of the 11 men and 11 women on

Canada's long-track speed skating team, six were born in Alberta, six in Manitoba (all from Winnipeg), five in Saskatchewan, two in Ontario, two in British Columbia, and one in Quebec; all but two of the long-track skaters lived and trained in Calgary. Similarly, if Canada's depth is in long-track skating, when one looks at the nation's most decorated long-track speed skaters—Cindy Klassen, Jeremy Wotherspoon, Michael Ireland, Catriona LeMay Doan, and Susan Auch—the trend is the same: they all lived and trained in Calgary at the height of their careers. Clara Hughes and Kevin Overland were exceptions. What does this trend mean?

Although the rugged, individualist, frontier culture of Calgary and Alberta might explain why athletes living and training there did so well in 2006, it is more likely that the opportunity to train and develop in the winter sport facilities that were part of the 1988 Calgary Winter Games legacy is the dominant reason for the significant overrepresentation of athletes living in Alberta standing on the Olympic podium for Canada. The presence of world-class training facilities and international-level coaches gives Calgarians and many other Albertans the opportunity to develop winter sport talents that they would not have in the absence of those amenities.

Contrast, for example, the opportunity enjoyed by a young Calgarian with that of aspiring long-track speed skaters living in Thompson, Manitoba (who would have to travel to Winnipeg to get access to a long-track oval), or living in Corner Brook, Newfoundland, or Nanaimo, British Columbia (who would both have to travel considerable distances into the Canadian mainland to skate on an oval). While each of those three aspiring long-track skaters has the opportunity to buy long-track skates and find ice on which to learn and progress, the opportunity to realize the goal of becoming an Olympic champion is very different for each. In Ontario, there are almost 30 speed skating clubs and some 3,000 registered participants, but there is not at this time an indoor, climate-controlled, long-track oval—although an initiative

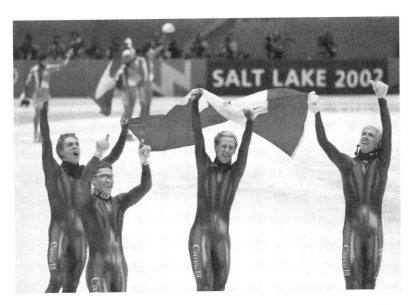

Canadian teammates and gold medalists (L to R) Mathieu Turcotte, François-Louis Tremblay, Jonathan Guilmette, and Marc Gagnon jubilate after the men's 5,000-metre relay final of the short-track speed skating at the Olympic Ice Center, February 2002, during the XIXth Winter Olympics in Salt Lake City. Canada won the event, ahead of Italy and China.

JACQUES DEMARTHON/AFP/Getty Images

in Lakefield, near Peterborough, should result in the province's first indoor oval. Until that time, Ontarians with Olympic long-track aspirations must travel to Calgary, Lake Placid, or Ste-Foy, Quebec. As a result, the equality—or, in this case, inequality—of opportunity has an important impact on who will be able to try a particular sport and develop the talents and abilities they possess.

In a country so geographically vast, the location of athletic facilities in only a few parts of the country has a tremendous impact on opportunities for young Canadians to realize their particular athletic potential and perhaps pursue Olympic dreams. Although long-track speed skating ovals may seem to be the exception and, given their expense, are correctly confined to a few very select places, there are lots of facility problems in Canada. While most cities have pools in which young Canadians can begin to explore their swimming talent, as one progresses upward in the competitive system the presence of 50-metre pools gains in importance. For young swimmers in the Toronto area and in many locations west of Toronto, the distance to the nearest 50-metre pool is manageable to many who have sufficient economic and parental support. An aspiring swimmer in Belleville, Trenton, Napanee, Kingston, Gananoque, Brockville, Morrisburg—any of the centres along the 401 corridor between Port Hope and Cornwall, to say nothing of those in Deep River, Petawawa, Pembroke, Kaladar, Bancroft, Sharbot Lake, and other communities north of the corridor—faces a much different situation. For those athletes, the only 50-metre pools they can train at lie in the areas of Toronto, Ottawa, and Montreal.

Inequality of opportunity is a significant problem in Canada's sport system, but it involves more than just facilities—it also involves, for some, the fundamental opportunity simply to take part. For much of the post-war period, one group of athletes was excluded from the stratification system in Canadian sport: athletes with special needs. Now, two different movements, both with Canadian connections, advocate on behalf of athletes with disabilities and showcase their athletic talents. The Special Olympics movement had its origins in the charity work of Eunice Kennedy Shriver, who in June 1962 opened a camp for 35 boys and girls with intellectual disabilities at her home in Rockville, Maryland. From that small beginning, physical activity and sport opportunities began to grow, leading to the inaugural International Special Olympics held in Chicago in 1968 that hosted 1,000 athletes from 26 states and Canada. The Special Olympics now involves more than 2.5 million athletes from 150 countries (Special Olympics, 2006).

The Paralympic Games had their origin in the International Wheelchair Games that Sir Ludwig Gutmann, an English neurosurgeon, organized to take place alongside the 1948 Olympic Games in London. The Paralympics, per se, were first held in Rome, Italy, in 1960 and involved 400 athletes from 23 countries (Hayden, 1996). Held every four years, coinciding with the Olympic Games, the Paralympics used the Olympic facilities in 1988, and by 1996 the athletes used the same village as the other Olympic athletes even though the Paralympics were still not integrated into the Olympic Games.

Despite the gains made by the Paralympics, it was really Canadians Terry Fox and Rick Hansen, friends and teammates on Canada's Paralympic teams in the 1970s, who genuinely transformed people's perceptions of disabled athletes' abilities and capabilities through their unparalleled achievements of elite physical performance. Fox began his "Marathon of Hope" in the Atlantic Ocean off St. John's on April 12, 1980, and over the next 143 days covered 5,565 kilometres—averaging just over "a marathon a day" (a marathon is 42 km, or 26.2 miles; Fox averaged 43 km a day) until his cancer spread to his lungs, ending the marathon in Thunder Bay on September 1, 1980. Inspired by Fox, Hansen began his around-the-world "Man in Motion" tour on March 21, 1985, at the Oak Ridge Mall in Vancouver and completed it two years, two months, two days, and an incredible 40,000 kilometres later.

From the perspective of sport and social stratification, the Special Olympics and the Paralympics raise several important issues. First, both events raise the question of how the public ranks different formal athletic competitions—are the achievements of Paralympians considered equivalent or even surpassing those of able-bodied athletes; are their sports simply different forms of highly competitive sports undertaken by elite athletic performers? The Special Olympics raise the question of performance versus performance *potential*—to what extent are the accomplishments of Special Olympic athletes recognized as equivalent to mainstream, high-performance athletes who are also seeking to maximize their athletic potential? These questions are important because they feed directly into institutional support, funding, and media coverage for Paralympic and Special Olympic sport. Without these things, sport for athletes with disabilities remains second-class—unequal in comparison to mainstream sports. How and why, given the artificial nature of all athletic competitions, can government, sports, and education leaders, and even the citizens of a country, justify ranking some elite international sport forms less worthy of resources, facilities, coverage, and interest than others? When sport forms are differentially ranked, what does that mean about the meritocracy of sport? On what basis is the hierarchy established?

The absence of long-track ovals in most locales in Canada, limited access to Olympic-dimension pools, and the limited number of fully accessible athletic facilities may not be the prohibitive barriers faced by African Americans in the southern United States from the 1890s to the 1960s, or those faced by Blacks in South Africa from 1948 to 1991 when apartheid was a legally sanctioned system of discrimination, but for numerous Canadians these inequalities of opportunity serve as serious barriers to the full development of their athletic talent. More important, inequality of opportunity was an issue that the federal government recognized in 1970, when it began to support sport in Canada. "We must face the fact," Munro (Canada, 1970) noted, that

> it's only fair, just as a dash in a track and field meet is only fair, that everyone has the same starting line, and the same distance to run. Unfortunately, in terms of facilities, coaching, promotion and programming, the sports scene today resembles a track on which some people have twenty-five yards to run, some fifty, some one-hundred, and some as much as a mile or more. (pp. 4–5)

Unfortunately, more than 35 years later the lack of access to fully accessible facilities and equipment, especially for athletes with disabilities, in urban and rural Canada means that some athletes are still metaphorically running 1,500 metres while others need only run 100, 50, or 25 metres or less.

Inequality of opportunity has important implications for sport in particular and for stratification theory in general. Canadians want to produce winners—they want to fully develop all of the talents of Canada's most dedicated athletes. Canadians seek inequality of outcome in athletic competition. The placing of athletes—the inequality or stratification of outcome—is the "object of inequality" under consideration. To ensure that the best athletes have the opportunity to develop all of their talents and abilities, it is imperative that Canada offer as equal an opportunity as possible to all of them rather than allowing those with certain advantages, such as the privilege of access to specialized facilities and coaching, to have an unfair head start over others. For Canadian sport to be genuinely meritocratic, there must be equality of opportunity so that every aspiring athlete may develop and demonstrate his or her true ability. It is a perfect example of how the support for inequality in one aspect of social life—here, the ranking of athletes on the basis of performance—requires support for equality in another aspect of social life—the equality of opportunity. While it may appear to be a contradiction to support inequality in one instance and equality in another, the two require one another insofar as inequality of outcome is the object of inequality.

The opportunity to develop one's athletic talents and the equality or inequality of opportunity to do so extends well beyond access to facilities; it also concerns the quality of one's experience. Because equality of opportunity is such an important issue, it is worthwhile exploring it further.

There are primary, secondary, and post-secondary schools throughout Canada; most of them are publicly funded, while some are privately operated. The opportunity to learn in the formal education setting is widespread, but do all Canadians have the same opportunity to master the formal educational curriculum?

The provincial governments and ministries of education develop and implement a formal curriculum for all students in the province. All Canadians have the opportunity to learn material in the formal curriculum, but sociologists have shown that the educational experience is far more complex than the opportunity to have access to the same formal curriculum—the educational experience involves a "multi-dimensional, enacted curriculum" (Weisz & Kanpol, 1990).

Although the formal curriculum is detailed and explicit, the actual, or "pragmatic," implementation or enactment of those documents is among the most decisive factors affecting students' opportunities to learn. The opportunity to learn is shaped by variables such as time, financial and material resources, the type and location of the school, teacher strengths and interests, and the amount of educational support a teacher can offer. All of these factors influence how much of the official curriculum a teacher, or teachers, can and will cover in the course of an academic semester. More important, they directly influence the quality of students' experiences and the opportunities they have to learn. Despite the formal curriculum's intentions and objectives, the actual delivery process involves real teachers and students in particular social situations and conditions.

The parallels between education and sport are instructive especially insofar as they influence athletes' opportunities to develop their full athletic potential and compete for the top spot in their sports. In exactly the same way that success in education rests on students' learning opportunities, success in sport depends upon the opportunity to learn. But, in exactly the same way that the opportunity to learn mathematics, language skills, history, or geography is not equally available to young Canadians, there is significant inequality of opportunity for different Canadians to learn sport skills and strategies. While not nearly as developed as the formal educational curriculum, Canadian sport leaders have developed elaborate technical-development programs for athletes and coaches alike since the creation of Sport Canada, the centralization of national sport organizations in Ottawa in the early 1970s, and the establishment and funding of the Coaching Association of Canada. These programs are the formal curriculum of Canada's sport system. The implementation of these technical programs—the development of athletes' skills—involves the same processes of enactment as the formal education system.

As a result, athletes who have a coach who is a former athlete and a formally trained teacher who is utilizing a number of learning modalities have a different opportunity to learn fundamental skills than those who have a parent volunteer with little experience in sport and none in teaching. The pragmatic dimension of those athletes' experiences will also be shaped by the local resources available—successful local athletes who can serve as an easily identified inspiration, for example, or better equipment or more opportunities to practise at optimal times in the day—as well as social-process experiences that enhance rather than obstruct athlete development.

The opportunity to learn is crucial to athlete development. For Canadians to enjoy a genuine meritocracy in sport, the significant inequalities of opportunity within the multi-dimensional, enacted sport curriculum must be reduced or eliminated. As long as they remain, some athletes enjoy privilege of opportunity that others do not: they have a significant advantage—to return to our metaphor, they have to run only 50 metres while others are running 100 and some 1,500 or more.

OPPORTUNITY, CULTURE, GENDER, AND SPORT'S MERITOCRACY

If resources and the social processes of learning influence opportunity, it is also shaped by culture. Canada has a culture that encourages sport involvement, but that encouragement is not the same for boys and girls; there are significant gender differences in Canadian culture and they impact upon the equality of opportunity faced by boys and girls in general, and among girls in particular. Although Chapter 6 examines sport and gender in detail, it is important to consider a few issues related to gender and opportunity within the context of social stratification.

There is no question that fewer Canadian girls and women take part in formal, organized sport than boys and men do. In hockey, for example, although girls' and women's hockey is one of the fastest growing sports in Canada, of the half-million Canadian children registered in organized hockey, girls constitute fewer than 15 percent.

The most common explanation for the different rates of participation is biology. It seems obvious to some that the XY and XX chromosome combinations distinguishing males and females must predestine boys and men to some activities—physically based, competitive, hierarchical ones of which sport would be a good example—while girls and women are predestined to less physical, non-competitive, "mutualist" activities. It is, according to conventional wisdom, because men and women are "opposites"; that their social activities are so fundamentally different.

The first problem with this explanation is that although the sexes differ in their reproductive organs and functions, those differences do not make them opposites. The reproductive differences between men and women complement each other rather than constituting an oppositional difference. More important, even though males and females play different but complementary roles in the biological process of human reproduction, if one is concerned with biology then, far from being opposites, males and females as biological beings are more identical than different—they share the same genes and chromosomes, for example. Moreover, although there is variation between the sexes, there is as much variation within each sex for virtually every biologically determined trait, and the distribution of different characteristics overlaps considerably. Furthermore, human biology and behaviour are not fixed and unchangeable. As the human brain is stimulated, neurons branch out and form different connections; as boys' and girls' senses are stimulated, hormonal levels change; exercise changes muscle shape, builds strength, and alters body composition in girls, boys, women, and men. Although it is tempting to link differences in behaviour to biology, it is clear that there is not a firm, biologically driven predetermination to human behaviour—human lives and actions are shaped by a complex mixture of biochemical, physiological, biological, psychological, social, political, and cultural forces.

The sociocultural forces that play a significant role in differentiating male and female behaviours stem from childrearing and family practices and experiences, from play and educational experiences, and from immersion within larger cultural influences. In contemporary Canadian society, parents still tend to spend more time interacting directly with girls while leaving boys more time to explore and experiment on their own. Boys are more likely to have computers than girls and they are encouraged, even pressured, more than girls to engage in physically active pursuits. Girls are either discouraged or not strongly encouraged to pursue physical activities (Kilmarten, 1994). Even the household chores children tend to be assigned reinforce dominant activity patterns—boys are asked to shovel snow, take out the garbage, and cut the grass, while girls work inside the house. Although it would be an exaggeration to see these patterns extending directly from the earliest interactions between mother and child, Connell (2005) and others have argued that because women give birth to babies and tend to be intimately involved with the child in his or her earliest days, weeks, and months, they form strong nurturing bonds with their children. The bond between mother and daughter tends to remain one of mutual nurturing, whereas dominant cultural patterns tend to separate boys from mothers much earlier, encouraging greater independence.

Added to these cultural factors are political and resource issues. In 1955, eight-year-old Ab Hoffman played in the Little OHA Junior "A" League for the St. Catharines Tepees. As the best goalie, Ab was chosen as the all-star goalie to play in a tournament in Toronto—but when league officials looked more closely at the registration form they noticed that Ab's full name was Abigail. Allowed to complete the season, Abby and almost 100 other girls turned out for practices in 1956 hoping to play in a girls' league, but the Toronto Hockey League executive shut it down, arguing that practice time for the girls would cost too much money (Canadian Broadcasting Corporation, 2004).

Despite a glorious pre–World War II history of involvement in sport, girls and women were marginalized in the post-war period and effectively excluded from the best opportunities to develop their skills until into the 1980s. The high-profile sport of hockey was a key catalyst in opening more opportunities for girls and women in Canadian sport.

Eleven-year-old Justine Blainey, who was already playing on an all-star women's hockey team, wanted to develop her hockey skills to their utmost by playing in a league where she would be continually challenged to develop. In 1981, Justine tried out for and made a team in the Metro Toronto Hockey League (MTHL). The MTHL refused to let her play by arguing it provided hockey only for boys. Justine challenged the MTHL's discrimination on the basis of the Ontario Human Rights Code. After five court cases, the Supreme Court of Canada—which in 1986 ruled that, except under special circumstances, discrimination on the basis of sex in athletic activities was unlawful—heard her appeal.

Seven years later, Blainey ran into a different roadblock to her hockey development. Despite their winning the provincial championship in 1992—the 13th in 15 years—the University of Toronto cut the funding for the women's team. By running a "Save the Team" fundraising drive, Blainey and her teammates kept the team alive by raising more than $8,000 (University of Toronto, 2004). More important, in 1995 the University's Board of Governing Council voted to provide equal funding for men's and women's sport. That decision was not binding on other universities and did not apply anywhere else in the education system. Symbolically, in point of principle, and from a public relations perspective, the Supreme Court decision and the University of Toronto's position, which was shared by a number of Ontario universities, created an important change in the political culture within which girls' and women's sport developed. While these represent important steps toward greater equality of opportunity, female athletes in the United States have much stronger protection and support.

In 1972, the U.S. federal government passed "Title IX of the Education Amendments of 1972," which declared that: "No person in the United States shall, on the basis of sex, be excluded from participation in, be denied the benefits of, or be subjected to discrimination under any education program or activity receiving Federal financial assistance" except for certain circumstances covered in the legislation (United States Congress, 1972). This legislation meant that educational institutions in the United States receiving federal financial assistance had to ensure that funds were equivalently distributed to men's and women's programs. While a number of inequities still exist and Title IX has not resulted in genuine financial equity between female and male sports, it has resulted in a number of significant changes for American girls and women. Notably, high school sports participation rose from 294,015 in 1971 to 2,784,154 in 2001; this increase and better funding of university sport created the talent and player pool that allowed the Women's United Soccer Association, the Women's National Basketball Association, and the Women's Professional Football League to develop into thriving enterprises.

Despite the gains girls and women have made in the United States, Title IX did not bring full equity to male and female sport. There are still more sport opportunities for boys and men than there are for girls and women (about 30 percent more), and boys receive $1.1 million more in support for high school sport and almost twice the resources for sporting opportunities from pee wee to professional sport outside the school system. There is also about $133 million more in athletic scholarships for males than females (Dworkin & Messner, 2002, p. 348).

The cultural institutions, formal political organizations, and personal family networks of contemporary Canadian and American society have changed considerably since the second wave of the women's movement in the 1960s. Girls and women today have opportunities that are much broader and far more equitable than their mothers or grandmothers experienced not so long ago, but the sociocultural forces that play a significant role in differentiating male and female activities still create inequalities of opportunity for females when compared to those for males—this is as true of sport as it is of education or work in the paid labour force. Like the inequalities in facilities or learning opportunities, the dominant sociocultural and political forces in Canadian society prevent Canada's sporting system from being genuinely merito-cratic; not all of the participants enjoy the same opportunity to compete for the positions at the top.

CONDITION AND SOCIAL STRATIFICATION

While the opportunity to take part in any activity—sport, education, or the labour force—is key, the *conditions* under which one enters into those activities is at least equally significant for the overall outcome of one's participation. To examine the differential conditions under which people engage in various activities, sociologists have employed different conceptions of strati-fication. Although they may seem to complement each other, they are all fundamentally dif-ferent and based on different, incompatible understandings of social inequality. The class theories that began with the work of early British political economists and were most sharply presented in Karl Marx's work indicate that social inequality and, thus, social stratification is fundamentally tied to the production and distribution of social wealth (see Marx, 1844; Ricardo, 1951; Smith, 1976). Marx argued that inequality was ultimately tied to who owned and controlled the means of production in society and that all of social history was character-ized by class struggle.

Writing in the early twentieth century, Max Weber (1946) argued that although class was a key factor, the social status conferred on particular positions in society, and the political influence that individuals, groups, and political parties carried, meant that there were addi-tional key factors to social inequality. By the mid-twentieth century, structural functionalists and industrial society theorists argued that with a growing complexity to the economy, a larger white-collar workforce, an increasing diversity of occupations, and a stratified structure of income, status, and consumption patterns, theories of class inequality were no longer appro-priate. Contemporary advanced industrial societies were increasingly open, allowing for greater upward (and downward) mobility on the basis of achievement and merit. Conceptions of social inequality were replaced with theories of social stratification based on a number of different indicators of "socioeconomic status," which was determined by a number of factors like educa-tion, occupation, occupational status, income, and wealth (see Parkin, 1978).

The persistence of inequality, and the failure to demonstrate that advanced industrial societies were truly open, led to further theoretical conceptualization in stratification theory. One key development was the work of Pierre Bourdieu (1984, 1998), who argued that human practices, including sport, are located in a multidimensional space. The key concepts are *field*, which is the "structural dimension" of social action, and *habitus*, which are "cultural structures" that exist in people's bodies and minds. It is through practice that habitus and field are brought together.

Drawing upon Bourdieu's work, Booth and Loy (1999) have argued that the habitus of the upper class—those whose field rests on inherited wealth of significant proportion, investment income, and perhaps the controlling ownership of a commercial enterprise—tends to lead them toward and afford them the opportunity to engage in sport for enjoyment and status confirmation. Riding, sailing, golfing, tennis, and squash at prestigious private clubs, helicopter skiing, or sojourns to elite ski locales in Europe are examples of upper-class sporting activities that result from the habitus and fields they bring together in their sporting practices.

Those in the middle class are concerned with appearance and health in their sporting practices, although they also seek to emulate upper-class sporting activities—sailing, golf, tennis, and squash (but in public facilities or inexpensive, mass private ones), and skiing at hills catering to a mass clientele. The field and habitus of the middle class result in practices that are carried out in very different social spaces than those of the upper class, and the overall intent of their sporting practices is qualitatively different than that of the upper class. The children and youth of middle-class families are exposed to and take part in more competitive-oriented sports than their upper-class peers. Very often the long-term goal of middle-class sport participation is social status and recognition from peers as well as the opportunity to underwrite some of the costs of social mobility through athletic scholarships. Track and field, gymnastics, figure skating, golf, rowing, basketball, football, hockey—all sports that can be undertaken through the school system or in local clubs—serve as potential aids in the pursuit of upward mobility via scholarships. Some middle-class participants try to turn their financial advantages over lower-class athletes into a competitive edge in gaining access to the lucrative opportunities that exist in mainstream professional sport: football, hockey, baseball, and basketball.

Children in lower-class families generally demonstrate low rates of participation because of the direct costs of sport participation as well as the time constraints of part-time employment. At the same time, the habitus of lower-class children and youth orients them toward more passive engagement with sport and physical activity—they tend to be spectators rather than participants (Sennett & Cobb, 1973; Young, 1997). Finally, lower-class youth will take part in free-time, non-mainstream sporting activities such as skateboarding because they provide feelings of group solidarity and carve out their own particular niche within a school or community setting (see Willis, 1990; Willis, Dolby, & Dimitriadis, 2004).

White and Wilson (1999) and Wilson (2002) also use Bourdieu's framework to examine the relationships among field, habitus, sporting practices, and class in the area of spectatorship and show the impact of stratification on sports consumption. Their analyses stress the importance of habitus over field with respect to spectatorship: lower-class males are more apt to watch and identify with the so-called "prole sports," like stock car racing and motorcycle racing, than are upper-class males because taste influences where one will spend one's time if money is not a barrier.

Two important points emerge from Bourdieu's approach. First, even when a person's field does not prevent him or her from pursuing a particular sporting practice, the tastes that are part of one's habitus influence one's sporting practice. As a result, the cultural component of sporting practice cannot be ignored with respect to interest in certain sports. Second, with regard to participation, the unity of habitus and field creates a further obstacle for the use of sporting practices by lower- and middle-class youth as a means of upward mobility. Sports such as golf, rowing, cycling, and even to a certain extent soccer given its particular structure in North America are not sports lower-class youth can use to break out of the lower class and into the financially rewarding world of professional sport at the highest level. Baseball holds some attraction as an affordable practice for some lower-class youth (although Black Americans no longer use baseball for upward mobility as much as in the past). Basketball, because of its tremendously individualist nature and low cost, affords the greatest promise of mobility and delivers often enough to make the promise even more enticing. Hockey for a small minority of Canadian males is still a field where lower-class youth can combine their field opportunities and habitus into a practice that might create some opportunities for upward mobility, although the competition for places at the highest levels has increased significantly with the expanding use of European players.

Nevertheless, even though it is true that the growth of consumer society has expanded the opportunities for all Canadians to take part in an increasingly wide array of sports, and previously excluded groups like the disabled now have opportunities to engage in competitive sport and physical activities, there are still important dimensions of one's social field that significantly impact upon the sporting practices of contemporary youth. It is the persistent inequality of condition that continues to prevent contemporary society from being one of open mobility, and inequality of condition stems first and foremost from the unequal income structure in Canada and the inequitable distribution and control of wealth in Canadian society. Two aspiring athletes—one whose family lives below the "low income cut-off" (LICO) (popularly referred to as the "poverty line") and one whose family is in the top 20 percent of Canadian earners or ranks within the top 20 percent of families in terms of wealth—do not enter the competition for spots in the Canadian sport meritocracy under equal conditions. One has a significant head start over the other.

There are numerous ways to examine income and wealth, and while there is no uniform approach, there are several basic features that stand out. As expected, studies of income or wealth in Canada show that the economic conditions of prospective athletes are highly unequal. Examining the Canadian income structure between 1980 and 1995, Soroka (2000) found an increase in income inequality in Canada, with the 1990–95 period showing the most pronounced growth in income inequality. The growing inequality applied to both males and females, with the greatest growth in Canada's larger cities. More important, contrary to public perception there was an absolute decline in both the average and median income levels in the 1990–95 period (see also Morissette & Bérubé, 1996). MacLachlan and Sawada (1997) reported similar findings, noting the trend toward increasing inequality applied to individual and household incomes. Kerr and Beaujot (2003) documented that, in 1981, about 16 percent of children in Canada lived below the federal government's LICO, with about 5 percent living in "deep poverty" (less than half the LICO). Conditions improved by 1989 (15 percent and 3.8 percent, respectively), but those gains were lost in the 1990s with 19 percent of Canadian children living below the LICO and 5 percent in deep poverty by the end of the decade.

Some argue that one's economic condition is best represented by wealth rather than income; Morissette, Zhang, and Drolet (2002) showed that wealth among Canadians parallels the findings on income. Between 1984 and 1999, the inequitable distribution of wealth in Canada grew. While a number of factors explained the growing inequality, the key factors seemed to relate to the control of existing assets, the growth of inheritances, the rates of return on savings, and the number of years in full-time employment. The study noted that the rates of return on savings and the strong growth in the stock market during the 1990s played an important role in the growing disparity of wealth in Canada.

All of these studies indicate that inequality of condition is a very real aspect of Canadian life and it has a predictable impact on sport participation. The cost of outfitting a minor hockey player in second-hand equipment can be as low as $200; outfitting the same player in new equipment can cost about $400 or more. For some those costs represent a prohibitive barrier to participation in organized sport. For a young teenager the cost of equipment varies from $400 for all second-hand to $1,000 or more for new, with the brand of skates and type of stick potentially driving the price far higher. Young adult players' equipment runs from $500 to $1,500, with skates, stick, and gloves having the potential to push costs significantly higher.

Fees for house league participation tend to range from $300 to $500; playing a step higher in an A or AA rep program will cost from $700 to $1,000; AAA team fees range from $3,000 to $6,000 per season. In the United States, the fees are as much as $1,300 for B-level and $3,500 for A- or AA-level hockey (Wolff, 2004). None of these fees include transportation costs, snacks, meals, hotel accommodation for tournaments, and extra tournament entry fees— or, as is the case in some jurisdictions, the admission fee parents and siblings must pay just to watch the young player's games. Sports like soccer and basketball are less expensive (although, depending on the brand, shoes can be very expensive); all the extras cited above will apply and can add up quickly even for house league players. These costs provide some insight into how economic circumstances influence the conditions under which a child competes with others for the prized spots at the top of the sport pyramid.

Only a few studies in Canada have examined the relationship between athletes' socioeconomic status (SES—a composite indicator of family income, education, and location in the labour force) and participation, but each of them has shown the same pattern of involvement despite federal and provincial governments' attempts to eliminate economic condition as a major factor in the exclusion of young Canadians from sport. Gruneau's (1972) groundbreaking study of Canada Games athletes showed that the competitors were drawn heavily from families where parents held professional and high-level white-collar occupations, while those whose parents were involved in blue-collar and primary industrial occupations were significantly underrepresented. The Canada Games athletes were also disproportionately drawn from families with higher incomes and educational achievement. Using Blishen scores that indicated a composite SES ranking, Gruneau found that 37 percent of the athletes came from the top three Blishen categories, while only 17 percent of the Canadian labour force ranked there. (Blishen scores were one of the most widely used—and generally accepted—composite rankings of socioeconomic status that sociologists employed in their studies of stratification patterns in Canada during the 1960s through to the 1980s.) Only 29 percent of the athletes came from the two lowest categories, although 63 percent of the Canadian labour force ranked in those categories.

Gerald Kenyon's (1977) study of elite track and field athletes and Barry McPherson's (1977) study of hockey players found similar patterns. Kenyon found that, with 63 percent of the track and field athletes coming from families ranking in the top three Blishen categories and only 29 percent from families in the bottom two, track and field was more exclusive than the sport system as a whole. McPherson's data on elite hockey players was comparable to Gruneau's—22 percent of the players' parents were located in the top three Blishen categories.

Beamish's (1990) study focused on national-team athletes in 1986. He demonstrated that despite more than 15 years of federal government support for high-performance sport and a number of strategies to reduce the impact of family background on athletic participation, patterns of significant exclusion existed among Canada's top athletes. Close to half of Canada's national team athletes (44 percent) came from families in the top 20 percent of Canadian income earners; only 10 percent came from the bottom 20 percent of income earners. Canada's best athletes were drawn from families with fathers in managerial positions at almost two and a half times the expected rate, and those whose fathers were employed in the professional and technical sectors of the economy were more than double their proportional representation. At the other end of the workforce, athletes with parents in farming, logging, mining, crafts, production, and unskilled labour were significantly underrepresented. The data on Blishen scores showed that since Gruneau's study Canada's national teams had become more exclusive—68 percent of the athletes came from families in the top three Blishen categories. White and Curtis (1990), using a completely different data set, found similar patterns of representation.

On behalf of Sport Canada, Ekos Research Associates (1992) performed the last comprehensive study of Canada's high-performance athletes. One of the key areas of concern was the sociodemographic profile of Canada's national team athletes that would address the extent to which there were sex, language, educational, or economic biases to accessibility in the sport system (Ekos, 1992). The results of this exhaustive study were the same as the earlier researchers'. Ekos found that there was an overrepresentation of anglophone athletes among Canada's best athletes. Canada's athletes did not come from "average" Canadian families. Forty-one percent of the athletes' fathers and 30 percent of their mothers had university-level educations (compared to 14 percent in the Canadian population as a whole). Like Beamish (1990), Ekos found that a significantly disproportionate number of athletes came from families with parents employed in professional, managerial, or administrative positions. Most important, Ekos concluded that the various funding and support programs in Canada's high-performance sport system had not reduced or eliminated inequalities of socioeconomic condition as a major factor determining who would rise to the top of the Canadian high-performance sport pyramid.

Inequality of condition, like inequality of opportunity, has a significant impact on who is able to enter into the sport system and stay within it long enough to pursue an Olympic dream. The Canadian sport pyramid cannot be a genuine meritocracy as long as inequalities of condition exist and act as a barrier to equal participation and equal competition for the uppermost ranks of the pyramid. All of the studies of Canada's elite athletes have shown that, on the whole, those who enjoy conditions of financial and economic advantage are disproportionately represented among the small group of athletes competing for spots on Canada's national teams, while others struggle simply to enter into the competition at all.

CANADIAN SPORT PERFORMANCE

Canada is the only country that has failed to win a gold medal while hosting the Olympic Games. When the IOC granted the 2010 Games to Vancouver, the COC, along with Sport Canada and some select commercial supporters, committed itself to improving Canada's performances at the Games. Torino's third-place finish (24 medals, 7 gold) was an improvement over the last three winter Olympiads—fifth in 2002 (17 medals, 6 gold), fourth in 1998 (15 medals, 6 gold), and sixth in 1994 (13 medals, 3 gold). It was a dramatic improvement over recent Summer Games rankings—twenty-first in 2004 (12 medals, 3 gold), twenty-first in 2000 (14 medals, 3 gold), and eleventh in 1996 (22 medals, 3 gold). To establish Canada as a world leader in high-performance sport, the COC launched *Own the Podium*, which explicitly commits the COC and Canada's athletes to the pursuit of gold. *Own the Podium* the COC notes, is a "technical program designed to help Canada become the number one nation in terms of medals won at the 2010 Olympic Winter Games, and to place in the top three countries overall at the 2010 Paralympic Winter Games" (Vancouver 2010, 2006).

Although *Own the Podium* was a dramatic change of philosophy within the Canadian Olympic movement, it did not happen overnight. In its 2004 annual report, the COC noted that while historically it had provided grants to each national sport federation based on a formula that focused on historical results and the number of potential participants to enter events, that philosophy changed in 2001. Over the 2001–04 quadrennial, the new "High Performance Support Program" allocated $14 million on the basis of the results achieved at the most recent Olympic or Pan American Games and a "comprehensive sport review process." "The Sport Review Process," the COC (2004) noted, "introduced the principle of performance accountability and return on investment as a requirement for COC funding" (p. 10). The COC had moved to a purely performance-based funding model. The approach is "a more targeted investment strategy," which the COC felt was imperative to build Olympic success.

Own the Podium targets sports and athletes in pursuit of more "podium finishes" in 2010. Since there is not much time between 2004 and 2010 to develop new athletes who might win medals, the key strategy is to improve the success rate of potential medal winners. This led to specifically targeted funding in the "flat ice sports" followed by "snow sports."

Is the approach consistent with the principles of a meritocracy? Clearly it is aimed at selected athletes—athletes who have proven international performances and athletes who are most likely to place among the top three in the world in 2010. Thus there is a strong merit or performance base to the program. What the program does not do is ensure that all athletes have an equal opportunity to draw upon the extra funding, coaching support, and access to world-class facilities, training opportunities, and competitions that identified athletes will have. The program seeks to increase the advantages enjoyed by established, successful athletes, while not directing additional funds to other developing athletes.

INEQUALITY AND MERITOCRACY

There is a final element in stratification theory that cannot be overlooked. Throughout the course of their lives, the "baby boomers"—Canadians born between 1945 and 1960 (though some extend it as far as 1965)—have had a tremendous influence on Canadian society (Owram, 1996). Their anticipated impact on the Canada Pension Plan and the Canadian healthcare system has been the subject of debate for some time (Fougère & Mérette, 1999). Scant attention, however, has been directed to the impact they will have on sport and recreation due to the influence they will exert on facilities and policies. There are four points of particular importance to note regarding the baby boomers and issues of social stratification in general and sport and recreation in particular.

First, the baby boomers have forced sociologists to explicitly think about age as a key factor in social stratification (Knickman & Snell, 2002). On the whole women outlive men, but because they have tended to work outside the paid labour force or have had careers interrupted by children they may have no, or very low, pensions, and most spousal pension plans result in a sharp decline in pension benefits if the husband predeceases the wife. As a result, age and poverty have become closely associated, especially for women (Nelson & Robinson, 1999). So age, in and of itself, seems to play a significant factor in where one resides in the social stratification system.

Second, because large portions of the baby boomer generation have enjoyed the benefits of consumer society and purchased a very wide variety of athletic and recreational gear, and have been exposed to a variety of media campaigns and continually reminded about the benefits of an active lifestyle, the baby boomer generation has been more active—and active at older ages—than previous generations. Physical activity is a significant enough part of the boomers' lifestyle to have a social impact (Hartman-Stein & Potkanowicz, 2003).

Third, because boomers have been more active and continued to be active into their 30s, 40s, and 50s, and appear ready to remain more active in their 60s than previous generations, they too are placing demands on athletic and recreational facilities. The demand is an important one, because despite the fact that the boomers are using sport for activity and entertainment, they are certainly not seeking upward mobility through sport. The facilities they want are user-centred, requiring little spectator seating but providing comfortable after-activity amenities. The sport and physical activity needs of boomers compete with the traditional youth and professional sport orientation in most facility debates. Most important, because the boomers are well established, have political connections, and are currently major taxpayers, they wield considerable municipal power in decisions over the building and use of athletic and recreational facilities.

This means, finally, that in view of their political and economic power and their own particular goals, the Boomers may significantly alter the orientation of organized sport in Canada. Their full impact is yet to be felt, but it could dramatically change the stratification system in Canadian sport.

Formally organized sport in contemporary societies is rooted in differential outcomes based on competitive excellence—sport is supposed to result in a hierarchy of outcomes on the basis of demonstrated performance. Sport is, ideally, a meritocracy.

As the object of inequality, Canadians tend to support a pyramid approach to high-performance sport—inequality of outcome is expected and the unequal allocation of rewards is accepted as part of the appropriate, meritocratic reward structure. But a genuine meritocracy relies on fundamental equalities in other spheres of social life. If the most talented, dedicated, hardest-working athletes are to compete for the top spots, everyone must have an equal opportunity to enter the race.

Unfortunately, whether one looks at the opportunity to benefit from comparable facilities, the opportunity to learn within the multidimensional, socially enacted sporting experience, or the opportunities presented through predominant sociocultural and political forces, there are significant inequalities of opportunity experienced by Canadians who might want to rank or have the potential to rank among the nation's best. Added onto those inequalities of opportunity are significant inequalities of condition.

As an object of inequality, a genuine meritocracy is premised upon and requires equality in other key spheres of social life—and those equalities do not exist in Canada in general, or its sport system in particular. Ironically, perhaps, the overall inequalities of Canadian society make a sporting meritocracy incredibly difficult to build. It would be only through a commitment to eliminate inequalities of condition and opportunity that Canadians could enjoy watching the very best athletes the nation could produce—as apparently contradictory as that may seem.

CRITICAL THINKING QUESTIONS

1. What is a meritocracy? Is the Canadian sport system a meritocracy?
2. What is meant by the term "the object of inequality," and why is it important to identify it in any discussion of social stratification?
3. What is meant by the term "equality of opportunity," and what factors in Canada prevent a true equality of opportunity in sport?
4. What are the key issues in social stratification that a discussion of the Special Olympics or the Paralympics must include?

5. What is meant by a "multidimensional enacted curriculum," and how is it significant to a discussion of social stratification in sport?
6. Is the mandate for equal funding in male and female sport consistent with the principles of a meritocracy?
7. What is meant by the term "inequality of condition," and how does it impact upon sport as a meritocracy?
8. Who are the "baby boomers," and what is their significance to discussions of sport and social stratification?

SUGGESTED READINGS

Gruneau, R. (1999). *Class, sports, and social development*. Champaign, IL: Human Kinetics Press.

Lemel, Y., & Noll, H. (Eds.). (2002). *Changing structures of inequality: A comparative perspective*. Montreal: McGill–Queen's Press.

Osmani, S. (2001). On inequality. In J. Blau (Ed.), *The Blackwell companion to sociology* (pp. 143–60). Oxford: Blackwell Publishing.

WEB LINKS

International Paralympic Committe (IPC)

http://www.paralympic.org/
Information on the IPC and its history, the Paralympic Games, the sports involved, the Paralympic Hall of Fame, contacts, and other information.

Sport Canada

http://www.pch.gc.ca/sportcanada/
Official website for Sport Canada, with information on its mission, policies, funding programs, and links to sports federations as well as the Ministry for Canadian Heritage.

Statistics Canada

http://www.statcan.ca/
Gateway to a vast array of official statistics collected by the Canadian federal government; studies arranged by subject; site is easy to search.

CHAPTER 5

RACE AND ETHNICITY IN CANADIAN SPORT

Victoria Paraschak and Susan Tirone

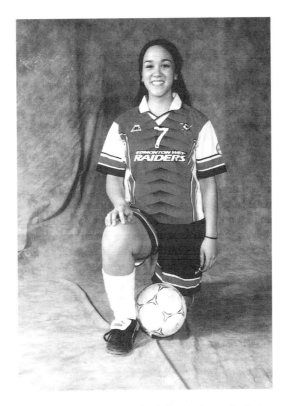

Katie Illnik, an Inuk from Yellowknife, Northwest Territories, moved to Edmonton, Alberta, to pursue more competitive soccer opportunities as part of her high school experience.

Reprinted by permission of Harvey Alberta Trophy/Elite Sportswear Awards

Pride in one's roots is essential to finding one's voice.

Spence, 1999, p. 17

We shall not cease from exploration
And the end of all our exploring
Will be to arrive where we started
And know the place for the first time.

T. S. Eliot, 1943, p. 313

We all have individual characteristics that differentiate us from, or connect us to others. Hair colour, gender, height, skin colour, ethnicity, and eye colour are a few examples of such characteristics. Think of how you would describe yourself for a minute. When we thought about this question, Vicky described herself as female, brown haired, hazel eyed, 5'4", urban Canadian, and white. Susan described her physical attributes in a similar way but she lives in a rural community. Yet as each of us live out or "do" our lives, those individual characteristics are continually reshaped by our experiences. For example, Vicky recollects how some children have considered her tall, while adults often claim that she is short. Her eye colour varies with what she wears, and her ethnicity has been shaped by years in the Canadian north and the specific cultural practices she learned there and continues to do. She is also often quizzed on her race, because of her research on First Nations peoples. Susan notes that her studies of Canadian immigrants and children in those immigrant families help her to reflect on what is meaningful in her own life, having been raised within a large extended Italian Canadian family. So while, when asked, we can each describe our individual characteristics, that description changes over time and from the perspectives of others. We continuously construct the ways we see ourselves, and that involves the social world in which we live. Our individual characteristics are much less definitive than we might, at first, think.

Some of these characteristics take on a particular social significance in our society. While eye colour remains unimportant at a social level, characteristics such as ethnicity and skin colour—or race—have become socially constructed markers of difference. Persistent patterns of unequal treatment have developed around them, in North American society broadly and in sport. Individuals assigned those characteristics get identified as part of a group that shares traits differentiating it from others. Our sense of ourselves is thus constructed in relation to groups we believe are similar to or different from us.

We know ourselves, and our culture, in part through our bodies. For example, as we "do" physical activities, such as sports, we shape, reinforce, or challenge the understanding we—and others—hold about our racial and ethnic identities. Students in a physical education class learning basketball all perform the same activities, but the ways those movements reinforce or challenge each individual's sense of his or her own race and ethnicity influences the meaning assigned to those movements, and the enjoyment felt or not felt within the class. After school, an Asian youth may head to a program where she participates with others from her ethnic background in activities tied to her cultural roots. Through this process, she reinforces the importance of her ethnic identity in a manner not possible in her earlier gym class on basketball. A Black male student, practising with the school basketball team at the end of the day, feels confirmed as a talented athlete as he emulates the playing styles of his favourite NBA players. Another student heads home to spend time with her family, having no interest in after-school athletics. Day after day, these students continue to know themselves and to represent themselves to others through their involvement—or non-involvement—in physical activities.

This chapter explores the relationships among movement, race, and ethnicity in Canada. It builds on two assumptions, which are captured in the quotes at the start of the chapter. Firstly, we believe that movement opportunities in Canada—such as sport—potentially provide the opportunity for all individuals to generate a feeling of pride in their cultural heritage. However, the sport system has been structured so that some individuals—specifically, Caucasians of European descent—are privileged to feel racial and ethnic pride more so than others. Secondly, we encourage our readers to enter into a reflective process through which they can better understand how race and ethnicity are constructed in our society and in sport. By doing so, they can more knowledgeably shape their own identities while honouring the individual identities desired by others; prerequisites for creating an inclusive sport system in Canada.

ETHNICITY AND SPORT IN CANADA

The Concept of Ethnicity

Sport is one of the most popular leisure activities Canadians enjoy. Whether we are involved as a spectator at a football game, a recreational swimmer, or an elite athlete, Canadians tend to be highly interested and invested in sports. Our ethnic identity shapes, and is shaped by, our sport participation. Ethnicity refers to the values, beliefs, and behaviours we share in common with a subcultural group to which we most closely identify based on common country of origin, language, religion, or cultural traditions (Hutchison, 1988). Ethnicity takes into account individuals' religious practices, their clothing, their language or accented English, the food they eat, and what they value as a result of their cultural heritage. Ethnicity, like race, has social significance in our society. To understand ethnicity and sport we need to know about ethnicity and how one's ethnic identity may influence decisions and preferences around sport participation. We also benefit from knowing about past trends and theory developed to explain trends or beliefs about ethnicity.

Everyone can be linked to at least one ethnic group, whether it is one of the dominant European-white, English/French speaking groups, or one of the more than 200 other ethnic groups known to exist in this country (Canadian Heritage, 2005a). The scope of our extraordinary national diversity was evident in the 2001 Census when almost half of all Canadians reported identifying with an ethnic group other than British, French, or Aboriginal (Statistics Canada, 2003). As new immigrants arrive in Canada from non-Western countries and as the number of minority ethnic people in Canada grows, ethnic diversity in sport is one of the many parts of social life that is changing.

Diversity Theories

With the passing of the Multiculturalism Act of 1988, Canada officially declared its support for cultural freedom of minority peoples. The term "cultural pluralism," first introduced in 1915 by Kallen, refers to the approach our country takes with regard to receiving and welcoming immigrants. It means that in Canada, we as hosts support newcomers in preserving their cultural identity if they choose to do so (Glazer, 1970). Our approach differs from that of our neighbours to the south. In the United States, immigrants are expected to shed their unique cultural practices, adopt new ones based on the values and beliefs of the host country, and as a result of this process of assimilation contribute toward building a better nation. This second approach is commonly referred to as the "melting pot" perspective (Glazer, 1970). Cultural pluralism, on the other hand, recognizes that for many newcomers, meaningful experience incorporates "'stubborn chunks' of cultural practice and preference, and is more like a chowder than a melting pot" (Bhabha, 1994, p. 219). Some aspects of life do change with immersion in the host culture. But other "chunks" remain intact and provide the basis on which some minority people create cultures "in between" that of the dominant majority and the cultures known to the migrant in their own homeland (Bhabha, 1994; Hollingshead, 1998). As a result of our legislation, Canadians officially support physical cultural practices like sport, dance, music, and religious expressions that are meaningful to people of all minority cultural groups and are meaningful to the experience of leisure. However, Claude Denis (1997) challenges this description of Canada, instead labelling it a "whitestream" society because it has been primarily structured on the basis of European white experiences. In keeping with his perspective, academics and practitioners have only recently begun to explore the meaning of leisure from the perspective of immigrant groups, as well as ethnic minority physical cultural practices and the challenges they face related to discrimination, racism, and indifference from dominant group Canadians in mainstream sport.

In spite of Canada's policy of multiculturalism that officially embraces diversity, many immigrants and ethnic minority people strive to take on characteristics of their host culture in order to improve the likelihood that they will "fit in." *Assimilation* is the term used when immigrants adopt the culture of the dominant group (Li, 1990). The underlying assumption of assimilation theory is that ethnically distinct cultural traditions are detrimental to one's ability to fit in and that it is not desirable to be different. This assimilationist approach is problematic because it normalizes mainstream cultural practices as the "appropriate" behaviour for all. As well, as new immigrant groups arrive in places like Canada, looking and sounding different from dominant groups, it is not always possible to fit in and become like the majority since race, culture, and behavioural diversity sets newcomers apart.

In trying to understand the behaviour of ethnic minority people, researchers have relied primarily on two theoretical perspectives: marginality theory and ethnicity theory. Marginality theory suggests that the differences in participation are due to the poverty experienced by many minority racial and ethnic people, a function of the discrimination they face in accessing training and education, as well as jobs. Therefore, under-participation in activities like sport is thought to be due to their marginalization in society. This perspective helps explain why some minority group Canadians do not choose the same sports as the dominant, majority population but it falls short when applied to those immigrants and ethnic minority people who are not poor, and who have somewhat different sport participation patterns, as is the case with South Asian Canadians who play field hockey, cricket, and other sports not popular among dominant group Canadians (Tirone & Pedlar, 2000).

Ethnicity theory is based on Washburne's (1978) thesis that differences in leisure between dominant and minority populations are the result of variations in the value systems and social norms of the minority groups. This approach suggests that ethnic subgroups interact with dominant cultural groups for school, jobs, commerce, and when needs cannot be met within the subgroup. However, many ethnic minority people maintain their distinct cultural traditions and pass them along to their children and subsequent generations. Using this approach, researchers compare behaviours such as sport participation patterns of ethnic minority people to the leisure experience of dominant groups. Problematic here is that the leisure of the white, Eurocentric majority is held as the norm and minority people are considered as "others" for the sake of comparisons, similar to the "whitestream" approach mentioned earlier. This approach fails to explore the unique opportunities for leisure evident in minority cultural groups as a result of their cultural heritage.

We have found that "whitestream sport" is a useful concept for analyzing race and ethnic relations in Canadian sport, because it emphasizes that the existing sport system is primarily structured by, and most effective for, individuals who align with white, European values. Additionally, *marginality theory* identifies that poverty plays a role in limiting access to mainstream sport for some minority ethnic groups. Finally, *ethnicity theory* emphasizes that the differing value systems of immigrant Canadians can lead to different preferences for sport and/or different ways of organizing and playing mainstream sports. The pattern of immigration trends in Canada helps to explain how whitestream Canadian society has been created, and also how it is challenged by increasingly diverse minority group Canadians.

Immigration Trends

In the early part of the twentieth century, Canada's economic, industrial, agricultural, and commercial growth and development was fuelled by many waves of immigrants seeking a better life than what was available in their countries of origin. Canada recruited its first large wave of immigrants from Great Britain, Europe, and the United States. The early immigrants from

Britain and France, recognized as the primary architects of our major institutions and communities, have expected other groups to assimilate to their ways. However, these groups were not ethnically homogeneous (Burnet & Palmer, 1988; Knowles, 2000). Among early French immigrants were distinct ethnic groups such as the Acadians in eastern Canada, les Canadiens in Quebec, and Métis people who were the children of French settlers partnered with First Nations peoples. British immigrants identified with diverse cultural practices of England, Scotland, Northern Ireland, and Wales and issues of social class also created distinct communities among British immigrants (Burnet & Palmer, 1988). For many decades the ideals that newcomers were expected to aspire to aligned with the values and beliefs of upper- and middle-class British settlers. Newcomers often found assimilation to these value sets difficult or even impossible to attain.

Changes to immigration patterns occurred in the last decades of the twentieth century and first years of the twenty-first century when migration flows shifted. New waves of immigrants tended to move from "east" to "west"; that is, from former Soviet Union and Eastern bloc countries to the United States, Canada, and Israel; and from countries of the "South" to countries of the "North"; such as from South Asia to Canada (Chiswick & Miller, 2002). The immigrants of the new millennium often look and sound different from the dominant groups and their distinctiveness in terms of skin colour, language, clothing, religion, and other cultural practices has often resulted in their marginalization.

To learn the language skills necessary for job attainment and to achieve a sense of belonging, immigrant groups may cluster into concentrated areas of similar immigrants or ethnic enclaves. Here they find important sources of social support, whether that be in employment opportunities, leisure such as sport participation, education, or shelter (Chiswick & Miller, 2002; Rosenberg, 2003). Ethnic enclaves and institutionally complete ethnic communities have been well established in Canada since the earliest minority group settlers arrived here (Breton, 1964). Communities considered to have high levels of institutional completeness are those in which a range of social supports and relevant services are available to minority people, and often these are delivered within well established ethnic enclaves. This is what happened in the case of early Jewish, Italian, and German immigrants who formed small communities or enclaves in some of the major Canadian cities. Within the enclaves, people were able to access culturally and ethnically relevant social services, familiar food, and familiar religious and cultural traditions, all delivered in the language of their homeland and by people with common ethnic roots. For example, late nineteenth- and early twentieth-century Jewish immigrants to Toronto settled primarily in the district known as St. John's Ward, where they experienced abysmal housing conditions but had the benefit of social support such as language, religion, food, music, and other cultural goods that were familiar to them and which facilitated their settlement (Rosenberg, 2003). Sport organizations operated by ethnic community associations provided youth important opportunities for affirming membership within their own ethnic group and for drawing together people from diverse ethnic groups around common sport interests (Rosenberg, 2003). Those who enter a host community without the help of friends and family members from their country of origin may find they have no alternative but to try to assimilate quickly into the dominant society, although that process is likely to be extraordinarily challenging (Chiswick & Miller, 2002).

Immigration trends in the early third millennium are quite different from those of the past 150 years. New immigrants reported in the 2001 census such locations of origin as Kosovo, Azerbaijan, Afghanistan, Yemen, Saudi Arabia, Nepal, Kashmir, Congo, Bolivia, and other countries in Central and South America (Statistics Canada, 2003). As these newcomers are immersed in Canadian society, their sport traditions and preferences will likely continue to have an impact on how sport is experienced in this country.

As well, many people report multiple ethnicities primarily due to intermarriage, as was the case for 38 percent of respondents in the 2001 census who reported identification with more than one ethnic origin (Statistics Canada, 2003). This identification with more than one ethnic minority group, sometimes referred to as *hybridity* or *part cultures* (Bhabba, 1994), is a growing trend that will undoubtedly affect the participation of Canadians in cultural activities and sporting events in years to come. For example, Dallaire's studies of youth participants in the Francophone Games in Alberta, Ontario, and New Brunswick found the youth tended to identify themselves as having hybrid identities or a "melange of francophoneness and anglo-phoneness" (Dallaire & Denis, 2005, p. 143). These youth, like the South Asian youth in Tirone and Pedlar's study (2000), construct and re-construct their identities drawing upon their inherited traditions and upon the cultural traditions of the anglo dominant group in which they are immersed for much of their school and social lives. While francophone youth in Dallaire's studies participated in the same sports as are offered at the Olympics, other minority youth draw upon the traditional sports they learned from their minority community. As minority youth "do" sports such as field hockey and cricket, common among youth in South Asia, and sports like dragonboat racing and martial arts that originated within minority communities, dominant group youth are also able to access these non-traditional sports, thereby changing the nature of some sport participation in Canada.

Not all immigrants and ethnic minority people choose to live in places where other minorities like themselves also live. Chiswick and Miller (2002) explain the value of immersion into dominant society where ethnic minority people gain exposure and social capital necessary for career development and economic success. Young immigrants and children of ethnic minority families are often immersed in or at least familiarized with dominant cultural practices, because they usually attend schools with peers from a vast range of ethnic and racial backgrounds. Schools therefore provide opportunities for learning the values and beliefs of diverse peers and for learning the priorities of the institutions with which minorities are expected to conform. Sport is very much a part of the Canadian school system; for many ethnic minority youth, school is the place where they first encounter sport participation.

Ethnic Minority People and Sport in Canada

Since many of the early-twentieth-century white settler groups were not British or French, they brought with them, as part of their distinct traditional cultural practices, a number of sports that were not familiar to dominant group Canadians. For example, Estonians, Finlanders, and people from the former Czechoslovakia introduced modern and rhythmic gymnastics to Canada after World War II, and Southeast Asians have made popular a number of their traditional sports such as tai chi and karate (Burnet & Palmer, 1988). In those early days, sports clubs and teams were sponsored by some ethnic communities and churches to engage the youth of the community in meaningful activity and to shelter participants from discriminatory practices of dominant sport and recreation associations (Kidd, 1996a; McBride, 1975). Exclusionary practices of dominant group sports associations gave rise to sports teams and clubs sponsored by workers' movements and political organizations whose membership was comprised of minority ethnic workers. These included sports teams supported by Canadian communists in the 1920s and 1930s (Kidd, 1996a).

Ethnic sport associations remain a valued part of institutionally complete Canadian ethnic communities, providing opportunities for youth to experience activity similar to that of dominant group peers within organizations their parents support. In a study of children of immigrants from South Asia, Tirone and Pedlar (2000) learned that during their school years prior to university, South Asian clubs and associations were an important venue for sport and physical activity for many of the youth. Several participants in that longitudinal study, which began in 1996, described how they and their families participated in sports such as badminton and volleyball with other South Asian families who rented public gymnasia space exclusively for use by their group (Tirone & Pedlar, 2000). Stodolska and Jackson (1998) describe a similar pattern of sports provision and participation in Polish Canadian ethnic clubs. Sport and recreation participation is beneficial for new immigrant youth, providing opportunities for social integration with other youth in their neighbourhoods. It is the source of both embedded and autonomous social capital. Embedded social capital refers to the connection between people based on trust and common values, which serves to unite people within an enclave or ethnic group. Autonomous social capital is the trust and respect that can develop between people of diverse backgrounds and which leads to opportunities for people from an enclave to interact outside of their homogeneous group (Woolcock, 1998). While high levels of embedded social capital mean people within a homogeneous group are well connected to one another, those connections may not provide group members with information and connections they desire to be recognized and to prosper outside of the enclave. Autonomous social capital is useful when people want to interact and be recognized for their skills and potential outside of an enclave.

There are several reasons why ethnic sport associations have continued to exist. Sports teams, music, cuisine, language, and other cultural traditions are an expression of group identity (Burnet & Palmer, 1988). These ethnic sport organizations also provide a supportive environment. For example, worker sport associations and ethnic clubs provided sports and physical activities for early immigrants who were ridiculed and excluded from mainstream sport associations (Kidd, 1996b). More recently, sports associations like those sponsored by Canadian South Asian cultural associations provide youth with the benefits of sport participation, as well as opportunities to meet other South Asian youth their own age in competitive environments their parents support (Tirone, 2000). Ethnic sport associations thus serve to protect participants from the harassment some people experience in mainstream sport.

The popularity of ethnic sports is no more evident than in the sport of soccer. Harney (cited in Burnet & Palmer, 1988) describes participation of ethnic groups in soccer in Toronto in the 1970s. His account describes the 78 teams in the Toronto District Soccer League at that time, more than three-quarters of which displayed ethnic emblems or the names of various countries as team names, such as First Portuguese, Croatia, Serbia White Eagle, Hungaria, and Heidelberg. In the winter of 2006, this multicultural approach was linked to hockey for the first time. An inaugural Canadian Multicultural Hockey tournament was held, where 16 teams of Toronto-area players competed for their "home country," such as Russia, Finland, Serbia, Japan, China, Korea, Native Canadians, Poland, Greece, and Italy. This tournament launched the new Toronto-based Canadian Multicultural Hockey League (Lewi, 2006).

Early ethnic sport associations valued competitive success as well as positive group identity. Ethnic sports teams that displayed ethnic insignia often recruited players based on ability and not ethnicity. Seeking the most skilled players, ethnic sports clubs often accepted players of diverse ethnic backgrounds—as was the case when Finnish Canadians, recognized for their skills, were encouraged to take up Canadian sports (Kidd, 1996b). Ethnic minority athletes have been and continue to be a source of pride for their ethnic group. Participation in sports by ethnic minority athletes provides them with opportunities to engage in and experience the values of other cultures, including those of dominant group members.

Ethnicity, Poverty, and Access to Sport

While few Canadians would argue the health and social benefits of most sport participation, especially for children, we have not been able to ensure that everyone can participate in sport.

Poverty has long been known to prevent many Canadian youth from participating in organized sports, and often children in poor families have little or no access to unorganized sport and recreation (Frisby et al., 2005). Recent Canadian income data and poverty studies report that ethnic minority families are failing to secure the same income levels as Canadian-born families (Kazemipur & Halli, 2001). Although 80 percent of new immigrants report that they found work in Canada during the first two years of residency in this country, only 42 percent of them found work in the fields in which they had trained, and many of these people work at jobs that provide little more than subsistence wages (Statistics Canada, 2003). A study of poverty among Torontonians indicates one-third of the immigrant families in Toronto in 2001 lived in higher-poverty neighbourhoods, and that number represents an increase of 400 percent between 1981 and 2001 (United Way of Greater Toronto, 2004). The same study reports that visible minorities were eight times more likely to live in poverty than they were in 1981. Statistics indicate far fewer children in low-income families participate in sport compared with children in high-income families (Frisby et al., 2005). Their participation is limited by lack of money for registration fees, equipment, and clothing. Ethnic minority youth in low-income families can also face additional limitations due to parental priorities that emphasize academic pursuits and discourage participation in sports (Rosenberg, 2003; Tirone & Pedlar, 2000).

Discrimination

Another barrier to sport participation that affects some ethnic minority Canadians is discrimination, both situational and systemic. In a study of leisure and recreation of teenagers who were the children of South Asian immigrants, racism and indifference were noted as reasons why some youth stopped participating in sports (Tirone, 2000). That group explained how when faced with overt racism or situations in which they were criticized or ridiculed because of skin colour, clothing, or religious practices, no one in a position of authority attempted to intervene in the situation. In another study of new immigrants to the Halifax area, a young university student who immigrated from the Middle East explained that he felt discrimination played a part in why he was not able to play soccer for his high school team. He had been an accomplished soccer player in his homeland prior to emigration, and when he arrived in Halifax as a high school student he attempted to try out for the school soccer team but was told that all positions were filled and he was not given a chance to demonstrate his skills. He satisfied his love for the game by volunteering as a coach for youth soccer, and upon entering university was recruited to play varsity soccer (Tirone, 2005) (see Box 5.1).

Ethnic identity has thus shaped and been shaped by sport participation in Canada. Oftentimes, barriers to sport participation based on ethnic identity are compounded by racism. The next section explores ways that racial identity shapes and has been shaped by sport participation.

RACE AND SPORT IN CANADA

The Concept of Race

"Race" is a term used to establish socially constructed distinctions between groups of people based on their genetic heritage. These distinctions, marked by skin colour, take on social significance because of differences assigned to members of these groups. For example, we could look at a group of people and assume that some are Caucasian, Black, Aboriginal, or Asian. It is, however, our belief that the colour of their skin indicates immutable differences between

---

Box 5.1   Problems Faced by Ethnic Youth in Sport

In several studies of new immigrants and second-generation Canadian youth the issue of sport was raised in the context of how important it is for youth development and how problematic it can be for some youth who are not able to gain access to the sports they prefer. The following quotes were provided by the participants in studies of young Canadians who identify with minority cultures.

Re: Parents Prioritize Education
Say you are a really good athlete, like my brother. Actually myself too when I was younger. We had the chance of going on and becoming, like for me, in swimming and my brother in whatever sport. And our parents said, "No." Once they found out we were good at something they took us out of it right away. Like they didn't want us, and they still say this. They don't want us to put our mind to sports and not to school. They wanted 90 percent school and 10 percent sports.

Re: Traditional Clothing
When we were really young it was hard for a lot of kids in elementary school. Because that is when you really get picked on, if you do [wear a turban]. But then I know some kids who have had a real problem with it and they have cut their hair because they can't take the teasing.

Re: Discrimination and Indifference
I remember being called all the racial things you can ever imagine . . .
     See I have been lucky. Like whenever I have played whether it was soccer or baseball, I guess a lot of it is, you have to prove yourself. Once you prove yourself, you are fine. If you don't prove yourself, like if she is playing tennis and she is really just learning for the first time, and she can't even hit the ball, well that is like a double whammy for her. But if she can smash that ball down the end line, they will look at her in a different light.

Question: But does she have to be even better than normal, because she is not white?
Yes. So that is where the racism comes in.

Re: Access to High School Sports
I played soccer ever since I was 6 years old and I was on varsity team (in Kuwait) when I was 13, and I wasn't even given a chance to get on the school team. I was cut before I even tried out.

Question: And it was because you didn't grow up in that school?
Yeah, I am totally a hundred percent convinced that that was what it was, that I didn't grow up here. I know it wasn't my skill level, cause I saw, like when I went to university after high school I got on the soccer team for [Ontario university] and I had no problem getting on the team. Yet, I had a problem getting on the high school team, so you know. It's just when you reflect back, you see things that you didn't see at the time. But, sometimes you just hope that they weren't there but they're there . . . I think the coach had his certain people, like they grow up from junior high and it's the same people and they don't change, some people don't like change so.

---

them that makes race a socially significant category in our society. We might look to Caucasians for leadership, Blacks for athletic talent, Aboriginal peoples for environmental guidance, and Asians for academic excellence. By assuming that race automatically gave individuals an advantage in some areas more so than others, we would be reproducing race-based understandings of human behaviour.

Skin colour has taken on social meanings in North America that privilege Caucasians over others. A hierarchy of privilege/discrimination has thus been created—commonly referred to as racism. Spence (1999, p. 15), quoting Carl James (1995, p. 37), explains it this way:

> Racism . . . is the uncritical acceptance of a negative social definition of a colonized or subordinate group typically identified by physical features. . . . These racialized groups are believed to lack certain abilities or characteristics, which in turn characterizes them as culturally and biologically inferior.

Racial classification systems and ideas about race emerged in the sixteenth and seventeenth centuries, while Europeans were exploring and claiming dominion over different parts of the world. As they encountered people who appeared and acted differently, these strangers were placed in an evolutionary hierarchy. Those most similar to Caucasians were judged to be the most evolved and civilized. Whiteness became the norm by which others were judged. The exploitation of people from other "races" thus became justified on the basis of their presumed inferiority relative to Europeans.

Social Darwinism extended Charles Darwin's theory of natural selection into the social realm. This theory provided British and American social theorists with a scientific tool for determining the superiority of some races over others, and thus with a justification for endorsing racial inequality (Coakley, 2001). The presence of slavery in Canada, beginning in 1628 (Spence, 1999), and the colonization and legislative regulation of First Nations within North America reinforced the subservient position of Blacks and Aboriginal peoples relative to Canadians of European descent in similar ways. This race logic eventually became institutionalized as a racial ideology involving "skin color, intelligence, character, and physical characteristics and skills" (Coakley, 2001, p. 247).

Identification by race is not, however, a straightforward process. What did it take, for example, for someone to be considered Caucasian, or Black, or Aboriginal, or Asian, and what were the consequences? The social constructedness of this process can be seen in the ways that race was defined for, and applied to, different groups in Canada. For example, historically, just "one drop of black blood" identified individuals as Black, even though they may have had white ancestors (Coakley, 2001).

In contrast to this, the British North America Act, which constituted Canada as a country in 1867, identified "Indians" as a race apart from other Canadians and placed them under federal jurisdiction. The Indian Act of 1876, which controlled almost every feature of Aboriginal social life, served to separate them further from other Canadians on the basis of race. Treaties were the third factor regulating native life. Here again, the underlying premise was that Aboriginal peoples had an "uncivilized nature" that must be altered before they could enjoy full civil rights. Everyday practices, such as performing traditional dances, were outlawed. It was not until 1960 that First Nations, as a race, could vote federally in Canada (Paraschak, 1997).

Chinese migrants were treated differently yet again. They were forced to pay a head tax to enter Canada beginning in 1885, and in 1902 a Royal Commission on Chinese and Japanese Immigration concluded that Asians were "unfit for full citizenship . . . obnoxious to a free community and dangerous to the state" (Wickberg, 1988, p. 416). Chinese and East Indian Canadians were not given the right to vote until 1947.

In contrast to these examples, being Caucasian in North American society has remained unmarked. White people rarely have to think of themselves in racial terms. They are privileged by race. They have access to opportunities in society without having to worry that their race will be a barrier. However, they may be treated differently because of their ethnic background. For example, on *Hockey Night in Canada* Don Cherry often comments on the differences among—and suitability of—professional hockey players who are francophone, anglophone, or European, even though all these athletes would be considered "white" by race (Langford, 2004).

Tiger Woods, a prominent professional golfer of mixed Black, Asian, Aboriginal, and white heritage, brought the complexity of defining individuals by race to public notice in 1997. After his successful first year on the tour, and his win at the Masters specifically, the press heralded him as a successful Black golfer. Tiger, however, eventually clarified publicly that he had developed a different racial description for himself as a youth, based on his actual background. He called himself a Cablinasian, to reflect his CAusasian, BLack, INdian, and ASIAN genetic heritage. In this way, he highlighted two important points: racial labels can be assigned to people without those labels being accurate, and the way individuals view themselves may be quite different from the racial category assigned to them by others.

Racial Patterns in Canadian Sport

Canada has an early history, in amateur sport, of discrimination by race. Cosentino (1998) argues that while "class" formed the basis of amateurism in England, in Canada "race" became the definer of who could compete. This was evident as early as 1835, when Black jockeys were banned from competing at the Niagara Turf Club. The first big regatta in Nova Scotia, in 1826, offered prizes "for first and second class boats and a canoe race for Indians . . . which was considered the most entertaining . . . [and] remained part of the Nova Scotian scene until at least 1896" (Young, 1988, pp. 87–8). In 1880, Aboriginal players were excluded, by race, from competing in amateur competitions for lacrosse—a game that had originated in Aboriginal culture! A special league for Black hockey players titled "The Colored League" was begun in Halifax in 1900, becoming the seventh league in that city—and the first one overtly defined by race (Young, 1988, p. 31). As late as 1913, the Amateur Athletic Association of Canada opted to ban Blacks, by race, from competing in Canadian amateur boxing championships, since "Competition of whites and coloured men is not working out to the increased growth of sport" (Amateur Athletic Union of Canada, quoted in Cosentino, 1998, p. 13). Even the first definition of an amateur in Canada, created by the Montreal Pedestrian Club in 1873, noted that no "labourer or Indian" could be given that designation.

Yet Canada is also a country where Blacks have, at times, found acceptance as athletes more readily than in the United States. Jackie Robinson broke the colour barrier in Major League Baseball playing for the Brooklyn Dodgers in 1947. However, the president of the Dodgers, Branch Rickey, actually signed Robinson in October 1945 to play professionally for the minor-league Montreal Royals. While Robinson played that first year, he experienced intense racism during games in the United States. In Montreal, however, he had great fan support. Scott (1987, p. 37) writes:

> Robinson's play made him a beloved sports figure in Montreal. Children hounded him for autographs, while adults poured into the ballpark to see him steal bases and score runs. As a Montreal sportswriter noted, "For Jackie Robinson and the city of Montreal, it was love at first sight."

Three decades later, Warren Moon was able to play professional football as a Black quarterback in Canada when that opportunity was not available in the United States. After being selected as the 1978 Rose Bowl Most Valuable Player, Moon was completely overlooked by the National Football League in its 1978 U.S. college draft. As a result, he came to play with the Edmonton Eskimos in the Canadian Football League and won five Grey Cups with them. In

1984, he became the highest-paid player in football when he joined the Houston Oilers of the National Football League (Mullick, 2002), and in 2006 he became the first Black quarterback inducted into the NFL Hall of Fame.

These examples demonstrate different ways that "race" has been given social meaning in Canadian sport. Such meanings are indicative of broader societal race relations. Frideres (1988), writing on racism in Canadian society, noted that "Racism in Canada from 1800 to 1945 was reflected in restrictive immigration policies and practices regarding non-white immigrants, particularly the Chinese, Blacks and Jews, and by the treatment of native peoples" (p. 1816). Racist sport practices during this time period would thus have reinforced, and been shaped by, broader understandings of race. Canadian attempts to address racial inequity through legislation coalesced in the Canadian Charter of Rights and Freedoms (1982), where equality rights in the public domain were entrenched. Section 15 stated:

Equality Rights

15. (1) Every individual is equal before and under the law and has the right to the equal protection and equal benefit of the law without discrimination and, in particular, without discrimination based on race, national or ethnic origin, colour, religion, sex, age or mental or physical disability.

(2) Subsection (1) does not preclude any law, program or activity that has as its object the amelioration of conditions of disadvantaged individuals or groups including those that are disadvantaged because of race, national or ethnic origin, colour, religion, sex, age or mental or physical disability.

Human Rights Commissions have also provided a legal avenue for addressing racial inequities in Canada. Participants and administrators who wish to make sport a more welcoming—and legislatively aligned—place for all can benefit by understanding the social construction of race and racism in sport.

Race and Ethnic Relations

In society, individuals always act in relation to others. The possibilities within which we live are thus formed through the "social relations" that exist between individuals and groups. Through social relations, rules are created concerning how things work and how resources can be distributed. They thus become "power relations," because those rules always provide for or privilege some people over others. Race and ethnic relations are a particular type of power relations—they privilege individuals on the basis of race and/or ethnicity. Gruneau (1988) defines power as "the capacity of a person or group of persons to employ resources of different types in order to secure outcomes" (p. 22). He then identifies three measures of power in sport: the ability to structure sport, to establish sport traditions, and to define legitimate meanings and practices associated with dominant sport practices. These measures of power, differently shaped by race and, at times, by ethnicity, can be seen when looking at mainstream sport, and at race-structured sporting opportunities such as all-Aboriginal sport competitions.

Whitestream Sport

As was mentioned earlier, Claude Denis (1997) uses the term *whitestream society* "to indicate that Canadian society, while principally structured on the basis of the European, 'white', experience, is far from being simply 'white' in socio-demographic, economic and cultural terms" (p. 13). Extending his term, the rules of mainstream or "whitestream" sport have been primarily shaped by individuals of white European heritage, in ways that privilege their traditions, practices, meanings, and sport structures. This is an example of "institutionalized racism," since the structure of the system, if followed, will always produce outcomes that discriminate against those who are not white—it will privilege Caucasians of European heritage over others.

Differential treatment of individuals, by race, occurred in whitestream sport in various ways. For example, the ability of George Beers, in 1860, to create and then institutionalize lacrosse rules in a manner that he found meaningful, as opposed to the ways the game was played by Aboriginal Canadians, demonstrates his privilege by race over the originators of the game of lacrosse (Cosentino, 1998, p. 15). As well, during this time period Black and Aboriginal athletes were banned, by race, from competing against white Canadians in a wide variety of sports. If they did compete, descriptors such as "Indian" or "coloured" were added after their name, to indicate that they were different from, and subservient to, white competitors.

When overt discrimination was eliminated in sport, other more subtle forms of racism remained. The organization of sport privileged those activities that were played in international competitions, including the Olympics and world championships. The federal government criteria for funding sports reflected this; physical activities that fell outside the whitestream model were not seen as legitimate and were denied federal funding. For example,

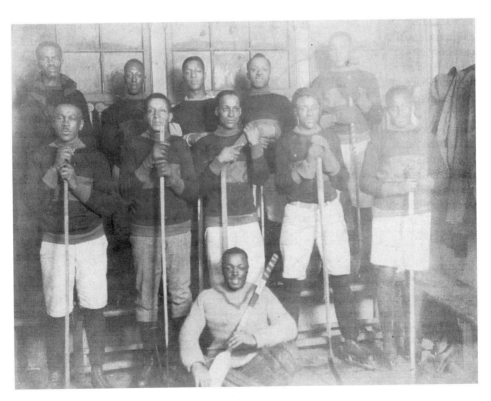

Champions of the "Colored League," early 1900s, Halifax.

From the Public Archives of Nova Scotia/Tom Conners Collection the Northern Games Association, which organized yearly Inuit and Dene traditional games festivals in the Northwest Territories beginning in 1970, was informed by letter in 1977 that their federal sport funding would be stopped. The letter pointed out that the Games activities, which had their origin in Aboriginal cultures, were not deemed to be "legitimate sport" according to the parameters of the funding agency. Aboriginal organizers argued that their traditional activities were also sports, but they had less power over defining "legitimate" sports, and thus lost their funding (Paraschak, 1997).

A third drawback to whitestream sport in Canada is the uncomfortableness experienced by marginalized peoples in mainstream sport experiences. Both individual and institutionalized racism in hockey were detailed in a 1991 TSN documentary, *Hockey: A White Man's Game?* Ted Nolan, an Aboriginal NHL player, spoke of the racism he faced from his teammates as a teenager, and the isolation he felt as a result. Other Aboriginal players spoke about the racial slurs they endured while playing. And they spoke about the structure of hockey in Canada, which took them far away from their families and support systems, and how that structure made it more difficult for them to succeed in light of their cultural practices. Since Aboriginal players were not able to structure sport in preferred ways, they found it difficult to feel part of, or to succeed in, professional hockey (TSN, 1991).

Another reason why some Aboriginal people feel uncomfortable in whitestream sport is the tradition of using Indian mascots for sports teams. This issue is laid out clearly in a 1997 documentary on American Indian mascots in sport titled *In Whose Honor?* (Rosenstein, 1997). Through looking at one case study—Chief Illiniwek, the mascot for the University of Illinois—the documentary points out the devastating impact this stereotypic Indian mascot had on Aboriginal children, and the efforts required to try to eliminate it. Relevant to our discussion on whitestream sport are the accounts of how the Indian mascot was created by white students at the university, how the actions of Chief Illiniwek are portrayed as "authentic" even though they are constructed by the performer and often degrade Native traditions, and the comments by white alumni and administrators about the importance of the Chief as part of "their" traditions.

Patterns of differential treatment based on race have been documented in various professional sports. The Centre for the Study of Sport at Northeastern University, for example, has provided a Racial Report Card for several years on discrimination within the various professional sports leagues operating in North America. They report on progress in the elimination of discrimination, both among the players and in the administration of sport. In Canada, research on professional sport has focused more so on ethnicity rather than race. The discriminatory treatment of French Canadians in the National Hockey League (NHL) has been explored in terms of salary discrimination, entry discrimination, underrepresentation at certain positions or "stacking," and underrepresentation on certain teams (Longley, 2000). For example, Longley (2000) completed a study that looked at all French Canadians playing in English Canada or the United States on NHL teams from 1943 to 1998. His analysis identified an underrepresentation of French Canadian players on English Canadian versus United States teams. After discounting many other explanations, Longley provides support for the thesis that French–English tensions may lead English Canadian teams to discriminate against French Canadian players. This explanation was strengthened when the degree of underrepresentation in English Canadian teams was shown to be greater during seasons when sovereigntist political threats in Quebec were highest.

Lavoie (1989), researching player positions in the NHL, highlighted how francophones were more numerous in the goalie and forward positions, while rarely playing as defencemen. He argued that discrimination against francophone defencemen stems from the more subjective nature of that position. He pointed to the primarily anglophone club management, who would prefer anglophone players when other talents were equal, and argued the Quebec-based teams likewise prefer francophone players (Hall et al., 1991). Lavoie has also documented entry discrimination against francophone players, as evidenced by their underestimation in draft position relative to their future offensive performance. In an examination of veteran players during the 1993/94 season, for example, he found the French Canadian players suffered from entry discrimination at the time of the draft. Although the two teams within Quebec did not discriminate against English Canadian players, the American teams did discriminate against French Canadians (Lavoie, 2003). All these studies point to the possibility of systemic discrimination, based on ethnicity, in the NHL.

Claims of discrimination in the Canadian Football League have focused on a different factor—nationality. As early as 1973, research suggested that Canadians in the CFL were stacked primarily on defence, and in supporting and reactive positions (Ball, 1973, cited in Hall et al., 1991). Meanwhile, American imports were placed in the more desirable positions, such as quarterback. In 1979, Jamie Bone, a former Canadian university quarterback, unsuccessfully tried out for the Hamilton Tiger-Cats. He subsequently complained to the Canadian Human Rights Commission that the CFL's designated import rule discriminated against him on the grounds of national or ethnic origin because it "prevented Canadians from being hired to play quarterback." The Commission concluded "that it was always in a team's best interest to select the most talented quarterback regardless of his national origin, and that although a particular CFL coach may mistakenly perceive the designated import rule to favour hiring imports to play that position, the rule itself does not" (Hall et al., 1991, p. 178).

Whitestream sport, then, provides varying opportunities for athletes depending on their race. This differential treatment can be overt, such as racial slurs that make participation uncomfortable for those groups. Discriminatory treatment is also, at times, built into the existing system of sport. In Canada, for example, francophones experience various types of discrimination in professional hockey, demonstrating that ethnicity, as well as race, impacts on sporting opportunities. Marginalized groups have thus had to look elsewhere for alternative sport opportunities—or to create some themselves.

Doing Race, Doing Racism

Race as a socially constructed idea becomes naturalized (i.e., accepted as "truth") as individuals, on a daily basis, behave as if it were true. West and Zimmerman (1991), in their discussion on "doing gender," point out that this process involves individuals behaving in appropriately masculine or feminine ways, "but it is a situated doing, carried out in the virtual or real presence of others who are presumed to be oriented to its production" (p. 14). Applying this to race, "doing race" means that individuals act in relation to each other in ways that confirm their socially constructed beliefs about race. It is through the acting out, the "doing" of race on a day-by-day basis, both in terms of our own race and the race we assign to others, that we maintain a society where race has social meaning and consequences.

Stereotypes—rigid beliefs about the characteristics of a racial group—take on importance as we live or "do" them into existence by operating as if they were true. Spence (1999), in his study of Black male athletes in a Canadian high school, heard from these youth that their teachers encouraged them athletically, but not academically. This treatment fit with the stereotype that Blacks as a race are athletically more and academically less gifted than whites. As these athletes worked hard on athletic competence, and gained status through their success, they had less time to give to academics, and thus their actions, in the end, reinforced the stereotype. All the while, they and their teachers were "doing racism."

"Doing race" can also be carried out in ways that offer positive race-connected meanings to members of a group, providing them with a form of cultural expression that is uniquely their own. Majors (1990), for example, identified "cool pose" as a creative way that Black men express their masculinity in a society where opportunities are limited and racism is institutionalized. Wilson (1999) describes the expression of cool pose in sport this way:

> Sport, particularly basketball, are sites where young Black males symbolically oppose the dominant White group and create [a positive race-connected] identity by developing both a flamboyant on-court language (now popularly known as "trash talking") and a repertoire of spectacular "playground" moves and high-flying dunks. (p. 232)

While this way of "doing race" was initially generated by Black male youth, Wilson (1999) also discusses ways that this style has been incorporated by sport marketers to sell to a mass audience, and in particular to sell the National Basketball Association Toronto Raptors. These advertising messages, he argues, undercut the resistant symbolic message that cool pose provides Black males, while potentially reinforcing stereotypic Black male images to Canadian audiences. Sport marketers were "doing racism."

Race-Structured Sport Systems

Opportunities for sport, created by and for racial groups outside mainstream society, have a long history in Canada. When Aboriginal or Black athletes were banned from whitestream sport, they often countered with the creation of their own leagues and competitions, limited to participants from a specified racial background. This provided organizers with the opportunity to assign their own meaning to sport and to develop traditions in keeping with Aboriginal, or Black, or Asian cultural understandings. And it created opportunities for marginalized groups to play sports when they did not have that chance in the mainstream sport system.

An example of a race-structured sporting event would be the North American Indigenous Games, first held in 1990 in Edmonton. These international Games, restricted to those of verifiable Aboriginal ancestry, "stress fun and participation while encouraging our youth to strive for excellence" (Aboriginal Sports/Recreation Association of B.C., 1995, n.p.). The Games were comprised of all mainstream sports, because the intent was to provide a stepping-stone to national- and international-level sport competitions; however, the cultural program showcased various traditional games and dances. The 2002 Games in Winnipeg had more than 6,000 participants celebrating Aboriginal culture as well as competing in sporting events organized by Aboriginal sports organizations.

Through this event, Aboriginal sportspeople experience more "power" in sport than is found in the whitestream system—they are in charge of its structure, its practices and meanings, and the traditions they will continue into the future. Unfortunately, these race-structured opportunities rarely qualify for the kinds of financial and material rewards given to "legitimate," whitestream sport, although the Canadian government has recently acknowledged the presence of the all-Aboriginal sport system in Canada through federal policy and funding (see Box 5.2).

People sometimes attach the term "reverse racism" to situations where normally privileged individuals—usually Caucasians—are excluded from opportunities on the basis of race. For example, non-Aboriginal people cannot compete in the North American Indigenous Games, even though Aboriginal athletes can theoretically compete in mainstream sporting events. As the Charter of Rights and Freedoms section 15(2) directs, however, efforts to address "the conditions of disadvantaged individuals or groups including those that are disadvantaged because of race" are seen as a necessary part of providing equality rights, because such efforts are required to help right the imbalance created by unequal privilege in the first instance. This section on racism in sport has documented the individual and institutionalized racism present in

---

Box 5.2   Federal Government Approaches toward Aboriginal Sport in Canada:
Continuities and Changes, 1972–2006

The federal government rationale for funding Aboriginal sport has remained fairly consistent throughout the past 35 years, since Sport Canada first funded the Native Sport and Recreation Program in 1972. Their hope is to prepare Aboriginal peoples for success in mainstream sporting opportunities. The government identified Aboriginal sport in Canada as a concern because of the marginalized status of Aboriginal athletes within the Canadian sport system. They have also been prompted to act when the success of prominent Aboriginal athletes, such as Sharon and Shirley Firth, Alwyn Morris, Steve Collins, Angela Chalmers, Waneek Horn-Miller, Jordan Tootoo, and Tara Hedican fostered an interest in Aboriginal sport talent potential more generally. Recently, potential benefits through healthcare savings, reduced numbers of youth at risk, and economic benefits from international competitions such as the North American Indigenous Games (NAIG) have also been cited as rationale for their involvement in, and funding of, Aboriginal sport.

Aboriginal sport organizations have likewise remained consistent in their rationale. They wish to create a system more aligned with Aboriginal values, as seen by the recent creation of National Coaching Certification Program (NCCP) coaching units on racism, holistic approaches to sport, and traditional foods. They are fostering all-Aboriginal teams and competitions that remain under Aboriginal control and represent Aboriginal peoples in their preferred manner, such as the Iroquois Nationals in lacrosse and Team Indigenous in hockey. They have thus increasingly developed Aboriginal sport premised on a belief in their separate nationhood. However, there has been an increased willingness by Aboriginal sport volunteers to work with/in the mainstream sport system. Examples include joint involvement in the NCCP and in elite athlete development, and the administration of the NAIG in conjunction with federal/provincial/territorial sport departments.

In May 2005, *Sport Canada's Policy on Aboriginal Peoples' Participation in Sport* was released. This policy signals a closer link between the vision of sport held by Sport Canada and by Aboriginal peoples. In the document, future developments in Aboriginal sport are aligned with the four goals of the 2002 Canadian Sport Policy—enhanced participation, excellence, capacity, and interaction—thus continuing federal emphasis on Aboriginal sport linkages to the mainstream sport system. However, the policy also acknowledges the existence of a separate Aboriginal sport system in Canada, noting that "An Aboriginal sport delivery system exists and it is important to work with the ASC, its national body, to identify and address the areas of priority to advance Aboriginal Peoples' participation in sport" (Canadian Heritage, 2005b, p. 6). This policy is thus an important step forward in the federal acknowledgement that Aboriginal participants may choose to enter into the mainstream sport system, but they may also legitimately opt to participate in an Aboriginal sport system under the control and aligned with the vision of Aboriginal peoples in Canada.

whitestream sport in Canada. Race has been, and remains, an indicator or "marker" that provides meaning in our everyday sporting practices. In order to ensure that all Canadians, regardless of race, have opportunities to find meaningful participation in sport, race-structured sporting opportunities are currently needed to ensure that the sport system in Canada provides broadly for the needs of all Canadians. Until whitestream sport broadens and becomes truly inclusive, alternative race-structured opportunities should be celebrated and supported as part of the Canadian sport system. In this way, the institution of sport becomes a more welcoming practice reflective of the cultural meanings and traditions of all Canadians, regardless of race.

CONCLUSIONS

Race and ethnicity are aspects of our heritage that take on social meaning in Canadian society. These constructed meanings become naturalized each time we "do" them in accordance with the dominant beliefs around us. Caucasians of European descent in Canada have been the most privileged in sport, with those from other racial backgrounds often discriminated against both overtly and through systemic racism. Whitestream sport has emerged, legitimizing select activities such as Olympic sports and marginalizing other activities that do not fit within such understandings. Segregated sporting opportunities have likewise emerged, enabling organizers and participants from marginalized groups to structure their own experiences in sport in ways that foster pride in their cultural heritage, while giving them opportunities to play that are not available otherwise. Legitimizing these sporting opportunities, and the alternative ethnic practices preferred by immigrants and their descendants, takes us one step further toward creating a sport system that is representative of all individuals in Canada.

A racial incident in hockey in 2005 reminds us that racism is still present in Canadian sport. Ted Nolan, an Ojibwa from Sault Ste. Marie, Ontario, has a storied career as a successful NHL player, coach of the NHL Buffalo Sabres, and NHL coach of the year. In 2005 he was the coach of the Moncton Wildcats in the Quebec Major Junior Hockey league. At a game in Chicoutimi, Quebec, on December 16, fans hurled racial slurs at him throughout the game. Nolan said the verbal abuse left him trembling after the game. "Some fans whooped and made tomahawk gestures at the aboriginal coach, prompting the Sagueneens to post an apology on their website" (*Halifax Herald*, 2005, p. C1). In this case, one of our most successful Canadian hockey coaches was inhibited from enjoying pride in his Aboriginal heritage and skills because of racist behaviours by others in sport. We need to reflect on incidents such as this that still happen in Canada. To begin to resolve the issue, we need a clear definition of racism and discrimination that everyone associated with sport can understand, along with clearly articulated ideas about how everyone should respond when these things happen. Our outrage at such occurrences helps to ensure that we are promoting an inclusive sport system that enables all individuals to foster pride in their ethnic and racial identity. Our silence, on the other hand, reproduces a sport system where particular individuals—those who are privileged by white skin and European heritage—too often benefit while the rest of Canadians do not.

The social construction of race and ethnicity as integral aspects of sport, and of leisure more broadly, needs to be recognized if we are to find ways to decrease discrimination based on these factors. At the same time, the positive ways that our cultural identities can be shaped by movement need to be facilitated equally for all, regardless of race or ethnicity. As we look to others, from different cultural backgrounds, to see how they know themselves through movement, we will expand the ways that we can potentially know ourselves. In this way, we can help to shape, as well as to be shaped by, the social meanings assigned to race and ethnicity in Canadian sport. And we will be more ready to help create equitable opportunities for all people trying to access meaningful sport in Canada, by providing activities that honour the racial and ethnic differences between participants rather than erase them.

CRITICAL THINKING QUESTIONS

1. Explore the sport interests of minority group residents, including Aboriginal, Inuit, Métis, African Canadian, and other minority ethnic groups, in the community in which you live and/or study. Prepare a table that outlines the various sports, the groups interested in each sport, and the values connected to each sport.

2. If you encounter children from a minority ethnic family—identifiable from their distinct clothing and accents—what are some of the questions you might ask them to determine if there are factors that may prevent or restrict their participation in sport or physical activity? If you determine that they do indeed have special needs, how might you facilitate their involvement in sports or physical activity?

3. What are two ways that a coach, teacher, or sports administrator might respond to an incident of overt racism, such as name calling directed at a teenager in a basketball program?

4. How do you "do race" in your life? In sport?

5. Write about an incident where the social meanings attached to race influenced your life, by either privileging you or providing a barrier to opportunities you wished to experience.

6. Write a code of conduct for sport that would align it with the Canadian Charter of Rights and Freedoms.

7. How do race-structured sporting events address discrimination in mainstream sport?

8. Outline examples of how sporting performances can provide opportunities for decreasing racial distinctions, and for increasing racial distinctions.

SUGGESTED READINGS

Cosentino, F. (1998). *Afros, Aboriginals and amateur sport in pre World War One Canada*. Canada's Ethnic Group Series, Booklet No. 26. Ottawa: The Canadian Historical Society.

Denis, C. (1997). *We are not you: First Nations and Canadian modernity*. Peterborough, ON: Broadview Press.

Dimeo, P. (2002). Colonial bodies, colonial sport: "Martial" Punjabis, "effeminate" Bengalis and the development of Indian football. *International Journal of the History of Sport, 19*, 72–90.

Jones, R. L. (2002). The black experience within English semiprofessional soccer. *Journal of Sport and Social Issues, 26*, 47–65.

Paraschak, V. (2007). Doing race, doing gender: First Nations, "sport," and gender relations (2nd ed.). In P. White & K. Young (Eds.), *Sport and gender in Canada* (pp. 137–154). Don Mills, ON: Oxford University Press.

Paraschak, V. (1997). Variations in race relations: Sporting events for Native peoples in Canada. *Sociology of Sport Journal, 14*, 1–21.

Paraschak, V. (1996). Racialized spaces: Cultural regulation, Aboriginal agency and powwows. *Avante, 2*, 7–18.

Spence, C. (1999). *The skin I'm in: Racism, sports and education*. Halifax: Fernwood.

Tirone, S. (1999–2000). Racism, indifference, and the leisure experience of South Asian Canadian teens. *Leisure/Loisir, 24*, 89–114.

Wilcox, R. C., Andrews, D. L., Pitter, R., & Irwin, R. L. (Eds.). *Sporting dystopias: The making and meanings of urban sport cultures*. Albany, NY: State University of New York Press.

Wilson, B. (1999). "Cool pose" incorporated: The marketing of black masculinity in Canadian NBA coverage. In P. White & K. Young (Eds.), *Sport and gender in Canada* (pp. 232–253). Don Mills, ON: Oxford University Press.

WEB LINKS

Lotus Sports

http://www.lotussports.com

Dragonboat racing clubs in Western Canada.

Ancient Future

http://www.ancient-future.com/

World dance and music; new cross-cultural music and dance is created by learning from the world's great ancient traditions.

Field Hockey

http://www.fieldhockey.com

Information about the game of field hockey, popular for men and women in many countries outside the United States and Canada.

Canadian Charter of Rights and Freedoms

http://laws.justice.gc.ca/en/charter/index.html

Provides the entire Charter, including the section on equality rights noted in this chapter.

Aboriginal Sport Circle

http://www.aboriginalsportcircle.ca

The federally funded national organization overseeing Aboriginal sport in Canada.

Ontario Council of Agencies Serving Immigrants

http://www.ocasi.org/index.php

Organization working with the city of Hamilton on developing recreation programs to meet the needs of immigrant youth.

First Nations Athletes in History and in the Media: Tom Longboat and Steve Collins

http://www.histori.ca/minutes/lp.do?id=12956

A class lesson plan that discusses First Nations athletes in sport and the challenges they face.

Sport Canada's Policy on Aboriginal Peoples' Participation in Sport

http://www.pch.gc.ca/progs/sc/pol/aboriginal/index_e.cfm

Contains the entire text of the 2005 Sport Canada policy.

CHAPTER 6

WOMEN'S ISSUES AND GENDER RELATIONS

Helen Jefferson Lenskyj

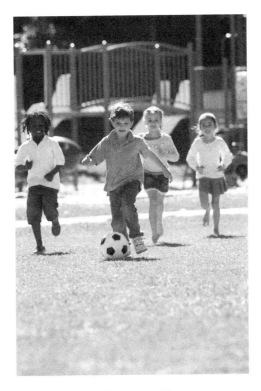

Children have fun and learn social skills through sport.

IT Stock Free/Picture Quest/Jupiter Images

You can't be a female athlete without addressing questions of femininity, sexuality, fear, power, freedom, and just how good you are compared with men.

Nelson, 1991, p. 196

Sport . . . can offer a privileged few [boys] that succeed the opportunities to develop a positive sense of identity and status, while, on the other hand, it can serve to exacerbate insecurities, poor self-images and lack of identity for the less successful.

Drummond, 2002, p. 42

At the beginning of the twenty-first century, with more Canadian girls and women enjoying the benefits of sport and physical activity, there remain significant barriers to full female participation. At the same time, there are many boys and men whose bodies or physical abilities prevent them from enjoying sport as it is currently constituted. This chapter begins with an analysis of various theoretical and political approaches to understanding gender inequality in sport and physical activity, with an emphasis on the impact of harassment and violence on girls and women, and on non-conforming boys and men. The social construction of femininity and masculinity through sport is examined, and feminist, antiracist initiatives that address inequalities based on gender, ethnicity, social class, sexuality, and ability are explored. Finally, recommendations based on human rights and health rationales are evaluated.

WAYS OF UNDERSTANDING GENDER, SPORT, AND THE "ISMS"

A critical sociological approach to understanding gender issues in the context of Canadian sport and physical activity aims at identifying the ways in which systemic barriers, including sexism, racism, classism, heterosexism, motor elitism, and ableism, work together to perpetuate longstanding, male-dominated sporting practices. A critical approach goes beyond simply describing current trends; it also seeks to explain why these conditions prevail, and to interpret the meanings behind the social relations of sport and physical activity (White & Young, 1999b). Finally, this kind of research often includes recommendations for educational interventions and policy innovations, with the goal of addressing social injustice and promoting social change. In other words, critical sociological research has an overt political agenda and offers a serious challenge to the status quo.

Sexism refers to discrimination based on biological sex, that is, maleness or femaleness; racism is discrimination based on ethnic identity and/or skin colour; classism refers to discrimination against people of low socioeconomic status. Heterosexism is discrimination based on the presumption that heterosexuality is the only acceptable expression of sexuality; the irrational fear and hatred of lesbians, gay men, and other sexual minorities is termed homophobia. Motor elitism refers to the practice of privileging and rewarding those who are athletically gifted, to the detriment of children and adults whose body size and type, fitness level, muscular strength, eye–hand coordination, and other physical traits prevent them from participating successfully in mainstream sport. People with physical or other disabilities are in this category, and the term ableism refers to exclusionary practices that fail to take disability into account, particularly the failure to make sport and recreation programs and facilities fully accessible. The targets of these various "isms" are girls and women; Black people; people of colour and ethnic minorities; working-class and poor people; gays, lesbians, and other sexual minorities; and people with disabilities or limited physical capacities.

It is important to recognize that there are significant numbers of Canadian girls and women who are doubly or triply disadvantaged; in addition to sexism, they experience discrimination as a result of their ethnic backgrounds, sexual identities, socioeconomic status, and/or disabilities. A study of Indo-Canadian females (Vertinsky, Batth, & Naidu, 1996) identified how sweeping generalizations and racist stereotyping of South Asian females as weak, passive, and uninterested in physical activity falsely implied that they were a homogeneous group and that they should adjust in order to fit into existing sport or educational systems. While recognizing that traditionally "feminine" physical activities were promoted over more demanding contact sports in some Indo-Canadian communities, the authors emphasized the need for systemic change, as well as for alternative, culturally appropriate programming strategies to enable young Indo-Canadian women to enjoy their physicality and participate in sporting activities of their choice.

Discrimination experienced by women and members of disadvantaged minorities ranges from exclusion and marginalization, to verbal and physical harassment, and even to violence. Such discrimination can be challenged under Canadian law; for example, courts have established that it is the responsibility of the employer or the educational institution to ensure discrimination- and harassment-free conditions. Unfortunately, this does not mean that discrimination and harassment have been eliminated from Canadian sport and physical activity contexts. In many situations, the process is complaint-driven, and therefore reactive rather than proactive—the burden falls on those who experience the problem to lodge complaints or lawsuits, often a costly and time-consuming process. Moreover, from their already disadvantaged position, many of those who are targets of harassment may correctly believe that it is futile to complain. In one example, professional football players, who were using university facilities for training, sexually harassed women at an Ontario university. The women were reluctant to pursue any formal complaint procedure for fear of reprisals from these men and from football fans on the campus.

LIMITATIONS OF LIBERAL APPROACHES

The more common liberal feminist approaches, which rely on psychological rather than critical sociological theories, tend to conceptualize a universal or generic Canadian girl or woman who, according to this line of thinking, simply needs opportunity and encouragement in order to become physically active. This approach is in evidence whenever sport administrators ask, "What can we do to get more girls and women involved in sport?" rather than asking, "What are the systemic barriers that keep certain groups of girls and women out?"

This generic female is generally assumed to be able-bodied, white, heterosexual, young to middle-aged, and middle-class. More specifically, it is assumed that she:

- has sufficient discretionary income to purchase clothing and equipment, and to pay registration fees and travel costs;
- has family members who will support, and not undermine or prevent, her efforts to become physically active;
- will not be harassed because of her gender, skin colour, ethnicity, body size, sexual orientation, disability, age, or any other characteristic;
- has ready access to transport and facilities that are safe and barrier-free;
- will enjoy Canada's mainstream sport and recreational activities and embrace their underlying value systems.

In reality, there are still significant systemic barriers to full female sporting participation in Canada. The values and practices in men's professional team sports—most notably ice hockey, football, and basketball—dominate most Canadians' understanding of the term *sport*. To the limited extent that amateur sport is recognized, the "faster, higher, stronger" Olympic model privileges male athletes who, as a gender group, are likely to be faster, higher, and stronger than females as a group (although it is important to acknowledge that there is significant overlap in the performance of males and females at all levels). Flawed assumptions about the actual context of Canadian sport and physical activity include the following:

- that it is a safe and welcoming place for all girls and women, regardless of their ethnic and social class backgrounds, sexual orientations, or abilities;
- that comprehensive anti-harassment policies and effective complaint procedures are in place in order to address sexual, racist, homophobic, and all other forms of harassment;

- that existing physical activities reflect a wide range of human values and priorities, including enjoyment, cooperation, and camaraderie, as well as winning and improving one's performance;
- that sport as currently constituted will not need to be changed; it is assumed that girls and women will have to change to fit into existing patterns and practices.

Liberal approaches have dominated women's sport advocacy and research in most Western countries, including Canada, since the 1960s wave of the women's movement. This approach defined formal equality primarily in terms of girls' and women's access to the same or equivalent sport and recreational opportunities as boys and men. The liberal agenda focused on removing policy and legislative barriers that prevented girls and women (mostly white and middle-class) from enjoying the same opportunities as their male counterparts. In addition to increasing female participation at the club and community levels, this approach called for more Olympic sports and events for women, more balanced media coverage of female athletes, and more women in coaching, officiating, administration, and the sport media.

These are all strategies that critics have characterized as the "add women and stir" approach. In other words, although the resulting mix was quantitatively different—there was more female involvement at all levels—it was not qualitatively different from the original. In fact, increased female participation did not necessarily bring with it an increase in leadership opportunities for women; unless organizations adopted an affirmative action policy, new positions were likely to be filled by male applicants who, as a group, were more experienced and qualified for coaching and sport administration than females (Lenskyj, 1994). The shortcomings of traditional male-dominated models of sport and physical activity were perpetuated, rather than challenged, by "add women and stir" initiatives, with the result that women's competitive sport was often indistinguishable from men's. For example, the 1997 National Film Board documentary *The Game of Her Life*, which followed the Canadian women's national ice hockey team as they trained for the 1998 Winter Olympics, revealed the same mainstream approaches to coaching, training, and winning that characterized men's competitive sport (see also Theberge, 2000).

There was little recognition in liberal feminist discourse that the male-defined model of sport might need reforming—or, indeed, transforming—to reflect the priorities of women and men who valued enjoyment, health, and social relationships more than corporatized sporting spectacles and winning at all costs. Despite their goal of promoting opportunities for girls and women of all ability levels, liberal sport advocacy organizations routinely highlighted the credentials and achievements of Olympic sportswomen, while failing to recognize the chilling effect that this kind of preoccupation with high-performance sport might have on girls and women whose abilities and aspirations were "average" rather than "Olympian"—in other words, the vast majority of the female population.

SHORTCOMINGS OF THE "ROLE MODEL" MODEL

Although liberal initiatives produced important gains in terms of policy and legislative changes, assumptions about a universal Canadian female resulted in insufficient attention being paid to the impacts of systemic racism, classism, ageism, ableism, and homophobia on girls' and women's lives. As a result, gains were not evenly distributed across the boundaries of race/ethnicity, social class, age, ability, and sexuality. Often relying on a few high-profile female athletes to serve as "role models," liberal approaches largely ignored interlocking systems of discrimination and oppression that made it impossible for the majority of girls and women to emulate the few who were successful when judged by mainstream standards of competitive sporting achievement. The "role model" approach rested on the assumption that a major barrier to female sporting participation was lack of imagination, inspiration, and aspirations: in other words, "it's all in our heads."

According to this way of thinking, girls and women simply needed to see real evidence—a successful high-performance athlete who, as a "role model," would inspire them to great sporting heights. Nowhere was it acknowledged that the role model's international success in a narrow range of physical activities classified as sport in contemporary Western society was largely dependent on her body type, socioeconomic status, geographic location, family activity patterns, and other interacting individual and sociocultural variables. Biological inheritance, for example, plays a major role in determining physical activity behaviours, while children with active parents and higher family incomes have significantly greater sport participation rates than those with inactive parents and lower incomes (Kremarik, 2000; Physical Activity Promotion, 1999).

This is not to suggest that positive examples of female athleticism in girls' and women's everyday lives (as opposed to sporting celebrities giving motivational talks) are unimportant. As discussed later in this chapter, girls and women enjoy the social side of sport and physical activity, and the presence of exercise partners or friends who share an interest in a particular sporting activity is highly valued.

Concerns about media underrepresentation and distortion of women's sport are often associated with the role model approach. It is valid, of course, to argue from a simple equality perspective that the full range of female sports and sporting achievements should be reported and recognized in the mass media. However, there is a longstanding media preoccupation with conventionally attractive female athletes and media neglect of those who are not. As a result, the only female athletes who achieve celebrity status, and hence role-model status, are those who satisfy male-defined standards of heterosexual attractiveness. The recent international trend of female athletes posing nude for calendars and soft porn magazines reflects the ultimate outcome of the hypersexualization of sportswomen.

In relation to the effectiveness of the "role model" approach, although it is valid to assume that very young children may have difficulty thinking in abstract terms and may need concrete evidence in order to understand some concepts—for example, the idea of a female athlete succeeding in a male-dominated sport—this is not the case from preadolescence on. Indeed, in 1985, 12-year-old Justine Blainey was quite capable of understanding injustice and sex discrimination, and equally capable of imagining herself playing at the top level of ice hockey competition—at that time, on a boys' team. Justine was barred from playing on the Etobicoke (Toronto) Canucks A team, despite her success at the tryouts, because she was a girl; sex discrimination in sport was specifically excluded from the provisions of the Ontario Human Rights Code. (Ironically, around the same time, the Ontario Ministry of Tourism and Recreation had established its own "role model" program, with Olympic sportswomen visiting schools to give inspirational talks to girls.)

The (male) Ontario Hockey Association fought all the way to the Supreme Court of Canada to keep players like Justine out of their leagues, but in the end the court ruled that sex discrimination in sport contravened the provisions of the Canadian Charter of Rights and Freedoms. The struggle for equality, unfortunately, did not end with this decision; accounts of qualified girls who were excluded from boys' teams regularly appeared in the Canadian media throughout the 1990s. On a more positive note, female involvement in hockey has increased steadily since the 1980s. And in 2003 Canadian national team member Hayley Wickenheiser joined a men's hockey team in Finland and became the first female to score points in a male league.

SOCIAL CHANGE, RADICAL ALTERNATIVES

Radical and socialist feminists recognized that the roots of women's oppression needed to be addressed. Lobbying for increased female access to existing male-defined sporting activities would not be successful if other, more deeply rooted social problems remained unaddressed: for example, the impact of male violence on girls and women's lives, the links between the sub-culture of men's team sports and violence against women, and the economic disadvantages experienced by women as a gender group.

Drawing on the concepts of accommodation and resistance, radical feminists examined not only the impact of male power and privilege on women's lives, but also women's capacity to resist discrimination and oppression. Hence, women were not portrayed as helpless victims, but rather as active agents who have developed a range of resistance strategies as well as cre-ative woman-centred sporting alternatives, such as community softball leagues organized on feminist principles (see, for example, Birrell & Richter, 1987; Lenskyj, 2003).

Sexuality issues were central to these kinds of analyses. Radical feminists examined the ways in which heterosexist assumptions, rigid definitions of feminine (that is, heterosexual) behaviour, and the chilly climate created by sexual and homophobic harassment discouraged female sporting participation. As was the pattern in other traditionally male-dominated domains, the sexual identities of female athletes and women in sport leadership routinely came under suspicion. Characterized as "intruders" in a male domain, they were accused of being "unfeminine," man-hating, and/or lesbian. "Feminine" girls and women, according to this line of thought, played gender-appropriate sports that enhanced their heterosexual attractiveness and at the same time posed no threat to the myth of male athletic superiority. Although women's international profile in competitive sports like soccer and basketball has recently challenged some of this thinking, the popularity of long hair and jewellery still suggests adher-ence to conventional femininity.

These ideological arguments had particular power over adolescent girls and young women who were experiencing family, peer, and media pressure to establish their heterosexual cre-dentials. In other words, to pursue sport, particularly traditionally male sport, through one's adolescence was to risk being labelled lesbian (Lenskyj, 2003). Needless to say, many women in sport, as in every other area of human activity, are in fact lesbian, and many male athletes are gay. With increasing acceptance of sexual diversity and the human rights of sexual minori-ties in other sectors of Canadian society, it is to be hoped that the longstanding issue of homo-phobic harassment in sport will eventually be resolved.

VALUES AND PRIORITIES: GENDER-RELATED DIFFERENCES

There is extensive research evidence that shows how girls and women tend to value the social side of sport, especially the fun and friendship, more than their male counterparts, who are more likely to name winning and beating their opponents as their top priorities. This does not mean that female athletes don't want to win, or that male athletes don't enjoy the camaraderie of sport. Rather, these findings indicate that there are gender-related patterns of values, inter-ests, and priorities (Lenskyj, 2003). It is important to remember, too, that the significance of winning is learned—it is not an innate characteristic of all women or all men—and it cannot be assumed that all participants, regardless of their ethnocultural backgrounds, attach the same value to this component of sport.

It must be recognized that these so-called female values are socially constructed and trans-mitted, and are not a necessary outcome of biological femaleness. In men's sport, there is historical evidence from Canada, the United States, Europe, Australia, and elsewhere to show that existing sporting systems and practices have long been compatible with socially constructed and biologically based notions of what it means to be male. In these countries, sport has been treated as an essential component of boys' physical development and socialization into manhood—but, until the last decades of the twentieth century, it was seen as largely irrelevant for female socialization and development.

Social and biological factors interact in the sporting context to contribute to the construction of gender identity. For example, physical training, in combination with male hormonal changes in adolescence, promotes muscular development, which is both an indicator of physical maturation in the young male, and an important asset for the aspiring athlete. In contrast, physical training may slow down the onset of puberty in girls, and it may delay the development of girls' breasts and hips, which are indicators of female maturation. Furthermore, girls' normal hormonal changes at puberty lead to increased body fat, which is a liability rather than an asset in most sports. Hence, sport fits neatly into both biological and societal definitions of desirable masculinity, but is incompatible with most definitions of femininity.

MASCULINITIES AND SPORT

Masculinity can be briefly defined as the *performance* or the *doing* of maleness. The plural, masculinities, is a more accurate term for thinking about the issue, because it captures the multiple and changing ways that performances of maleness are defined in different sociocultural contexts and different sporting subcultures. For example, the masculinity of a Canadian Football League player is very different from that of an Olympic-level diver.

Critical sociologist R. W. Connell explained the ways in which hegemonic masculinity is inextricably linked to men's bodies and has come to mean "to be inherent in a male *body* or to express something about a male *body*" (Connell, 1995, p. 45, emphasis added). With hegemony understood as ideological control, hegemonic masculinity refers to the taken-for-granted, ideologically approved characteristics of a *real* man in a specific sociocultural context. A narrow range of behaviours that reflect common-sense assumptions about the normal and natural gender order characterizes hegemonic masculinity: men are the breadwinners, men prefer sport to opera, men don't do housework, and so on.

Feminist sport sociologist Pat Griffin (1998) identified five central ways in which sport maintains traditional power relations between men and women—specifically, the presumption of male superiority and female subordination. Firstly, sport defines and reinforces traditional definitions of masculinity. To this way of thinking, to be a real boy or a real man requires aggression, suppression of emotions, and the desire to dominate others who are weaker or less athletically skilled. In the Canadian context, the sports that promote these characteristics are typically team sports like ice hockey, football, and basketball. Boys and men whose athletic abilities lie in a non-traditional activity like figure skating exemplify a less desirable, often stigmatized type of masculinity. Moreover, they often experience pressure to establish their heterosexual credentials in the face of homophobic assumptions that males who prefer figure skating to ice hockey must be gay. In terms of self-presentation, the leather-and-studs outfits worn by some male figure skaters are intended to convey a tough, heterosexual identity. Regardless of the skater's actual sexual preference, this image is intended to counter rumours of a gay identity.

Secondly, sport provides "an acceptable and safe context for male bonding and intimacy" (Griffin, 1998, p. 20). Most boys raised in traditional families learn at a young age not to express physical affection toward male family members or peers. Despite this general taboo on

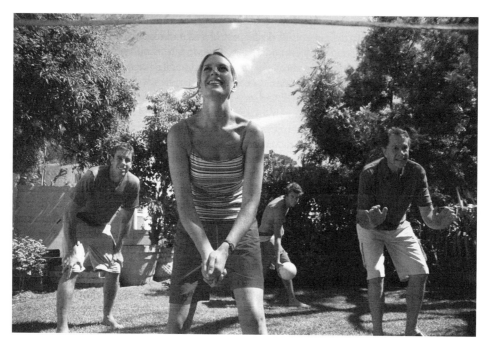

Mixed team sports challenge gender stereotypes.
© Royalty-Free/Corbis

touching other males, physical contact and emotional intimacy in sport are permitted without necessarily incurring homophobic rumours or harassment. However, the nudity and touching that are normalized in male locker rooms present problems for boys and young men who are experiencing same-sex attraction, as well as for those men who are, in fact, gay (Pronger, 1990). These boys and men must monitor their behaviour toward other males in order to avoid disclosing their gay identities.

Thirdly, sport reinforces male privilege and female subordination. Victories on the playing field, particularly in men's professional team sport, serve to symbolize men's physical dominance over women. Cheerleaders further reinforce women's proper place in sport. Literally on the margins, they serve a decorative, heterosexy role that is subordinate to men in every way. Moreover, as demonstrated by recent examples of male opposition and overt hostility to women playing on men's ice hockey teams, or to women joining men's golf tournaments, masculine identities rely heavily on sporting ability. In 2003, Vijay Singh stated unequivocally that Anneka Sorenstam should not be allowed to play on the Professional Golfing Association tour because she was a woman. According to this line of thinking, if male sport is "contaminated" by the presence of girls or women, it loses its power to define what it takes to be a man. And, one might add, professional sports like golf and tennis offer significantly higher prize money to men, and the ignominy of losing both the status and the money to a woman would be intolerable.

Lastly, sport establishes status among other males and reinforces heterosexuality. Hegemonic masculinity relies on using women and gay men as negative reference groups: real men are not female, not feminine, and not homosexual. Homophobic stereotypes portray gay men as sissies: effeminate men who are more interested in culture and the arts than in the rough, tough world of sport. It is generally accepted, based on Kinsey's American research and comparable studies in Europe, that about 10 percent of the adult male population is gay, and that significantly more than 10 percent have had some same-sex sexual experiences (Schneider, 1988, 18–19). In cities like Toronto, Montreal, and Vancouver that have large gay-friendly neighbourhoods and communities, the figures may be higher. Despite these patterns in sexual orientation, the myth persists that all male athletes, especially in professional team sport, are heterosexual. This is, of course, a circular argument: in a social context that views sporting prowess as a defining feature of heterosexual masculinity, how could a male athlete not be heterosexual?

Homophobic harassment poses a serious threat to gay athletes who disclose their sexual orientation, with the result that the majority remain "in the closet" as a survival strategy. Few, if any, professional male athletes have come out as gay during their sporting careers, citing genuine fears of violent physical reprisals from their own teammates, as well as from other players, if they had done so. Exceptions include internationally successful divers Greg Louganis and Mark Tewksbury, both of whom have been open about their gay identities since the 1990s.

In the sport context, the notion of male superiority is defined solely in terms of physical strength and power. Missing from this simplistic definition are the diverse criteria used to measure human performance and achievements outside of sport contexts—qualities such as intellect, artistic or musical ability, creativity, empathy, interpersonal skills, and so on. Non-conforming boys—especially those whose body size and shape, strength, coordination, and physical skills do not meet prevailing standards—face particular challenges in their adolescent peer groups. As one critic explained:

> Unless boys are cool, macho or sporty, their lives can be hell . . . until boys are free to be geeks, nerds and gays, without retribution, they will not fulfill their potential—at least not until they leave their school days behind. (Horin, 2005, p. 27)

In short, physical strength preempts other abilities in establishing hegemonic masculinity and the gender order. This does not, of course, mean that all males are physically stronger than all females, but even if this were true it is a flawed premise on which to organize an entire society. Yet in Canada and most other Western countries sport remains the last bastion of male supremacy, as sport sociologists since the 1970s have demonstrated (see also Burstyn, 1999; Messner, 1992).

HUMAN RIGHTS RATIONALES

Women's sport advocates use the two related rationales—human rights and health—to support arguments for equality in sport and physical activity. The human rights approach argues that discrimination against girls and women, and against ethnic or other minorities, contravenes the Canadian Charter of Rights and Freedoms, as well as most provincial human rights codes.

Because boards of education, municipal recreation programs, provincial sports organizations, and colleges and universities are subsidized either fully or partially with public money, they are required to operate on equitable principles. It is unfair, for example, for a disproportionate amount of university students' compulsory athletic fees to be spent maintaining the men's football team; in this common scenario on Canadian university campuses, female students are in effect forced to subsidize sports in which they themselves are ineligible to participate. Similarly, since property tax revenues support the building and maintenance of municipal ice rinks and baseball diamonds, it is unfair to girls and women if boys' and men's leagues receive the best timeslots and the bulk of the playing time. With allocation policies often giving priority to longstanding users, women trying to establish new leagues are at a distinct disadvantage under this system.

As noted above in relation to the Blainey case, human rights strategies have achieved some noteworthy successes. It could also be argued that it is preferable to base a complaint on justice and human rights rather than on health or other utilitarian arguments. In other words, discrimination and injustice have no place in a democratic society.

HEALTH RATIONALES: PROS AND CONS

The health approach emphasizes the benefits of regular physical activity on population health and the negative impacts of inactivity: chronic health problems, increased burden on health-care systems, absenteeism, and decreased workplace productivity. Since there is ample evidence to show that Canadian girls' and women's physical activity participation rates are below those recommended for optimal health (to be discussed in a later section), the health argument is particularly relevant for women.

There are both strengths and weaknesses to this approach. Pragmatically, it is clear that, in these times of drastic cutbacks to health, education, and social services budgets, as well as the generally right-wing political climate across Canada, provincial and federal governments are more likely to be persuaded by health arguments than by appeals to human rights, equity, and social justice in relation to female exclusion from the full range of sporting and physical activity opportunities.

However, if the emphasis is solely on the economic costs of inactivity, there is the danger of reducing the full humanity of women and men, so that they become cogs in an economic machine rather than citizens in a democratic country with well-founded expectations that social justice and equity, as well as health and economic security, should prevail.

The 1998 Canadian Heritage subcommittee's report (Mills, 1998), titled, appropriately, *Sport in Canada: Everybody's Business*, provided a good example of the dangers of economic reductionism. Mass participation in sport was identified as "one of the best ways to achieve our social and economic objectives"; a 10-percent decrease in the number of inactive Canadians, the report claimed, would produce a $5-billion saving in healthcare costs. Increased youth participation, particularly among "at-risk" youth, would "develop better potential for this growing human resource"; reduced rates of unwanted pregnancies, drug use, and crime were also listed among the benefits. Low female participation rates were treated not only as a health issue—because inactive females, the report claimed, were at higher risk of cardiovascular disease, osteoporosis, breast cancer, colon cancer, adult-onset diabetes, and hypertension—but also as a problem for "the vitality of the sport sector in Canada"; that is, "sporting goods manufacturers and the overall sport services sector" (Mills, 1998).

With regard to the question of research evidence to support its rather sweeping health-related claims, the subcommittee generally relied on reports or briefs submitted by sport organizations, including Sport Nova Scotia, the Canadian Association for the Advancement of Women and Sport (CAAWS), and the Canadian Association for Health, Physical Education and Recreation (CAHPER). For example, while Sport Nova Scotia was cited as the source for the reference to reduction in unwanted pregnancies among young women who are active in sport, this was in fact an American research finding popularized by Nike advertisements and probably attributable to self-esteem rather than sport itself.

It is possible, however, to examine the health benefits of physical activity from an equity and social justice perspective without reducing women or men to mere economic assets. There is no doubt that regular physical activity is essential for girls' and women's physical and psychological health and well-being, and that in a democratic society every effort should be made to ensure that barriers to full participation are removed. Conversely, since it is widely known that there is a strong correlation between physical exercise and the prevention of many chronic diseases, there is an obvious injustice at work when diseases related to inactivity produce or exacerbate health problems, pain, and suffering in the female population. Black women and Native women, for example, are particularly vulnerable to certain chronic, and ultimately life-threatening, conditions, with a sedentary lifestyle constituting a significant risk factor for heart disease, stroke, and type 2 diabetes (Healthy Weights, Healthy Lives, 2004; Wells, 1996).

All children require regular physical activity to ensure cardiovascular benefits, good bone development, healthy weights, and long-term health promotion. Childhood activity is a key element in the prevention of chronic disease and obesity in adulthood, and regular activity patterns established in childhood are likely to be maintained in adulthood (Ganley & Sherman, 2000; Summerfield, 1990). Psychological benefits for children include overall emotional well-being, positive self-concept, and lower levels of tension, anxiety, and depression (Psycho-Physiological Contributions, 1998).

An Ontario survey of overweight and obesity trends since the 1990s showed gradual increases in the adult (18+) population, with almost half in this category by 2003: 57 percent of men and 42 percent of women. Across Canada a similar gender difference was found, although for men overweight and obesity rates increased with income, whereas for women low income was associated with higher rates. Among Ontario adolescents, too, more boys than girls were overweight or obese (Healthy Weights, Healthy Lives, 2004).

Although the lower overweight and obesity rates for girls and women may seem to be a positive trend, it is important to recognize the price that many females pay for thinness. Female preoccupation with weight loss through exercise and/or dieting is, in most instances, an unhealthy result of societal, family, peer, and media pressure on girls and women to achieve an ultra-thin body in order to be seen as heterosexually attractive. Although exercise is a healthier strategy than dieting, the emphasis on weight loss often leads to dangerous eating behaviours. About 25 percent of women who suffer from anorexia nervosa (self-starvation) engage in high levels of physical training, and about 50 percent use exercise for weight-loss purposes. Indeed, surveys have shown that more than 50 percent of the general Canadian female population (aged 10 and over) exercise in order to lose weight; since only about 30 percent of Canadian females are at risk due to obesity, these figures demonstrated that significant numbers of girls and women of average or below-average weight were trying to lose weight (Stephens & Craig, 1990).

Formerly a health concern only among young, middle-class, white females, eating disorders are prevalent among ethnic minority females as well, and effective interventions are urgently needed. The "body equity" workshops developed by Toronto educators Carla Rice and Vanessa Russell (1995, 2002) are an excellent example of a feminist and antiracist initiative that addressed the ways in which oppressions are embodied and interconnected. By politicizing weight prejudice and connecting it to other systems of oppression, the workshops provided a much-needed alternative to the more common, individualistic "body-image" approach.

HEALTH AND FITNESS INITIATIVES: IMPACTS ON GIRLS AND WOMEN

Various provincial and national initiatives of the 1970s and 1980s—the Canada-wide ParticipAction campaign, and CAHPER's Quality Daily Physical Education (QDPE), for example—were aimed at increasing Canadians' regular participation in sport and recreational activities. With girls and women having lower participation rates at the outset, physical educators and sport leaders anticipated that these programs would prove particularly beneficial for females. Despite some initial successes, however, gains were not sustained, and the inactivity levels of Canadian adults have not dropped since the mid-1990s (CFRLI, 1999). The QDPE program, which required 30 minutes of daily physical education, was followed in only 10 percent of Canadian schools. Equally disturbing, recent figures from British Columbia for enrolment in year 11 and year 12 physical education courses show a generally steady decline for both male and female students since 1992, a growing gender gap, and an unprecedented low rate of approximately 10-percent female enrolment in 1999/2000 (Deacon, B., 2001).

Routinely in recent years, the release of statistics on child obesity has prompted renewed calls for compulsory physical education from kindergarten through high school, with only a minority of voices pointing out that this proposal does not fully address the problem. They argue, often from personal experience, that the girls and boys who most need regular physical activity are least likely to enjoy and benefit from school PE as it is currently conducted. As one woman explained, "They learn that they are inferior, incapable and disgusting . . . they will usually be picked last for teams . . . they learn humiliation" (Hughes, 2005). In other words, programs, not children, need to be changed if they are to be successful in promoting a lifelong, healthy, and enjoyable exercise program.

Statistics Canada's 1998 report *Sport Participation in Canada* showed that, between 1992 and 1998, adult (aged 15+) sport participation rates declined by almost 11 percent, and the gender gap widened by 3 percent. The 1992 figure of 38 percent regular female involvement in sport dropped to 26 percent, compared to 43 percent of men. Some of the general decline, according to the Statistics Canada report, could be attributed to the rising popularity of "Internet surfing" as a "relatively inexpensive" leisure activity when compared to the increasing cost of transportation, sporting equipment, and registration fees.

This explanation failed to take into account the economic disadvantage experienced by women as a gender group during an economic recession and a national housing crisis, and the limited likelihood that women with minimal discretionary income would consider the purchase of computers and monthly charges for Internet servers even "relatively" cheap.

Socioeconomic disadvantage interacts with race and gender discrimination in limiting female access to sport and recreation. Activities such as tennis, golf, figure skating, gymnastics, and skiing are frequently organized and practised in expensive and elitist ways—in private clubs, for example—with the result that working-class and minority girls and women are often excluded. With the growing trend toward charging user fees for admission to community recreation centre facilities and for basic instructional programs, even activities like swimming and fitness classes, which used to be free and hence accessible to low-income women and their children, are now beyond the reach of many. Similarly, a recent Ontario survey showed that 43 percent of publicly funded high schools charged a fee for instructional physical education, and 61 percent had an athletic fee ranging from $5 to $90; in the majority of schools, subsidies were available for students unable to pay, but it is likely that the fee requirement would be a deterrent for many students (People for Education, 2001).

Age is another significant factor for both male and female participation rates, with a clear decrease for both sexes over the life span. The age group 15 to 18 years participated in sport at twice the national rate: 68 percent were involved in sport at least once per week, compared to the overall rate of 34 percent. For adults 55 and over, the rate dropped to about 20 percent. Female rates were lower than male rates in every age category, with the most dramatic gap in the 15 to 18 age group, where 80 percent of males and only 55 percent of females reported regular participation. Although the gender gap decreased as age increased, some of this trend was attributable to men's more dramatic drop in participation over the life span. However, even in the 55+ age group, male rates were 10 percent higher than female (CFLRI, 1999; Sport Participation in Canada, 1998).

With women having a longer life expectancy than men, they are more likely to experience both health problems and economic deprivation in old age, and hence they face additional barriers in accessing affordable recreational activities. A physical recreation program for seniors, mostly women, sponsored by the University of Alberta and featured in the 1991 National Film Board documentary *Age Is No Barrier*, demonstrated an effective alternative approach to promoting physical activity among older women. Fun, friendship, and collaboration were emphasized over competition and achievement of external standards of success. The program showed, too, how personal relationships were central to women's learning and enjoyment.

The CFLRI and Statistics Canada findings demonstrate the importance of introducing regular and enjoyable physical activity into girls' lives from a young age. The barriers to starting a new sport or recreational pursuit increase with age, particularly for those who cannot build on a foundation of basic skills and physical competence and confidence that they have developed in their youth. Research indicates that inactivity poses a widespread threat to children's health, with two-thirds of Canadian children not sufficiently physically active for optimal growth and development. The 1999 CFLRI Physical Activity Monitor found that girls continued to be less active than boys; only 39 percent of girls, compared to 52 percent of boys, met the required level, and the figure for girls aged 13 to 17 dropped to 32 percent. In terms of regular sporting participation, the figures were 61 percent for boys aged 5 to 14 years, and only 48 percent for girls (CFLRI, 1999). Two earlier Canadian surveys also indicated the risks for girls and young women: their self-image and confidence declined during adolescence (Canadian Teachers' Federation, 1990; Holmes & Silverman, 1992), and there was a corresponding drop in their physical activity levels (Stephens & Craig, 1990).

BEHIND THE STATISTICS: CAUSES AND EFFECTS

Three related variables—education level, family income, and labour force participation—all had clear impacts on female participation. Female students (high school, college, or university) and women with part-time or full-time employment were more likely to be active in sport than women who were not in the labour force, with the latter group including women doing unpaid housework and childcare in the home. Women with family incomes of $80,000 or more had almost double the participation rates of those with incomes under $20,000 (Sport Participation, 1999).

Lack of time for physical activity was identified in earlier surveys as a major barrier for women (see, for example, Stephens & Craig, 1990), and the 1998 survey confirmed this finding, with both lack of time and lack of interest cited as equally important reasons for women's low participation. (Men, particularly those in the 20 to 24 and 25 to 34 age groups, also reported lack of time as the major barrier.) This is an interesting finding in light of the female labour force participation figures noted earlier. Many women who work full time experience a double workday; that is, if they have traditional male partners, and/or if they are mothers of young children, they probably complete several hours of domestic and childcare work at the end of each workday. It might be assumed these women would have less time for sport or physical activity than their unemployed counterparts. However, given the correlation among educational attainment, earning capacity, and sporting participation, it appears that, for many fully employed women, their (relative) financial independence enhances their leisure choices. In other words, they do not have to use family finances to pay for recreation-related expenses. See Table 6.1 for more on gender issues in sport participation.

Table 6.1   Highlights from the Canadian Economic Gender Equality Indicators, 2000

- Women aged 15 to 24, when compared to their male counterparts, work 18 percent more; although the share of paid work done by young women is high, their share of unpaid work is even higher;
- Income imbalances between women and men are declining, but women's after-tax income is only 63 percent of men's;
- Women work an additional 15 minutes a day, or the equivalent of more than two additional weeks per year;
- Women are making slow, steady progress into fields that have been heavily male-dominated;
- Yet women are also increasing their share in female-dominated fields and men are staying away from these areas.

Source: Economic Gender Equality Indicators 2000, 2002. Reproduced with the permission of the Minister of Public Works and Government Services, courtesy of Statistics Canada and Status of Women, 2006. Statistics Canada, "Canadian Social Trends," Catalogue 11-008, Spring 2001; no. 60.

Power relations in traditional families give men ultimate authority over women and children, especially daughters, and men's controlling of women's time and activities extends to their leisure pursuits. The prospect of women engaging in sport and recreation purely for their own enjoyment is antithetical to traditional expectations that women should put others' needs before their own. As a result, women may arrange their leisure activities to fit with family expectations, or they may try to combine childcare with a physical activity such as walking or swimming. These kinds of creative individual solutions do not address systemic problems such as power relations and the sexual division of labour in the family, or the absence of affordable childcare in the community.

Despite these obstacles, there is some evidence that Canadian girls and women engage in physical activities that are not usually defined as sport. When questioned about their exercise frequency in Statistics Canada surveys (1994–95), females aged 12 years and older reported much higher participation rates in the categories of walking for exercise, home exercise, and aerobics or fitness classes than did males, and slightly higher rates for swimming. Similarly, a 1998 Statistics Canada survey showed that men and women preferred different sports: swimming, baseball, and volleyball were women's top choices, while hockey, golf, baseball, and basketball were men's. In the 1997/98 cycle of Health Canada's National Population Health Survey, walking remained women's most popular leisure-time physical activity, with gardening, home exercise, social dancing, and swimming high on the list, even for women in the "inactive" category (see Table 6.2).

Survey findings also reflected girls' and women's tendency to value the social interaction that accompanies physical activity, and to view competition as a lower priority. For example, among active Canadians, 40 percent of males took part in competitions or tournaments, compared to 29 percent of females, although the latter figure represented an increase of 5 percentage points over the 1992 findings. With regard to the sport preferences of children aged 5 to 14, however, some new trends were identified: although hockey was the favourite for boys and swimming was the top choice for girls, both boys and girls put soccer in second place, followed by baseball and basketball.

Surveys that examined physical activities rather than sports produced somewhat different results. A fitness survey conducted in 1988 reported that walking was the top physical recreation choice for both males and females aged 10 years and older, while gardening was the second (Stephens & Craig, 1990). The 1999 CFLRI report found that 81 percent of adult Canadians listed walking as the most popular activity, 70 percent gave yard work and gardening as second choice, and 54 percent said swimming. Women are more likely than men

Table 6.2   Active and Inactive Women's Participation in Physical
Activities: Most Popular Choices

Activity	Active Women	Inactive Women
Walking	91%	61%
Gardening	52	27
Home exercise	52	21
Bicycling	43	10
Swimming	40	14
Social dancing	40	15
Jogging/running	32	<5
Weight training	21	<5

Notes: Active women: energy expenditure >3.0 kcal/kg/day
        Inactive women: energy expenditure <1.5 kcal/kg/day
        An average of 3 kcal/kg/day is recommended for optimal health benefits

Source: Based on data from the Statistics Canada National Population Health Survey, 1996.

to take part in yoga, tai chi, exercise classes, and walking for exercise, while adolescent girls are more likely than boys to list walking, social dancing, ballet, and exercise and dance classes.

Although the sex differences in the 1998 survey might well reflect discriminatory practices in access to facilities and programs, it is important to avoid using the male yardstick to judge female sporting achievement, preferences, and practices. This "female deficit" model upholds traditional male values and attitudes in sport as the ideal. Female perspectives are judged by the male standard and found lacking, and girls and women are then blamed for having an "attitude" problem—for example, they don't understand that winning is all that matters!

SYSTEMIC BARRIERS

Violence against Women

The threat of harassment and violence poses a serious obstacle to women's sport and recreational choices. Minority women experience additional problems of harassment or discrimination on the basis of their race/ethnicity, social class, or sexuality. Women as a group, and adults over 65, are more likely than men and younger adults to avoid walking or cycling for exercise because of safety concerns (CFLRI, 1999). Working-class and/or minority women may live in areas of the city where personal safety is a particularly serious concern, and parents of young women may justly fear for their daughters' welfare when walking or travelling on public transit to community recreational programs. Expectations in some traditional families, where domestic and childcare chores are expected to take priority over recreation, may further constrain girls' and women's options (see, for example, Borowy & Little, 1991).

There was growing recognition in the 1990s that many male sporting practices actively promoted woman-hating attitudes and violence against women (Lenskyj, 2003). Football coaches, players, and fans, for example, use misogynist and homophobic insults and obscenities to motivate the home team and to put down their opponents (Pronger, 1993). Such practices served as powerful symbols of the marginalization and brutalization of women. Statistics from American university campuses showed that male intercollegiate athletes were overrepresented among students convicted of sexual assault, including date rape and gang rape (Bausell, Bausell, & Siegel, 1991; Warshaw, 1988). Similarly, some prominent professional athletes were accused, and in some cases convicted, of sexually assaulting female spectators, sports journalists, and cheerleaders. The mythology surrounding male sporting heroes and the sense of entitlement that comes with their status makes it difficult for victims of sexual assault to report to police and to testify in court, particularly when the perpetrator is a millionaire sports figure (Benedict, 1998; Robinson, 1998).

The connection between wife assault and major male sporting events like the Super Bowl began to receive public attention in the early 1990s. The numbers of women who were victims of sexual or physical assault increased at the time of major North American sporting events, especially after men had watched their favourite team win (White, Katz, & Scarborough, 1992). In 1993, NBC-TV, the network that broadcast the Super Bowl, agreed to air a free public service announcement during the pre-game program, and American and Canadian television stations and newspapers also carried announcements and reports on the links between domestic violence and major sporting events in an attempt to raise public awareness.

The "Chilly Climate" Problem

Analyses of gender equity issues in education and employment recognize the problem of the "chilly climate" or "poisoned environment" and its role in deterring female participation, and there are clear parallels in the sport and physical activity context. An unwelcome, unsafe, or even threatening environment can be created by men's verbal or physical harassment, by nonverbal behaviour, and by the physical surroundings. It is important to note that concepts such as chilly climate and poisoned environment are recognized in legal contexts as forms of sexual harassment. For example, the first sexual harassment complaint lodged at the University of Toronto in the 1980s involved a male professor who was alleged to have persistently leered at women using the swimming pool. A current problem involves men "surfing" pornography sites on computers in the athletic centre. Although these practices are permitted under the university's computer policies (in the interests of freedom of sexual expression), the location of the terminals in a public area near the women's locker room is a cause for concern.

The "dripping tap" experience—sexual innuendoes, intrusive touching, unwanted and persistent requests for dates or sex, and displays of offensive images of women—erodes the morale and resistance of many women who work, study, or train in these settings (Dagg & Thompson, 1987). Alternatively, they may develop a high level of tolerance for sexual harassment in order to survive. If a woman experiences sexually harassing behaviour at the hands of a male coach, or is threatened with reprisals if she does not have sex with him, she may be forced to give up her sport. Even the less serious forms of harassment, including coaches' inappropriate criticism of girls' or young women's body size and shape, may contribute to dangerous eating patterns such as self-starvation, bingeing, and purging, with sometimes fatal consequences (Davis, 1999; Lenskyj, 1993). In most situations, the coach has significantly more institutional power and privilege than the athlete by virtue of his status as coach, his gender, race, age, social class, and sexual orientation, and so the odds are stacked against the female target of harassment.

The Sexual Abuse Problem

In 1993, CBC television aired a groundbreaking public affairs program called *Crossing the Line* that examined the problem of sexual harassment and sexual assault of girls and young women at the hands of male coaches. Many of the men whom they named as harassers were pursuing successful careers as coaches of female athletes, in some cases with the complete approval of the athletes' parents and the university administrations, while their female victims had abandoned their sporting careers and were hurt and disillusioned by the experience. The fact that two of the documented cases involved university sport was particularly disturbing, since at that time most Canadian universities and colleges, unlike community sports clubs and organizations, had harassment policies in place. Psychological abuse was clearly illustrated in the CBC documentary. The young women's perceptions of coaches' complete control over their lives were both illuminating and disturbing:

- "He owned your body and he owned your mind"
- "He could have asked us to do almost anything"
- "He was always in your head"

Coaches achieved this psychological control through some clichéd but effective messages:

- "No one remembers who comes second"
- "I can replace you—I made you and I can break you"

It was clear that the powerful "win at all costs" mentality and the young athletes' overwhelming dedication to training made it even more difficult for them to report the abuse. Time after time, a powerful, charismatic male coach would persuade a young woman that his abusive actions were "for her own good" and that reporting the harassment would cause him to lose his job and thereby ruin her chances—and the team's chances—of winning. CBC reporter Hana Gartner's response was illuminating: she had difficulty believing that these girls had remained silent when their silence served to protect the men who were abusing them. Like many viewers unfamiliar with the everyday world of high-performance sport, Gartner seemed baffled that a young woman would tolerate this kind of abuse, just because of a game. What was missing from the documentary was an analysis of the subculture of competitive sport—women's as well as men's—where the drive to win at all costs transcends other considerations. The CBC documentary succeeded, however, in raising public awareness, and some national sports organizations subsequently took action and formulated harassment policies and procedures (see Donnelly, 1999, p. 119). Ironically, it was a crisis in boys' hockey, when news of sexual abuse cases involving male coaches became front-page stories in 1997, that prompted Canadian sport administrators to take the most dramatic and far-reaching policy initiatives to address the problem of sexual harassment and abuse in youth sport (Donnelly, 1999). This is not to diminish the seriousness of any incidents of sexual abuse, for boys as well as girls. Indeed, given the generally homophobic climate of male sport, young male victims face additional challenges when they come forward to report abuse at the hands of a male coach.

CONCLUSIONS

The preceding analysis examined the roots of existing inequalities both inside and outside the context of sport and physical activity. Strategies for change must take into account the broader social context, most notably the powerful impacts of interlocking systems of oppression. Liberal strategies that simply "open the door" by introducing more programs, classes, or teams for females or minorities rarely address the problems of marginalization and exclusion experienced by those who suffer the effects of racism, classism, homophobia, ableism, and violence. Feminist and antiracist initiatives hold more promise of empowering females and minorities through challenging systemic barriers.

This chapter has presented an analysis of the social construction of femininity and masculinity, and various theoretical and political approaches to gender equality in sport and physical activity, including liberal and radical feminist approaches, human rights arguments, and health and fitness rationales. The emphasis has been on systems of oppression, including harassment and violence against women, and gender-related differences in values, priorities, and activity choices.

CRITICAL THINKING QUESTIONS

1. What changes could be made to high school physical education programs to make them more welcoming a) to girls? b) to students from ethnic minority backgrounds? c) to overweight students?
2. Debate the following statement: "Violence is an essential component of contact sports." Discuss the implications for female participation in contact sports.
3. What are the pros and cons of sex-integrated sport for a) children under 12, b) adolescents, and c) adults?
4. Select a particular government sport department, sport organization, or recreation centre, and discuss the following questions in terms of gender, ethnicity, and social class:
   • Who allocates the resources?
   • Who makes decisions?
   • Who operates the programs?
   • Who has access to power?
   • Who participates in the programs?
   • Who works in the office?
   • Who cleans and maintains facilities?
5. Debate the following statement: "People who enjoy sport and value democracy would be ill-advised to support any aspect of the Olympics . . . their energies would be better directed towards other regional, national and international sporting competitions that are currently conducted in more ethical and less exploitative ways" (Lenskyj, 2000, 195).
6. During the 2006 Winter Olympics, with the Canadian women's hockey victory and the men's defeat, a cartoon showed the men's coach telling them, "Play like girls." Discuss the hidden messages in this cartoon.

SUGGESTED READINGS

Brackenridge, C. (2001). *Spoilsports: Understanding and preventing sexual exploitation in sport.* London: Routledge.
Griffin, P. (1998). *Strong women, deep closets: Lesbians and homophobia in sport.* Champaign, IL: Human Kinetics.
Hall, M. A. (2002). *The girl and the game: A history of women's sport in Canada.* Peterborough, ON: Broadview Press.
Lenskyj, H. (1986). *Out of bounds: Women, sport and sexuality.* Toronto: Women's Press.
Lenskyj, H. (2003). *Out on the field: Gender, sport and sexualities.* Toronto: Women's Press.
Theberge, N. (2000). *Higher goals: Women's ice hockey and the politics of gender.* Albany NY: SUNY Press.
White, P., & Young, K. (Eds.). *Sport and gender in Canada,* 2nd ed. Don Mills, ON: Oxford University Press, 2006.

WEB LINKS

Canadian Fitness and Lifestyle Research Institute, Ottawa
http://www.cflri.ca
Annual statistics on Canadians' participation in sport and physical activity, and other research findings, with breakdowns by gender, age, income levels, education, and so on.

Sport Information Resource Centre, Ottawa
http://www.sirc.ca/
Leading bibliographic database producer of sport, fitness, and sports medicine information.

Status of Women Canada, Ottawa
http://www.swc-cfc.gc.ca/
A national organization committed to improving women's economic autonomy and well-being, eliminating systemic violence against women and children, and advancing women's human rights; information on gender-based analysis, and other research tools.

Tucker Center for Research on Girls and Women in Sport, University of Minnesota
http://www.education.umn.edu/tuckercenter
Follow links to "Resources" for excellent bibliographies on specific topics—a valuable research tool.

University of Toronto, Graduate Collaborative Program in Women's Studies
http://www.utoronto.ca/wgsi/
"Collection of Women's Resources on the Net": links to dozens of feminist websites in Canada and internationally.

Outsports.com
http://www.outsports.com
News and views on experiences of gays and lesbians in sport and recreation.

Women in Sport and Physical Activity Journal
http://www.aahperd.org/wspaj/
An interdisciplinary, international forum for woman-centred issues and approaches to sport and physical activity.

CHAPTER 7

CHILDREN, YOUTH, AND PARENTAL INVOLVEMENT IN ORGANIZED SPORT

Ralph E. Wheeler

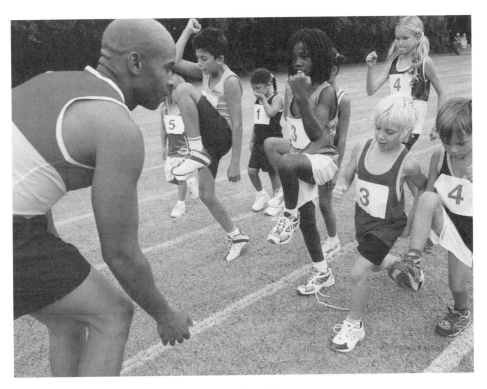

Today, organized adult-controlled sports for children are flourishing.

Bigshots/Photodisc Red/Getty Images

Play is basic to all normal, healthy children. It provides pleasure and learning and a minimum of risks and penalties for mistakes.

C. Schaefler and H. Kaduson, *The Quotable Play Therapist*

The rise in popularity of organized sports programs for children is still a relatively new phenomenon in comparison to the history of organized sports for adult populations. The focus on formal games for children may have had its earliest beginnings in North America with the founding of Little League Baseball in the United States in 1939. In the decades since, minor sports programs, as they are often referred to, have grown at a phenomenal rate. These programs offer a wide range of sport activities and encompass many levels of expectations for both participants and organizers. For many boys and girls in Canada, participating in minor sport is a normal part of their everyday lives.

Today, nearly 3 million Canadian children and youths between the ages of 5 and 18 participate regularly in organized sports programs. In fact, in a study of physical activity levels among Canadian children, the Canadian Fitness and Lifestyle Research Institute (CFLRI, 2004) found that the majority of parents in Canada (63 percent) indicated their child "participates in some organized sport" (p. 3). These programs are offered by a number of organizations and groups that serve to govern and control these activities in order to ensure children receive optimal benefits from their experiences. However, critics would argue that the initial vision and objectives of organized sport for children might have become lost in a highly institutionalized sport model that has emerged—a model that calls into question whether the needs of children are in fact being met. This chapter will review the organizational structure of children's sport in Canada; examine some of the reasons why children participate in youth sport and the benefits gained from this involvement; and, finally, explore a number of issues and concerns related to organized sport programs. This chapter will consider a number of areas relevant to children's sport participation that will serve as a framework for our examination and discussion. These include

- ethics in youth sport
- why children quit organized sport
- overemphasis on performance and winning
- sport specialization limiting children's choices in organized sport
- parental involvement in kids' sports, and
- coaches' influence in children's sport.

In order to guide our discussions of the issues emerging from these areas, this chapter will employ a number of theoretical approaches introduced in Chapter 2. These theories provide contrasting views of organized sport for children. It is only by viewing sport from a number of alternative perspectives that we can begin to interpret and understand the diverse effects of institutionalized sport on youth and to raise questions of our own as to the role sport should play in the overall development of young children. As beginning sport sociologists it is important to have a firm understanding of the major sociological theories used to study organized sport, such as functionalist theory, conflict theory, symbolic interactionism, and critical theory. While no one theory can fully answer all our questions about sport, the theories do provide us with the tools that help us in our examination and discussion of modern sport and its role in society.

THE ORGANIZATION OF MINOR SPORT

In the ensuing discussion of sport for children, it should be noted that sport in this chapter will be discussed in the context of those activities that are organized around a structured, competitively based model of sport, such as the type of programs seen in minor hockey programs, age-group swimming, or gymnastics programs. Other popular recreational-based activities such as bicycling, skateboarding, or street hockey—while having some of the characteristics of organized sport—will not be considered, as the primary distinction for our discussion is the competitive model of organized sport.

In Canada, organized sport for many children and youths very often begins in the preschool years and is organized and delivered through four main separate agencies or institutions. These include publicly funded community sport and recreation organizations; local sports clubs; service agencies and special-interest groups; and school-based sports. These groups offer a plethora of sport programs and provide diverse experiences through various levels of training and competitive activities. Many of these programs, while they may have different rules for participation than adult programs, typically reflect many of the characteristics of adult-based sport, complete with training schedules and competitive seasons that include playoffs and championships.

Publicly Funded Community Sport and Recreation Organizations

Community-based sport and recreation programs have become extremely popular activities for children in all parts of Canada. Statistics from the 2004 report by the CFLRI suggest that upward of 32 percent of children participate in sport through local community parks and recreation programs. It is not unusual, for example, to find both boys and girls playing a wide variety of sports such as hockey, soccer, baseball, basketball, and tennis as part of community-organized leagues. These programs are publicly subsidized and offer sport opportunities within a range of competitive levels. Coaches, officials, and league organizers, who are responsible for setting up and running all aspects of the program, often include both paid staff and volunteers. Programs are typically organized around "house leagues," which may loosely represent local neighbourhood boundaries. Because these programs are publicly supported, registration fees are usually modest and children who register are assigned to teams on a more or less random basis, the emphasis being on fun and participation. House league participants may practise and play one or two times per week. In addition, many programs support "all-star" teams selected from among a pool of talented players in a particular age group or division. At this level, competition takes on a more serious focus, with teams conducting tryouts, running regular training sessions, and competing in both league and tournament competitions. Teams from a community all-star league may also compete for the right to represent their respective communities in regional, provincial, and inter-provincial championships. Unlike house leagues, which usually play during the weekdays, all-star teams attend practices during the week, with competitions generally held on weekends. In this organizational structure, it is not unusual to find children participating simultaneously on both house league and all-star teams.

Local Sports Clubs

While community-based sports programs encourage wide participation and are relatively inexpensive, more and more children are opting to take part in local sports clubs or associations. The CFLRI 2004 report suggests that 35 percent of all children participating in organized sport are involved through the local club system. One reason for the emergence of local sports clubs is to provide a higher level of training and competition not usually available through school and community-based sport. While these two programs may serve to identify talented youngsters, privately run clubs are perceived as having the potential to develop young, talented athletes to a more elite level. Sports programs operating under this model tend to focus on a specific sport and require a far greater time commitment from the participant.

Many of these programs are highly structured, with scheduled daily training sessions. Because emphasis is on the development of athletic talent and the promotion of competitive prowess, children are often carefully groomed for success at each of the various levels or stages of competition. Private sport clubs operate in both public and privately owned facilities and offer training and competition in such popular individual sports as swimming, gymnastics, figure skating, martial arts, tennis, track and field, cycling, wrestling, and rowing. These clubs also run programs for team sports such as hockey, basketball, and soccer. Operating costs to run these programs may range from several thousand dollars to hundreds of thousands and employ full- and part-time coaches, instructors, and administrators. Club membership fees can range from a modest several hundred dollars annually to registration fees of more than a thousand dollars; in addition, participants are often expected to cover their own travel costs to competitions. Examples of young athletes who have come through this system and risen to stardom in sport abound—notable are the tennis-playing Williams sisters, who were groomed at an early age through private lessons and coaches for success at the professional level.

Service Agencies and Special Interest Groups

Co-existing and often sharing the same facilities with these organizations are a number of other groups that also promote sport activities for children. These include YM/YWCAs, religious organizations, boys' and girls' clubs, The Boy Scouts and Girl Guides movements, and independent sport groups. As in other organizations that offer sport programs, a wide variety of activities and competitive opportunities exist for the participant. A main focus of sport programs among these groups is to use sport as a vehicle to promote their particular set of values and beliefs. For example, children who participate in a church-run program may also be introduced to the underlying values espoused by that particular religion.

School-based Sports

Sport at the high school level has long been an integral part of Canadian educational institutions. Organized sport at the elementary and junior high school level, however, is a relatively new phenomenon initiated originally by physical educators concerned about the low physical activity and fitness levels among children in this age group. According to the 2004 CFLRI report, fewer than 10 percent of children receive their sport experiences through school-sponsored programs. School sports programs were an attempt to address this concern and originally involved sport activities on a more or less informal basis. Today, programs can involve inter-school games on a regional level and may be organized around several weekends or run over a two- to three-month season. These programs rely on coaches and officials, who are usually volunteers from the school staff or from within the community.

Because of a number of obstacles, elementary school sport has not achieved the potential outcomes envisioned by its early advocates. The absence of adequate resources such as suitable facilities, qualified coaches, and sufficient funding have continued to prevent sport at the elementary school level from having any significant impact on increasing overall student activity levels. Coupled with this is the fact that many of the schools that do sponsor sports programs tend to mirror a high school model, which traditionally has catered to a minority of a school's student population. As well, even though costs associated with school sports programs are usually low compared to community-based programs, student participation is limited based on the number of teams sponsored by a particular school. This has caused many physical educators to consider alternative activities to organized sport such as adventure and outdoor experiences, fitness pursuits, and other non-competitive experiences including co-ed and cooperative games activities.

In Canada, organized sport associations for children exist for a number of reasons. At the school level, sport is tied to educational objectives and is seen as a way to motivate children to become involved in an active lifestyle. Community programs promote sport opportunities for children for similar reasons while keeping costs at a reasonable level for the participant. Increasingly, however, there is a growing trend for children who aspire to become successful athletes to join private clubs that provide opportunities for children to excel at a high level within a particular sport. As many of these clubs must operate on income generated through membership fees and corporate sponsors, they resemble in many ways the practices and structures found in adult sport organizations.

Clearly, minor sports organizations have become an integral part of the social fabric of many Canadian communities. With few exceptions, every province that has a sport association responsible for governing and promoting that particular sport will likely have youth programs in place, often starting as early as age five for many children. As Leonard II (1998) noted, "What is remarkable and unprecedented is that there are sport leagues for children who have not even entered the primary grades" (p. 123). The significance of these programs with respect to the psychological, social, and physical effects on the participants will be discussed in another section of this chapter.

FACTORS DETERMINING CHILDREN'S INVOLVEMENT IN SPORT

While children still gather in community playgrounds and neighbourhood parks to enjoy spontaneous, informal games, an increasing number of boys and girls are now engaged in adult-controlled, sport-related activities. A 1998 Statistics Canada survey found that more than half of all Canadian children aged 5 to 14 (almost 2.2 million) reported that they regularly took part in some kind of organized sport activity. Table 7.1 shows the 10 most popular sport activities for children in this age category.

The survey also examined some of the underlying reasons for the increase in the participation rates of children in organized sport. Of the 2,220 families surveyed, the majority of children involved in sport were from middle-class to upper-class households. The study found that 73 percent of children from families with annual incomes over $80,000 were enrolled in organized sports programs; this dropped to 49 percent when the family income was below $40,000.

Table 7.1   Top 10 Sports among Canadian Children Aged 5 to 14

Sport	Percentage of Children Active in the Sport
Soccer	31
Swimming	24
Hockey	24
Baseball	22
Basketball	13
Downhill skiing	7
Figure skating	6
Karate	6
Volleyball	5
Cycling	3

Source: Based on data from the Statistics Canada General Social Survey, 1998.

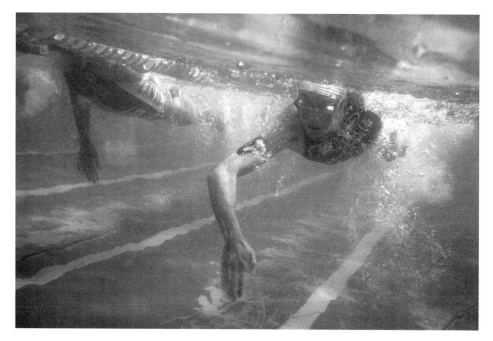

Youth sports programs should focus on what is best for the athletes.
© Clifford White Photography

Nevertheless, results revealed that in households where parents were involved in sport activities, children were four to eight times more likely to participate in sport than in families where parents had no athletic involvement, regardless of income levels.

Results from another study conducted by the CFLRI (2000), which examined the popularity of physical activities, found that bicycling was the top activity for children aged 5 to 12. Other sport or sport-related activities among Canadian children included swimming, walking, winter play such as tobogganing, skating, soccer, in-line skating, running or jogging, and basketball. It also found that boys and girls in this age group have different activity interests, with boys preferring to play golf, snowboard, or skateboard and engage in the team sports of soccer, football, hockey, and basketball. Girls, on the other hand, are more likely to participate in social dancing, skating, gymnastics, ballet, or other dance classes and engage in play activities on swings, slides, and teeter-totters.

The literature related to participation in minor sport programs offers many reasons for the increased involvement of children in organized sport. In a review of studies in this area, Welk (1999) identified five categories or determinants of physical activity for children. These included personal, biological, psychological, social, and environmental. Welk concluded, "the most commonly identified determinants were self-efficacy, perceived competence, enjoyment, some degree of parental influence and access to programs and equipment" (p. 11).

Coakley (2004) suggested that changes associated with family structure and the perceptions parents have about the role sport can play in their children's development has had a major impact on participation levels in organized sport. Perhaps one of the biggest changes, he contended, is the increase in the number of families with both parents working. For working parents, after-school and summer sport programs offer a safe, adult-supervised environment where children may acquire valuable social and athletic skills. In fact, many parents have concerns about their children's safety when they're playing in unsupervised situations. The 2000 CFLRI report found that about half of all parents surveyed had "moderate to serious concerns about their children's safety when they are playing outdoors in the local neighborhood" (p. 9). Coakley also suggested that parenting ideology has changed in terms of what it means, in today's society, to be a "good parent." Parents are now expected to be more accountable for the behaviour and whereabouts of their children. This makes sport a highly attractive alternative to "hanging out" at the mall, the video arcade, or on the street corner.

Several other factors also play a role in determining involvement for children in organized sport. Nixon and Frey (1996) identify both social background and status factors such as social class, gender, race, and ethnicity as influential in determining participation. They also point out that regional considerations such as where one lives, for example whether in an urban or rural area, may also affect sport involvement based on available opportunities. Likewise, for many children living in small rural communities, programs that are available may be more accessible and affordable than for children in larger urban centres with more sport opportunities but with greater associated costs such as higher program and coaching fees, transportation, and facility rentals.

Perhaps the single biggest factor for an increase in sport participation for children is the realization among the public that many children are leading inactive, unhealthy lifestyles and that something needs to be done. Alarming research results that have become strikingly familiar has jolted practitioners in recreation, education, and allied health fields. A rather gloomy picture emerges when we look at the physical activity levels among young Canadians. The Canadian Community Health Survey conducted in 2004 reported that the single largest increase in obesity rates was among youth aged 12 to 17, where the rate tripled from 3 percent in 1978 to 9 percent, an estimated 500,000 children. More recent research findings are pointing toward an obesity epidemic. Today, with that trend continuing, both provincial and federal government agencies are under greater pressure than ever to address the problem. Coupled with this is the perception that physical education programs across the country are having little or no influence on changing the long-term fitness and activity levels of children. Particularly disturbing is the trend for schools, once seen as the focal point for the overall development of the child, to reduce physical education opportunities for students. It is not surprising that many parents, in an attempt to provide a suitable alternative to this situation, look for other opportunities to enroll their children in organized sport programs.

MOTIVATING FACTORS FOR PARTICIPATION

It is clear from the literature that most playful activities, including sports, are appealing to children for a number of reasons. In fact, people of all ages share similar perceptions about the benefits of participating in sport. The Conference Board of Canada, Household Survey (2004) reported that active participants indicated the following benefits of their sport involvement:

> improved physical fitness and health
> fun, recreation and relaxation
> sense of achievement
> opportunities for family and household activities
> improved social, analytical and life skills
> opportunities to socialize and make new friends; and preparedness for sport competitions
> (Sport Canada, 2004, p. 1)

In comparing these benefits and motivating factors to the reasons children give for participating in sport we also find that many of these are both intrinsically and extrinsically rewarding. A study by Klint and Weiss (as cited in LeClair, 1992) reported that the top 10 motives for participating in youth sport were

1. learning new skills,
2. getting in shape or getting stronger,
3. improving skills,
4. having fun,
5. staying in shape,
6. being challenged,
7. using the equipment,
8. competing at higher levels,
9. being physically active, and
10. the teamwork (p. 94)

The National Coaching Certification Program, an educational program for coaches in Canada, also suggests that participants in sport are motivated by both intrinsic and extrinsic considerations, such as

1. a desire for achievement—a wish to improve, master new skills, and pursue excellence,
2. a need for affiliation—a desire to have positive and friendly relations with others,
3. a desire for sensation—a desire to experience the sights, sounds, and physical feelings surrounding a sport or the excitement in a sport, and
4. a desire for self-direction—a wish to feel a sense of control, to feel in charge (NCCP, 1988, pp. 2–9).

Clearly we can surmise from this that sports for children can and do have some perceived positive features. While children are drawn to sport for a variety of reasons, the challenge for parents, coaches, and sport organizers is to ensure programs continue to provide activities in a context that motivates and encourages children to participate.

BENEFITS OF ORGANIZED SPORT FOR CHILDREN

For many children today, involvement in organized sport activities begins at an earlier age. Youth sport has come to occupy an important place in the amateur sports system in Canada along with community, school, and intercollegiate sport. The Canadian Sport policy endorsed by the federal government in 2002 took a multi-year commitment toward the development of sport, in particular those initiatives that would encourage broad sport participation. Those initiatives included increasing the practice of sport in schools, enhancing community-based sport programs, and strengthening sport participation opportunities for targeted groups. As long as government funding and community support continue, we will very likely see an expansion of these youth sport programs in the future.

The proponents of early and continued participation in sport activities point to the benefits to be gained through this involvement. For example, Lumpkin (2005) suggests that

people of all ages enjoy playing games, engaging in recreational activities and exercising to maintain good health. Competitive, rule-bound sports provide opportunities to test one's skills against opponents. Through these programs, the all-around development of the individual is enhanced during activity. The purpose of these programs is to optimize quality of life through enjoyable physical activity and sport experiences. (p. 30)

The health-related outcomes from vigorous physical and sport activities are thoroughly documented and supported in both the medical and physical education research literature. National reports from both the U.S. and Canada provide overwhelming arguments in support of the health benefits of physical activity. Both the Healthy People report (2000) and the Improving the Health of Canadians report from the Canadian Institute for Health Information (2004) suggest that a number of areas need to be addressed in terms of increasing activity levels among the general population. These include development and improvement in muscular strength, flexibility and endurance, regulation of body weight, decrease in the risk of heart disease, and the release of tension and anxiety. Some of the social and psychological benefits of sport include the promotion of a positive attitude toward physical activity, the improvement of self-confidence, increasing self-esteem and self-control, as well as providing an avenue for fostering social competence.

The Canadian Centre for Ethics in Sport (2002) sees community-based sports promoting "a number of positive values in youth, with teamwork and commitment at the top of the list" (p. 3). Furthermore, it found through its 2002 Public Opinion Survey on Youth and Sport that Canadians think that sports benefit their local communities in a number of ways. "This is seen most broadly in terms of providing a great source of fun and recreation, but many also believe sports help to reduce crime and delinquency, bring people together, build community pride, and even provide positive values and character building in youth as they feel it should be doing" (p. 3).

Despite the overwhelming evidence supporting the benefits of sport and physical activity for youths, numerous studies have been published that show alarmingly low fitness levels among young people. Siedentop (2004) contends that this is not a recent concern and suggests that "the general notion that children are not fit has been argued in both the professional and popular literature since the 1970s" (p. 196). Given that the habits we take into adulthood are often formed during our youth, the overall physical benefits of youth sport participation is clearly one of the most significant outcomes for children's involvement in sport.

CONTROVERSIES AND ISSUES IN CHILDREN'S SPORT

As the popularity of children's sport has grown, so too have the scrutiny and the criticism of children's sports programs. Critics have come to question the merits of organized sport participation for children as young as four or five years of age with respect to a number of areas of concern. Many of the professionals involved in physical education and sport remain convinced of the need for changes to be made in minor sport if children are to reap the benefits that sport has to offer. This section will review a number of the interrelated issues associated with children and youths in minor sport. These include ethics in youth sport, withdrawal from sport, overemphasis on performance and winning, sport specialization, parental interference, and the role coaches play in youth sport.

It is important to understand at this point that there can be opposing or competing views to many of the observations and arguments that are discussed in the ensuing pages. While these points of view may be driven by widely varying factors, it is important to realize that many events and experiences serve to shape one's reality. As was discussed in Chapter 2, Sociological Theories of Sport, our different views of social reality or alternative perspectives are supported by various sociological theories. It is perhaps useful at this point in time to revisit Chapter 2 and examine the essence of Ian Ritchie's discussions around functionalist theory, conflict theory, and symbolic interactionism, along with a review of some of the critical social theories outlined in the chapter.

Ethics in Youth Sport

The often highly competitive and achievement-oriented nature of organized sport for children can create many dilemmas for participants, coaches, administrators, spectators, and officials who make decisions that can affect the outcome of a competition. In many of these instances, emotions such as resentment, anger, fear, and frustration are likely to play a role in the decision-making behaviour of an individual. Examples abound in sport where one's moral values and ethics are put to the test. "Ethics is concerned with issues of right and wrong in human conduct. It is concerned with what is good and bad; what is authentic and not authentic. Ethics is also concerned with the notions of duty, obligation, and moral responsibility" (Malloy, Ross, & Zakus, 2000, p. 46). One of the most obvious examples where ethical values are tested in children's sport is the overemphasis and importance placed on winning. For a coach or player, after countless hours of practice in preparation for a competition, to suggest that winning isn't important is both naive and unrealistic. Competition represents a way to measure athletic skill or prowess and can be used to express that measure of achievement in a healthy way. If excellence in sport is defined as winning, what lengths might one go to in order to win? Does winning become more important than acting within the rules of the game or treating your opponents fairly? If winning is important, how does this affect our definitions of strategy, rule bending, and cheating? Can we remain honest, fair, respectful, and unselfish if the ultimate goal is to win? These and other questions call for us to consider the ethical dimensions of our behaviour. The erosion of ethical behaviour and high standards of those involved in sport is perhaps the overarching concern with respect to many of the current issues facing youth sport today. Particularly disturbing for some involved in youth sport is the notion that sport may actually serve to promote moral insensitivity. For instance, coaches sometimes use the argument that "everyone is doing it" to rationalize their rule breaking or using questionable tactics.

Sport organizations throughout the country have begun to take steps aimed at improving or maintaining ethical standards of fair play, sportsmanship, and the conduct of individuals involved in their programs. Numerous documents, codes of conduct, fair play rules, and coaches' and players' creeds have been developed that attempt to prescribe guidelines to serve as the basis for making reasoned judgments related to sport activities. Most notably, the Canadian Centre for Ethics in Sport (CCES) has adopted as its mandate the "promotion of ethical conduct in all aspects of sport in Canada and to build a fair and ethical sport system that embodies respect, fair play, safety and non violence" (Centre for Ethics in Sport, 2002, p. 1). In the meantime, a number of provinces have instituted programs aimed at fostering fair play and ethical standards in sport. The fair play programs in Nova Scotia and Ontario are quickly becoming models other provinces are using to develop their own programs to address the issues related to ethics in sport. While these efforts should be applauded as a positive step in raising awareness and addressing the situation, we still do not have to look very hard to find examples of cheating, abuse of officials, violations of rules, and outrageous behaviour of parents to conclude that these disruptive practices are still widespread. Almost daily we are reminded of this issue in youth sport with media accounts of athletes, coaches, parents, and fans engaging in behaviour ranging from foul language, to coaches behaving badly, to incidents where brawling and out-of-control parents assault and injure young referees in minor soccer and hockey games.

Withdrawal from Sport

Even though many children enjoy their participation in sport and continue this participation well into adulthood, a large percentage discontinue their involvement at an early age for a variety of reasons. According to Ewing and Seefeldt (1990), the most commonly reported causes for children to quit playing sport are

lost interest
not having fun
took too much time
coach was a poor teacher
too much pressure
wanted more sport activity
was tired of it
needed more study time
coach played favorites
sport was boring
overemphasis on winning (reported in Bompa, 1995, p. 30)

Other studies have found that pressure on children can be a significant contributing factor; a reported 70 percent of youth athletes quit organized sport, outside of school programs, by the age of 13 (Engh, 1999). This pressure can originate from a number of sources such as coaches, teammates, and parents. Hecimovich (2004), in a review of sport specialization in youth, noted, "sport psychologists have determined that a lack of fun and enjoyment is the number one reason children leave organized sport" (p. 36). He also attributed overinvolvement and high parent expectations as playing a significant role in their child's decision to withdraw from organized sport. Some children, following a disappointing sport experience, simply move on to another sport or activity of interest. However, some experience the serious consequence of burnout. This phenomenon will be discussed further on in the chapter. It would appear that while children participate in sports for a number of reasons, it also remains clear that when their motivations for participating in sport are not met, they are likely to lose interest and discontinue their involvement. This is supported by the 2002 Public Opinion Survey on Youth and Sport in which parents reported that the three main reasons their child's expectations were not met in minor sport were lack of interest/participation, poor coaching/supervision, and too much emphasis on winning. Parental interference, lack of financial support, and a lack of quality programs were also given as reasons for being disappointed in their child's sport experience.

Overemphasis on Performance and Winning

One of the most controversial areas of organized sport for children is the highly competitive nature of some programs and the overemphasis placed on performance and winning. It is not unusual for sport clubs, and in some cases community-based sport programs, to promote their programs in order to recruit new members in an effort to boost registration numbers. By highlighting their dedication to excellence and showcasing the previous competitive successes of their athletes and teams, these clubs are able to present a very enticing picture. Parents perceive this to be an attractive feature of a program as it is seen to develop values and norms in their children that will be important to them in real-life competitive situations. However, many sport professionals and physical educators feel that the emphasis in youth sport should not be one of a highly competitive nature but rather the enhancement of physical, cognitive, and affective development of the participants. Wuest and Bucher (2003), in a criticism of youth sport as it currently exists, surmise that "this development is particularly critical during the child's younger years. The fun of playing (rather than dominating an opponent) should be emphasized, participation opportunities for many children of all abilities should be provided (rather than limiting participation to the gifted few), and the development of skills within the sport and in other sports should be stressed (rather than specialization)" (p. 342). As training guru Tudor Bompa (1995) pointed out, "it is important for us to provide more opportunities for children to learn the fundamentals of sports in a fun, low-stress environment. This is difficult to do if winning is the primary objective" (p. 26).

Sport Specialization

Directly linked to the emphasis on the competitive aspects of sport for children is the emphasis on developing highly skilled athletes. The process for identifying athletic talent in Canada is typically based on a sport model that provides a feeder system designed to progressively target and train athletes for the elite levels. While some sports such as swimming, gymnastics, and figure skating have traditionally been known to start training kids as early as 5 and 6 years, this has now become the norm to follow for other sports such as soccer, hockey, and basketball. Children who show promise are systematically moved through a series of skill development stages, introduced to more intense competitions, and engaged in longer, more frequent training sessions. Because of the amount of effort, time, and resources involved in this development phase, promising athletes are inevitably urged by a coach or parent to choose one sport in which to participate. Parents are persuaded that their child's progress and chances for success at the elite level of the sport will be enhanced if there is year-round commitment to that sport. The prospect of becoming an age-group champion, or the dream of making a national team, becomes a powerful enticement for both parents and their children. Parents can be easily lured into the "Tiger Woods phenomenon," believing that focusing on one sport early—like the world's best golfer, who reportedly started putting when he was three years old—will give their son or daughter a better chance to "make it to the big leagues." Early specialization in youth sport is still a contentious issue. While studies have suggested that the development of athletic expertise is linked to early specialization (e.g., Ericsson et al., 1993), some researchers have argued that a diversified approach to sport is not necessarily a disadvantage. Baker (2003), in his review of a number of studies, pointed out that "play-like involvement in a number of sports is beneficial for developing the intrinsic motivation required during later stages of development when training becomes more structured and effortful" (p. 89).

Critics of specialization also contend that programs that revolve around elitism and specialization undermine many of the positive aspects of sport. Regimentation, routine, and adherence to a long-term training program increasingly influence and shape the experiences of children in organized sports programs. The values that emerge from programs based on competitive success can be in conflict with, and in some cases act to subvert, the avowed ideals of children's sports. Furthermore, physical educators would argue that young children need to learn to value the aesthetic dimensions of physical activity and that, rather than focus on competitive games at an early age, the emphasis should be toward a movement-education approach that provides opportunities for kids to experience the joy of physical movement as opposed to objective performance (Siedentop, 2004, p. 247).

Specialization within a Sport

While some parents want to give their kids the advantage of an early start by supporting a decision to specialize in a particular sport, there is another interrelated dimension to this trend that sees children taking on an even greater level of specialization. Some programs are so highly structured that emphasis is placed on children to specialize in a particular position within that sport. For example, it not unusual for children to refer to themselves by their playing position: a soccer player is now a "striker" or a "fullback," and the age group swimmer is a "butterflyer" or a "freestyler." The athlete comes to view his or her role in the sport from the perspective of the relative status of the position, thus further limiting and detracting from the fundamental purpose of sport for children. Experts would suggest that such a deliberate structured approach to improve a child's sport skills places them under enormous physiological and psychological stress as well as robbing them of opportunities for developing important social skills.

A number of negative consequences arise from this trend. As children advance from one level of sport to the next, participation becomes progressively more selective for those who remain in the programs. The most promising players are often children who physically mature earlier than their peers and consequently have a greater chance for athletic success in their age group. Under this system the so-called "late bloomers" soon become discouraged, as limited playing time and fewer opportunities are made available to them. Related to this is the fear some children may have of physical injuries, particularly in such sports as soccer, hockey, and football when greater physical contact is introduced and permitted. As well, other sports such as gymnastics, diving, and figure skating have some element of risk and can be perceived as dangerous to children. The exclusionary model, which serves to "weed out" the less talented athletes, also serves to make sport less attractive to children as they get older. Minor hockey in Canada serves as a prime example of a sport based on a system that promotes and caters to the talented as they move through the various levels. Statistics show that registration for minor hockey programs has remained steady, with hockey continuing to be one of the most popular sports for Canadian children (Macpherson et al., 2006). However, an editorial piece in Canada's national newspaper *The Globe and Mail* cautioned that "kids 8, 9, and 10 years old, kids with no plans of making the NHL, are forced to treat hockey from an early age like a job. Seventy-five percent of those kids who start playing hockey at age 5 or 6 have dropped out by the time they hit 15" (reported in Donnelly, 2000, p. 192). While such reasons as the desire to pursue other interests, a lack of facilities, and rising costs may be contributing factors in the dropout rate for hockey, an equally significant factor appears to be related to who gets to play. Children who show promise in the sport are being selected at an earlier age for specialized treatment. Kids who fail to make travel teams or who aren't selected to play in an all-star league soon find themselves on the sidelines. This system of screening out the less talented is not limited to team sports, either, as is evidenced by the high numbers of children who quit or drop out of such individual sports as swimming, gymnastics, and figure skating.

The process of dropping out of sport was examined as early as 1976 by Donald Bell, who found that athletes, apart from not getting to play, may be "induced" to quit because of a continuing series of degrading or humiliating experiences. For example, "being yelled at, criticized, or ridiculed by coaches, parents, or teammates" are frequently reported as negative experiences that serve to drive children from a particular sport (cited in Nixon & Frey, 1996, p. 91). In a 10-year study on withdrawal from competitive sports Butcher et al. (2002) concluded that "lack of enjoyment" was one of the main reasons given for transferring to another sport or for withdrawal from sport altogether. Other factors causing children to leave a sport may be related to performance anxiety, forming new friendships outside the sport, or simply losing interest in the sport. It is worth noting that children who drop out of one sport activity often take up another sport that might be perceived to offer a more enjoyable, challenging, and satisfying experience.

Another negative consequence associated with an emphasis on specialization and the demands placed on young athletes to succeed is the possibility of burnout in children who pursue sport at a high level. This is not a new occurrence; as Figler and Whitaker (1991) explained early on, the phenomenon is the result of "too much participation, success, and pressure at too early an age. The causes may be physical, psychological, or a combination of elements" (p. 122). Coakley (2004) reports that this condition occurs when "age-group champions with the potential to succeed in their sport felt they had lost control over their lives and were unable to explore and develop their identities apart from sports. As stress increased and fun decreased, they burned out" (p. 89). Research has shown that children who leave sport at an early age because of burnout and the unrealistic pressure from coaches, parents, or peers are unlikely to become participants in any other sport activity in the future. Many burnout situations can be avoided; however, coaches and parents need to recognize burnout symptoms and provide programs that protect young athletes from having excessive demands placed on them at such an early age.

Limiting Children's Choices in Organized Sport

A further consequence with respect to specialization in organized sport is that it limits children's opportunities in other sports and non-sport activities. Exclusive participation in one sport activity at an early age can have physical and emotional implications for a child. One of the most alarming effects of sport specialization has been the increased risk of injuries due to overuse. Physiologically, injuries associated with overtraining or improper technique or conditioning are far more frequent when a child engages in a single sport over a long period. Repetitive movements that cause impact or strain to the joints can lead to damage in the fragile growth area of the bone and can result in permanent disability or can impair normal growth patterns. The American Academy of Pediatrics (2000) recommends that children be "encouraged to participate in sports at a level consistent with their abilities and interests. Pushing children beyond these limits is discouraged as is specialization in a single sport before adolescence" (p. 5). Limiting intensive involvement in sports that are physically demanding and providing children with a choice of less strenuous or more skill-oriented activities may help reduce the risk of overuse injuries.

Sport medicine professionals have also begun to raise a concern related to the likelihood of head injuries occurring in contact sports. Until recently, severe contacts resulting in head injuries during sporting events were classified as concussions only when a player exhibited typical symptoms, such as disorientation or loss of consciousness. Doctors are now cautioning that any blow to the head, even if it does not appear severe enough to cause the classic symptoms of a concussion, can still have long-term health consequences. Marchie and Cusimano (2003) concluded from their research on bodychecking and concussions in ice hockey that "repeated mild brain injuries in youth and adults occurring over months or years could result in cumulative deficits. The younger developing brain is at an even higher risk of injury" (p. 3). What this suggests is that young athletes in such sports as hockey, football, rugby, or soccer where contact is permitted may be exposed to even greater harm than was previously thought. Added to this dilemma is the fact that as sport begins to assume a greater place in a child's life, there is the danger that young athletes will continue to train and compete despite undergoing an injury and may in fact avoid reporting injuries for fear of falling behind in their training and risking loss of their place on the team.

Parental Interference

For the majority of parents who enroll their children in organized sport, their participation is limited to driving the kids to and from practices or games. In between, they are content to sit in the bleachers or along the sidelines and play the role of fan and supporter, encouraging and enthusiastically cheering their kids along. On other occasions, they may volunteer in a coaching or officiating capacity. This scene is played out in hundreds of communities across the country each day. These parents are more concerned with supporting their children and making the sport experience fun than in keeping track of their child's playing time or scoring statistics. Most parents who are involved at this level are interested in the redeeming benefits

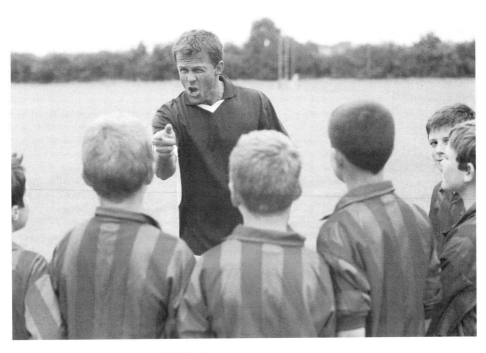

An irate coach depicts the dark side of children's sport.
© BananaStock/SuperStock

sport has to offer their children. Recently, however, a negative element of this involvement has emerged that is a major concern for both critics and supporters of minor sport.

The issue appears to be the sometimes overzealous nature of a minority of parents who engage in displays of unacceptable and sometimes outrageous behaviour before, during, and after their children's sport events. These go beyond well-intentioned parents cheering and rooting for a team or player to include verbal and even physical abuse against opponents. In some cases these abusive behaviours are directed toward their own children. James Deacon (2001), in an article for *Maclean's* magazine, noted that the bad behaviour of some parents in hockey "is so common it even has its own name—rink rage." He also suggested that "hostile behavior at youth games is far more pervasive and sometimes violent than it was a generation ago" (p. 22). A survey of recent newspaper articles seems to support this view as reported incidents of abusive parents threatening coaches, assaulting opposing players, and taunting officials appear to have reached epidemic proportions. In an effort to focus attention on this issue, the National Alliance for Youth Sports, an advocacy group for "promoting positive and safe" sport experiences for children, has posted on its website newspaper accounts of many other incidents where parents have acted violently or have been out of control and abusive.

In what is perhaps one of the most abhorrent and blatant examples of a parent's involvement having dire consequences, a hockey father attacked another parent after becoming incensed over rough play during a kids' summer recreational hockey game. As the children watched, Thomas Junta from Reading, Massachusetts, attacked and fatally injured Michael Costin, who had been supervising games between two groups of children. Junta was charged with manslaughter, subsequently found guilty, and sentenced to a six- to ten-year prison term.

Still other incidents of a far less serious nature than this terrible tragedy occur on a daily basis in children's sport. While parents involved in team sports appear to be the most culpable, individual sports are not immune to abusive parental behaviour. Incidents of a pushy parent who attempts to influence the judges in gymnastics, or a father who becomes enraged when his child is disqualified at a swim meet seem to be occurring more frequently. Regardless of the sport, evidence strongly supports the charge that parents are taking their kids' sport involvement more seriously than ever before. There are a number of reasons for this rise in parental interference in sport.

For parents with aspirations or dreams of their child becoming a top-level athlete or making a national team, sport is not about playing games or having fun. These parents willingly make sacrifices in order to give their youngster every chance to succeed. The possibility of having their child "make it to the top" despite the odds is an underlying motive for many parents involved in minor sport. Parents with this goal in mind are often prepared to do whatever it takes. This ranges from buying the most expensive equipment and paying exorbitant club fees to relocating the entire family closer to a training facility or sending a young child to live and train elsewhere in the country. Parents are also often expected to commit a great deal of their own time to club-sponsored activities such as fundraising projects or serving on committees. It is not unusual to see parents spending large amounts of time with other parents, either during practices, at games, or on road trips, and developing social bonds with these parents. Consequently, a greater sense of prestige may be associated with their child's athletic success. In effect, a parent's "bragging rights" are heavily influenced by their child's success or failure in sport. It comes as no surprise, therefore, when parents feel they have a stake in what happens and attempt to exert undue influence over their child's sport experience.

A second reason for increased interference by parents in children's sport may be an implicit desire to experience sport vicariously through their children. Parents who may have had unsuccessful athletic experiences in their youth sometimes unwittingly pressure their children to succeed in an effort to make up for their own lost opportunities. Even the most restrained parent can lose perspective when faced with the dilemma of giving a child "the chance I never had."

A third reason for parents becoming overly involved in their kids' games is the prospect of future financial rewards. The tantalizing possibility of a college scholarship, endorsements, or a professional contract can become more than just wishful thinking for some parents. It is not unusual to see parents with inflated hopes registering their children in gymnastics, track and field, or figure skating immediately following an Olympic Games. The publicity surrounding these events and the million-dollar contracts for medal winners can become a powerful, if unrealistic, motivator for some parents.

While much of the literature on parental involvement focuses on the overly involved or "pushy" parent, there are a number of dangers associated with parental under-involvement. Children may be more likely to quit sport when parents fail to take an active interest in their child's sport involvement. The support and encouragement are needed most at the initial stage of participation. Children need to feel their efforts are appreciated, which is implicit through their parents sharing the sport experience with them. A lack of parental support and involvement may inadvertently open the door for the development of an unhealthy coach–athlete relationship: "Where the athlete is distanced from the parent(s), because of a perceived absence of emotional support or because of family conflict or problems, she may turn to her coach or other authority figure to take on the role of substitute or surrogate parent. She may even fantasize that this person is, in fact, her substitute father or mother" (Brackenbridge, 2001, p. 72).

In spite of the negative consequences of parents' involvement in their kids' sport, parents can do much to positively influence children's sport experience. Parents need to provide supportive and stable family structures while encouraging involvement in sport. Parents also need to understand and appreciate the child's expectations as opposed to their own or the coach's expectations for the child.

The Role Coaches Play in Youth Sport

While parental involvement in sport has come under heavy criticism for the negative consequences this involvement may produce, it is the coach who has perhaps the greatest potential to influence children in minor sport. The youth sport coach is in a position to provide an atmosphere in which children can realize the many positive benefits of sports participation. Whether these benefits exist for the participant depends to a large extent on a coach's understanding of the purposes and goals of youth sport. One program that has played a significant role in providing education for coaches in this area is the National Coaching Certification Program (NCCP). Since 1975, coaches in Canada have had the opportunity to receive formal training in coaching through the NCCP. This five-level program, a collaborative venture among the provinces, sports governing associations, and the federal government, is designed to provide fundamental coaching principles and skills in addition to the particular techniques of each sport. To date, thousands of volunteer coaches from every level of sport in Canada have taken advantage of this program. In fact, many local sport organizations now have requirements in place that specify only certified coaches are permitted to coach in their league or program.

However, despite the best efforts of these and other educational programs to ensure qualified coaches, a number of issues and concerns related to coaches continue to plague youth sport. Nixon and Frey (1996), in discussing the aversive effects of sport programs for children, reported that while children lose interest and drop out of sport for a number of reasons, problems related to coaches were major factors in their decision to quit. These problems were often associated with "punitive activities by coaches, unrealistic expectations, and harsh and unfair treatment of players" (p. 91). In the past several years, there have been numerous incidents of youth sport coaches who have resorted to unethical, exploitative, and oppressive practices in order to produce a winning team or an elite athlete. Reports of falsifying birth certificates, using ineligible athletes, tampering with equipment, and flirting with starvation diets are just some of the disturbing stories that have made their way into the headlines in recent times.

Perhaps the most frightening and repulsive phenomenon related to organized youth sport to emerge in the past decade has been that of sexual harassment and abuse of young athletes. In a 1999 *Sports Illustrated* special report entitled "Who's Coaching Your Kid?" William Nack and Don Yaeger point out that "after decades of being ignored, minimized, or hidden away, the molestation of athletes by their coaches is no longer the sporting culture's dirty little secret" (p. 43). The report revealed that "although child molestation is by no means confined to sports, the playing field represents an obvious opportunity for sexual predators." With few background checks carried out and little supervision of coaches, "youth sports are a ready-made resource pool for pedophiles." In an exposé in *Maclean's*, James Deacon (1997) revealed the true extent of this behaviour. Quoting from a Canadian study undertaken by Kirby (1996) that examined incidents of sexual harassment and abuse among national team athletes, he reported that Kirby had found some disturbing results: nearly 9 percent of the athletes who responded to the survey reported having been previously subjected to a sexual assault by a coach or team authority figure, and most went unreported. Of the athletes who reported assaults, one in five were under 16 of years of age (p. 54). Nack and Yaeger (1999), in an 18-month review of newspaper stories, found "more than thirty cases of coaches in the U.S. who had been arrested or convicted of sexually abusing children engaged in nine sports

from baseball to wrestling" (p. 43). According to Sparkes (2000), a number of common circumstances relating to the athlete–coach relationship are found to exist in all of these sexual
abuse cases. These include being "under the coach's direct control, often lonely and isolated,
sometimes 'romantically' attached to the coach, threatened and/or bribed with regard to their
future in sport, and generally unable to report what happen to them to their parents, police,
sport administrators" (p. 110). In the wake of new revelations of sexual improprieties
involving minor-sport coaches, sport organizations at all levels have come under increasing
pressure to take measures to ensure the safety of young athletes. Consequently, Sport Canada,
along with a number of individual sports, has developed national guidelines for dealing with
sexual assault and harassment incidents. An immediate response by many sport organizations
across the country to these shocking incidents has been to implement policies that require all
coaches to submit to a police background check.

Unfortunately, these measures may not be enough to keep sexual predators out of sport,
particularly in the larger urban centres where thousands of volunteer coaches would need to
undergo screening. It could be argued that police departments that would normally be responsible for reviewing the backgrounds of these coaches simply would not have the time or the
resources to do so. Regardless, several precautions need to be taken on behalf of children in
organized sport programs to help safeguard them against sexual exploitation. First, where it is
feasible, organizers should insist on a background check by police. Where this is not practical,
volunteer coaches should, as a condition to coach in a league, be required to submit to a check
of their conduct, either through an employer or from previous coaching positions. Second, parents need to be aware of the danger signs that might suggest a sexually abusive or a harassing
relationship and take steps to protect their children. As Nack and Yaeger (1999) point out,
parents should be concerned when a child's interest in a sport suddenly diminishes. Parents
should try to be present at their children's practices and games, as unattended children are seen
as easy targets. Parents also need to be wary of coaches who lavish expensive gifts on players or
spend an unusual amount of time with a child. Perhaps most importantly, parents need to talk
to and inform their children about what is considered inappropriate behaviour by a coach and
to reassure them about reporting any improprieties that may occur between athletes and
coaches.

CHANGING CHILDREN'S SPORTS

While it is clear from this chapter that children's sports appear to be dominated by problems
and issues, it is just as evident that much needs to be done to address some of these concerns.
Firstly, parents must begin to take a more proactive stance toward changing the culture of
youth sport. The drive for excellence must be balanced with a greater regard for the overall
development of the child. There should be a focus not just on athletic performance but also
one that considers social, emotional, and intellectual development.

Secondly, organizers responsible for providing youth sport programs need to meet the
challenges facing sport as a result of these disturbing trends by instituting sound policies on
the ethical conduct of those in decision-making positions. As well, the codes of conduct of
sport governing bodies should carry penalties that are severe enough to be real deterrents to
those who might choose to act in an outrageous or unethical manner. Finally, coaches need
to be made aware of the potential for damage caused by early specialization and overtraining
in young athletes and to encourage and support involvement in a variety of sport activities
rather than placing primary emphasis on exploiting a child who shows athletic promise at an
early age.

CONCLUSIONS

The original objectives of organized sport for children have become obscured or replaced in many programs with an overemphasis on elitism, performance, and the pursuit of athletic glory. The current sport system in Canada comprises school, community, and private agencies. These serve to promote and maintain an exclusionary model in which young athletes are often pressured to succeed by overzealous parents and domineering coaches. As a result of this inappropriate pressure and interference, more and more children are expressing the view that sports are no longer fun. This is reflected in the research that shows nearly three-quarters of all children in organized sport drop out before they reach the age of 15. While it can be argued that parents and coaches have the most influence on a child's sports experience, all too often this influence has taken on negative overtones. The consequences of this shift in attitude about the objectives of youth sport in recent years has led to a much less harmonious environment than ever before.

CRITICAL THINKING QUESTIONS

1. What has led to the increase in the popularity of organized sport for children over the past several decades?
2. What are the dangers associated with early specialization for children in organized sport?
3. Parents and coaches appear to be mainly responsible for putting unrealistic expectations on children who are involved in organized sport. Is this an accurate statement? Are there other people and/or factors involved that contribute to the pressure felt by these children?
4. Studies have shown that more than 75 percent of all children who participate in organized sport drop out by the time they reach the age of 15. What suggestions and changes would you make to the way youth sport is currently structured in Canada that would encourage children to remain in sport?
5. As a parent of a child involved in organized sport, what precautions would you take to ensure that children remain safe from unethical coaches who might seek to exploit them?
6. Assuming that you are in charge of organizing a new sports program for children in your community, what steps would you take to ensure all children in the program receive equal participation opportunities?
7. Discuss what the three major stakeholders (parents, sport governing bodies, and coaches) need to do to resolve some of the problems associated with children's sport.

SUGGESTED READINGS

Donnelly, P. (2000). Part 8, Youth, chapters 26–29. In *Taking sport seriously: Social issues in Canadian sport.* Toronto: Thompson Educational Publishing, Inc.

Eitzen, D. S., & Sage, G. H. (2003). Children and sport. In *Sociology of North American sport,* 7th ed. Toronto: McGraw-Hill.

Hall, A., Slack, T., Smith, G., & Whitson, D. (1991). Youth and education. In *Sport in Canadian society.* Toronto: McClelland & Stewart Inc.

LeClair, J. (1992). How children become athletes. In *Winners and losers: Sport and physical activity in the '90s.* Toronto: Thompson Educational Publishing.

Malloy, D. C., Ross, S., & Zakus, D. H. (2000). *Sport ethics: Concepts and cases in sport and recreation.* Toronto: Thompson Educational Publishing.

WEB LINKS

Canadian Centre for Ethics in Sport (CCES)

http://www.cces.ca

Provides articles and relevant documents on the ethical conduct of all aspects of sport in Canada.

The Center for Sports Parenting (CSP)

http://www.sportsparenting.org

Provides practical advice for coaches, parents, educators, and others involved in youth sports.

National Alliance for Youth Sports

http://www.nays.org

Contains information related to children and youth in organized sport.

Sport Information Resource Centre

http://www.sirc.ca/online_resources/sportquest.cfm

A search engine and directory providing a wide variety of sport and fitness information.

CHAPTER 8

SPORT AND SOCIAL PROBLEMS

Kevin B. Wamsley

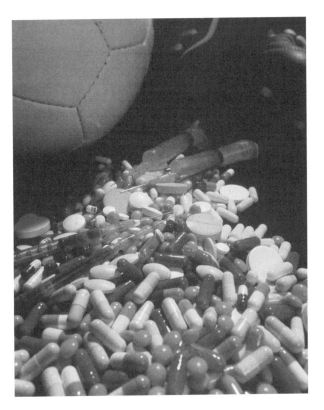

Drug use continues to plague sport today.

© Dimitri Iundt/TempSport/Corbis

I never met a man I didn't want to fight.
> NFL defensive lineman and Oakland Raider Lyle Alzado, poster-boy for aggressive masculinity, who in 1992 died at age 43 of cancer from what he claimed was the abuse of anabolic steroids

I am not a cheat. I do what I am supposed to do to win. Most of the people here in Canada still look at me as the fastest man alive.
> Canadian sprinter Ben Johnson, 2006

For almost two centuries, Canadians have played and watched sports in various social contexts—formal/informal, professional/amateur, major events and championships/minor events and local leagues. Governments, national and provincial associations, clubs, educators, church leaders, various forms of media, coaches, and athletes have encouraged Canadians to play sports or to celebrate the achievements of athletes and teams in order to promote the positive aspects of playing or enjoying the spectatorship of sport. We are often reminded that sport is an activity that promotes health, should encourage patriotic sentiment, and defines the Canadian identity—or, more implicitly, promotes positive interactions between players and fans alike. Historically, educators and sport leaders promoted competitive sports as a moral, character-building enterprise (Howell, 2001; Kidd, 1997; Morrow & Wamsley, 2005). Successful athletes became role models for twentieth-century youth. The Canadian media, through newspaper, television, and Internet coverage, position athletes—professional, Olympic, national team—as cultural icons, celebrities, even heroes. Consequently, for recent generations of Canadians sport participation has been viewed as part of the necessary and proper upbringing for children. Hierarchies of talent development invoked by parents, teachers, and club coaches operate in community and regional networks to identify young athletes and provide encouragement and incentives for them to progress through the ranks of competitive sport to achieve the highest levels of performance possible at all ages. This broad-based cultural identification with competitive sport derives its meaning from the highest levels of competition in professional and Olympic sport, cementing a naturalized order of low-level to high-level sport. Canadians understand, very well, the social, physical, and economic hierarchies that are sustained and celebrated through sport. These relationships generally are viewed as being natural and mostly positive. They also understand that sport has unique features, enclaves, and codes of conduct that are unlike other facets of social life.

Consistent with the global politics that emphasize the importance of winning world championships and Olympic gold medals, Canadians, too, place significant importance on winning and avidly follow the country's standings in world sport competition. During the Cold War period (post–World War II to 1991), sport became one of the most important cultural signifiers of international supremacy. Nations established systematic training centres and programs and invested millions of dollars into athlete training and development. The Canadian sport system—funded, promoted, and centralized—emerged from the Cold War significance placed on elite sport and from the internal politics of developing national unity and identity through sport (Macintosh, Bedecki, & Franks, 1987). Disciplines such as biomechanics and exercise physiology gained momentum during this period, offering training enhancement and principles of movement efficiency as the sport sciences became an integral part of the athletic training regimen. As athletic victory became more and more significant to Cold War posturing and to national identification—and, consequently, to individual achievement—athletes and staff became more willing to employ illicit techniques to improve physical performance (Hoberman, 1992). The ingesting of performance-enhancing substances or doping became, individually and systemically, even state-sponsored (Spitzer, 2004), more widespread. Other serious issues creating harm and suffering to athletes and fans have also plagued sport.

From time to time, we observe newspaper reports about elite athletes or experience events or incidents in community sport that are not positive. Indeed, there is cheating, violence, harassment, injury, intentional harm, and even death in sport. Through sports pages and sports channels and the mainstream news outlets, and depending on the severity of the incident, the media generally provide full and repetitive coverage as a matter of information but, increasingly, as forms of news and sports entertainment with shock value. As a globally popular and stringently rule-bound enterprise, sport receives significant media attention when extremely negative events occur. Conversely, however, sport has emerged as a rather well-protected and highly valued institution; thus, it has been relatively exempt from judicial interventions and guarded more broadly from serious and sustained challenges to its privileged social place. It is not often argued, for example, that people should not play sport or that significant changes should be made when an athlete is killed or seriously injured. Rather, these events are viewed as being an unfortunate part of participating in activities with high degrees of risk. This form of cultural and legal protection has served to situate sport in a unique position of authoritative insularity. Sport, itself, then, as a set of hierarchal relations among people, historically has been protected from sustained and destabilizing criticism in times of crisis or serious incidents. Consequently, athletes or fans are usually blamed for transgressions of rules or the law and the sports process per se, or sports institutions, are not frequently challenged. Some social problems in sport are, in part, the result of the systems of meaning that athletes, management, and consumers actively support or celebrate. Harmful aspects of sport are often viewed as integral components of play or training. Indeed, spectators at times take pleasure in the spectacle aspects of bodily harm (Dunning, 1999). Abusive training techniques or relationships between coaches and athletes reinforce hierarchies of power and/or the logic of high performance that pervade in a deeply politicized and commercialized sports process. The profound economic nexus of global sport notwithstanding, sport is governed primarily by structures of power, authority over meaning, value, and information, which emerged during the twentieth century. This has a direct influence on how athletes and fans relate to one another and how athletes conceive their own bodies.

This chapter explores some of the serious social problems extant in sport such as doping, injuries, and violence, exploring how such issues are in part a result of the ways that sport is organized and understood by participants, sport leaders, and spectators or consumers and how these issues are often interconnected. I argue that we must understand how athletes make choices about their behaviour and their participation in sport and how our model of sport—as it is historically constructed, culturally understood, and mostly preferred—contributes to these problems.

DOPING AND SPORT

Part of the twentieth-century fascination with sport for spectators, which continues in the twenty-first century, is the capacity of athletes to break the records of those who came before them. During the early portion of the 2006 Major League Baseball season, for example, the U.S. and Canadian media continued to follow the quest of San Francisco Giants hitter Barry Bonds to break Hank Aaron's career home-run record. Critics argue that Bonds does not represent a legitimate challenge to the records of Aaron and the legendary player Babe Ruth because, following the revelations of the Burlingame, California, Bay Area Laboratory Co-Operative (BALCO) drug scandal inquiry, Bonds was an alleged user. Other well-muscled, power-hitting baseball players such as Mark McGwire, Sammy Sosa, Jason Giambi, and Jose Canseco have created much excitement for fans, while at the same time raising the ire of baseball purists. Critics accept the fact that athlete nutrition, weight and exercise training, physiotherapy, and sports medicine support have changed markedly; the general physique of the latter-twentieth-century athlete has become an important part of sport iconography. But the use of so-called performance enhancers such as anabolic steroids and artificial stimulants has been widely rejected in the mainstream media. The use of drugs and supplements has been identified as unfair, unhealthy, and detrimental to sports competitions generally. It is important to note, however, that these criticisms speak more to how sport is promoted in society than to the sentiment of the general public. Indeed, Hoberman (2005) surmises that there is no homogeneity in public opinion on athlete doping. Although there is a significant following for the high-profile, American-based baseball leagues and players, Canadian athletes and spectators, too, have been more directly confronted by doping and performance enhancement.

On September 24, 1988, Canadian Ben Johnson reached the finish line of the men's 100-metre race at the Seoul Olympic Games in the record-breaking time of 9.79 seconds. This first Olympic sprinting victory since Percy Williams in 1928, and much-anticipated climax in Johnson's longstanding rivalry with the American sprinter Carl Lewis, signalled to Canadians that they could compete with the mighty American athletic giants. Prime Minister Brian Mulroney congratulated Johnson in a telephone call broadcast over national television, calling his performance a victory for Canada. Celebrations erupted across the country. Three days later, the International Olympic Committee (IOC) announced that Johnson had been stripped of his gold medal and record performance because he tested positive for a banned substance—stanozolol, an anabolic steroid. This story became a major world news happening, given that the men's 100-metre race had been the marquee spectator event at the Olympics since the celebrated photograph captured American Charlie Paddock's flying finish at Antwerp in 1920. In 1988, positive drug tests at elite sporting events were not new; however, the magnitude of Johnson's disgrace was exacerbated by a concerted media frenzy, in part generated by the newly corporatized Olympic Games and which reached billions of satellite television viewers, and in part due to the usual significant attention accorded to the world's fastest man. The shock was particularly felt in Canada, where the celebrations of fans, athletes, sports leaders, and politicians were quickly reduced to national embarrassment. Reactions were so severe that the Canadian media virtually disowned Johnson (Jackson, 1998b). The incident heightened a growing awareness that, worldwide, elite athletes took drugs to improve their performances. Canada responded with the comprehensive and lengthy Dubin Inquiry, commissioned by Prime Minister Mulroney, which eventually revealed that athletes routinely ingested banned substances to improve their performances. The Dubin Inquiry handed down 70 recommendations to deal with the issue of drugs in sport. For Canada, MacAloon (1990) concluded that the Inquiry was a matter of saving face for the Canadian government and the Canadian sport system. The Johnson doping incident and the Dubin Inquiry essentially placed Canadian athletes under the drug-testing microscope for some time.

Ben Johnson's positive test and public humiliation at the Olympic Games created a temporary crisis in sport beyond the borders of Canada—athletes and their handlers were employing a systematic regimen of ingesting drugs and masking agents to avoid detection. Yet why were people so concerned about preserving the sanctity of sport and special standards for athletes when, for decades, men and women of all ages had routinely ingested drugs for all sorts of physical ailments and improvements—to enhance performance at work, to sleep, to enhance social life, or to improve sexual performance (Kirkwood, 2004)? Canadians have consumed tobacco and alcohol regularly for centuries; caffeine consumption in the form of coffee, tea, and soft drinks is a normalized part of daily life for most Canadians. We live in a drug-taking society. People ingest vitamins, dietary supplements, protein shakes, and over-the-counter medications to improve their quality of life; musicians take beta-blockers for the calming effect. Why are we surprised or concerned that athletes take drugs to enable them to train harder or perform better? Hoberman (2005) asks, "[w]hy would a civilization bent on maximizing performances of various kinds require certain performers to exercise self-restraint?" (pp. 202–3). Although this issue is very complicated, there are typical explanations for our concerns with drugs: that sport was once drug-free and is now in a period of crisis; that drug consumption is harmful to athletes; that drugs challenge the notion of fair play in sport.

The Myth of Substance-Free Sport

Part of the crisis that performance-enhancing substances create for contemporary sport is that they place the integrity of athletic achievement in question (Hoberman, 1992). As mentioned previously, sport has been widely promoted and accepted as a moral and educative enterprise. Gaining advantage through the ingestion of drugs creates several problems within this paradigm: not everyone has access to or is willing to take drugs; drugs create "unnatural" physiological advantages and patterns of human growth; unsupervised doping creates health risks. Of course, each of these issues can be refuted by a simple critical analysis of the sports process itself. The access to material resources, expertise, facilities, and participation, for example, has historically prevented sport at all levels from existing on a level playing field. Athletes have always attempted to gain advantages through other technical means, including variations in equipment or even by taking shortcuts during races. "Corked" bats have been a problem in Major League Baseball; overly curved sticks and oversized goaltender equipment in hockey, the use of plasma on runners in bobsledding, and the clap skate and Fastskin swimsuit have also endured contentious introductions to sport competition.

A rather complicated point of departure on this issue of cheating is the broad assumption that sport competitions *used* to be fair and that performance enhancement is a recent phenomenon. In fact, the literature clearly demonstrates that athletes and handlers have looked for advantages in competition and in exercise recovery since the outset of international competition in the modern era, during the late nineteenth century and throughout the twentieth century; even in the ancient worlds of Greece and Rome some 2,000 years ago athletes adopted idiosyncratic diets and ingested substances thought to improve physical performance. Whether explicitly ingested for enhanced performance or to achieve particular results for scientific experiments, athletes once took doses of strychnine, brandy, cocaine, heroin, oxygen, testicular extracts, hormones, and, later, ultraviolet radiation (Hoberman, 1992), synthetic testosterone, and amphetamines (Hoberman, 2005). Further, in addition to the experimentation with doping and athletes in the immediate post–World War II era, politically inspired, state-sponsored, compulsory doping occurred in at least one nation, East Germany, between 1961 and 1988 (Spitzer, 2004). Techniques of performance enhancement are as old as sport itself (Todd & Todd, 2000).

As evident from some of the examples in Table 8.1, for more than a century athletes have ingested substances to provide competitive advantages. Doctors and trainers have convinced some, while others had no knowledge they were being doped. The factors behind this phenomenon are varied and complex: from simply seeking advantages to win for the symbolic or material value, to the obsessive Cold War nationalism of sporting nations, to the broader notions of bodily performance encouraged by science and medicine. Hoberman (2005) urges us to view the problem in its wider contexts: "while doping scandals invariably focus on individuals, doping is in fact a social practice that involves political institutions, international federations, professional networks, and powerful commercial interests—including corporate sponsors, media companies, pharmaceutical and supplement manufacturers, and the sports journalism business itself" (p. 237).

Table 8.1   Sport and Doping in the Modern Era*

1886	British cyclist Arthur Linton dies during a race. His death is attributed to drug use.
1904	Olympic marathon winner Thomas Hicks collapses at the finish line after trainers supposedly provided brandy, strychnine, and albumen.
1923	70-year-old John Pearson finishes second in the 50-yard dash at the San Quentin prison Thanksgiving Games, following the implant of a third testicle extracted from a deceased prisoner. It is reported that Olympic athletes are irradiated with ultraviolet light.
1930	Female athletes are given hormone treatments to delay menstruation before competition.
1945	Researcher Paul de Kruif publishes a study reporting that male subjects showed increased muscle mass following doses of testosterone.
1952	Soviet Olympic weightlifters use anabolic steroids.
1953	American weightlifting team physician John Zeigler observes the Soviets and returns home to begin testing the effects of testosterone on himself and American athletes.
1950s	Cyclists use amphetamines or "pep" pills.
1960	American Olympic weightlifters use steroids.
1960	Danish cyclist Knud Jensen collapses during a road race due to the use of a stimulant, fractures his skull, and becomes the first Olympic athlete since 1912 to die in competition.
1960	IOC establishes first Medical Committee.
1967	IOC develops regulations for athlete testing and a list of banned substances.
1967	British cyclist Tommy Simpson dies during the Tour de France from complications due to amphetamine ingestion.
1968	IOC Medical Committee introduces urine testing at the Olympic Games.
1968	Soccer player Jean-Louis Quadri and cyclist Yves Mottin die from complications due to amphetamine ingestion.
1972	American swimmer Rick DeMont tests positive for ephedrine at the Munich Olympic Games and is disqualified.
1975	European Cup Track and Field tests athletes for steroids.
1976	East German women's swimming team cited by the media for muscle size and deep voices.
1976	Seven male weightlifters and one female field athlete test positive in Montreal.
1983	15 athletes at the Pan American Games test positive.
1984	Olympic pre-testing reveals 86 positive tests on United States athletes prior to the Los Angeles Olympics.
1987	Blood doping scientifically reported to enhance aerobic potential.
1988	First anti-doping conference held in Canada.
1988	Ben Johnson tests positive in Seoul.
1989	A United States study reports that 6.6 percent of high school males use steroids for athletic enhancement and personal appearance.
1989	Canada's Dubin Inquiry begins.
1990	IOC reports that during 1988, 1,150 Olympic-sport athletes tested positive for banned substances.
1991	*Sports Illustrated* publishes the story of NFL star Lyle Alzado, who is dying of lymphoma he believes is directly attributable to his steroid use.
1997	Olympic swimming champion Michelle Smith tests positive.
1998	Canadian snowboarder Ross Rebagliati tests positive for marijuana.
1998	Mark McGwire breaks Roger Maris's home-run record in a race with Sammy Sosa—both are accused of using steroids.
1999	Supplies of EPO are found during the Tour de France and an investigation leads to evidence of widespread doping in cycling.
2002	Blood doping equipment and syringes found in Salt Lake City at Olympic residence.
2004	Greek sprinters Kostas Kenteris and Katerina Thanou miss drug tests at the Athens Games.
2005	BALCO drug-supply scandal.
2006	Barry Bonds chases the home-run record amid accusations of drug use.
2006	Tour de France winner Floyd Landis tests positive for synthetic testosterone and is disqualified.

* See also Hoberman, 1992; Kirkwood, 2004; and Todd & Todd, 2000.

HEALTH AND SPORT

The current organization with responsibility for Olympic athlete testing, established in 1999 and with headquarters in Montreal, has its own rationale for a concerted campaign against doping in all sports. The World Anti-Doping Agency (WADA) cites a number of reasons to eradicate doping in sport:

> Doping in sport is the complete antithesis of the Spirit of Sport. Doping destroys all that is good and noble about sport. Doping jeopardizes the health and well-being of athletes and erodes public confidence. In addition to risking serious health consequences, athletes who test positive for doping ruin their good name and reputation, and may lose their employment. (WADA, 2003)

With respect to the issue of doping and health, certainly Hoberman's (1992) brief description of the death of West German heptathlete Birgit Dressel and NFL football player Lyle Alzado's descriptions of his steroid-induced symptoms are horrific. Even more graphic is the plight of bodybuilder Gregg Valentino, whose misuse of steroid and synthol injections is captured in the Learning Channel documentary *The Man Whose Arms Exploded* (see photographs on his website: http://greggvalentino.net/). Valentino's already muscular arms reached enormous proportions after six years of injections, until a serious infection led to his hospitalization. Such cases represent a long-term abuse of performance-enhancing substances leading to serious health problems—even death. However, the results of some studies are ambiguous on the health risks of steroids and even suggest that low doses in controlled circumstances present minimal risks (Schneider & Butcher, 2001). Part of the problem is a matter of evidence, in that long-term studies examining the health of former steroid-using athletes have not been conducted and that current evidence is anecdotal. Others report that steroid usage significantly increases the risk of contracting some 50 diseases and physical disorders (Kirkwood, 2004). The literature is also not clear on the behavioural effects of steroid consumption. It has long been suggested, for example, that steroids make people aggressive or anti-social. However, Kirkwood (2004) suggests that we need to pay more attention to what attracts people to drugs, what problems they seek to address by using steroids, and what roles the media play in influencing our perceptions about performance, size, and aging.

WADA contends explicitly that sport is noble and healthy without doping. A critical analysis of these assumptions raises questions about how sport is promoted in broader political projects and through the media. There is ample evidence to show, for example, that sport is not a healthy enterprise, particularly when played or experienced at elite levels or at extreme levels in non-competitive settings. Since full-time, systematic, scientifically supported training was introduced during the early Cold War period athletes have spent inordinate amounts of time training, and a now–taken for granted network of training and rehabilitation infrastructure supports them. Sport became a full-time enterprise during the mid-twentieth century. Athletes in most elite sports place extreme levels of stress on their bodies, as much as they can handle physiologically and psychologically. Teams of trainers, coaches, physiologists, physical therapists, and doctors routinely ensure that athletes are training at maximum capacities. Moreover, similar to other high-risk occupations, muscle tears, bone fractures, acute and chronic pain, and injuries are routine, if not expected, in sport. Once studied purely for its positive contributions to society and to the promotion of exercise, sport is now being assessed by scholars for the physiological and social consequences of athletic injuries (Young, 2004). There is ample evidence to suggest that injuries, pain, and suffering are a naturalized part of modern sport; further, studies show that there are subcultural values within sports that celebrate athletes' ability to endure pain, and that athletes, managers, and coaches routinely expect players to play through injuries and significant pain. As a result, athlete peer groups understand their injuries as badges of courage and dedication and expect their teammates to share cavalier attitudes about risk and safety in sport (White & Young 1999a; Young, White, & McTeer, 1994). Young, White, and McTeer (1994) found that in 20 sports, including both the traditionally rough football and hockey and others such as skiing and squash, athletes preferred to conceal their pain. These researchers conclude the pressure from coaches, parents, and peers to play through injury is ubiquitous throughout sporting culture as represented in a particularly telling memory from one athlete:

> With my femur, I remember vividly just going up the wall and kind of having my head down and getting hit from the side. I know it was my left leg and all I felt was my left leg wrapping around my right leg. Then I fell down. I tried not to show pain and lay there on the ice. I was trying to get up and I remember just falling back down again. And then I remember the coach coming up and trying to help me up and he said, "Come on you can get up," "You're tough," or whatever, and just trying to stand on it, but there was no way. I remember my dad even giving me shit. Even going through the dressing room no one would help me take my equipment off. And we were in a small town and there was no stretcher, so I had to get put in the back of our van and taken to the nearest hospital. (p. 185)

Other standards and pressures to conform within the logic of twentieth- and now twenty-first-century sport include the alteration of body weight, shape, and appearance. The alteration of muscle size and rates of recovery, through doping, to enhance training abilities and to achieve greater performance results parallels widespread modifications in form and body composition to attain more biomechanically efficient and aesthetically pleasing athletic bodies through long-term dietary restrictions and the phenomenon of "making weight" immediately before competitions. Both behaviours, evident in gymnastics and bodybuilding in the first instance, and in wrestling, boxing, and rowing in the second (Johns, 2004), represent serious health risks to athletes. While it is clearly evident that the qualitative or judged sports, such as gymnastics, have changed markedly—introducing child athletes at the highest competitive levels where fully grown women once competed—the social problems accompanying such changes, including eating and body-image disorders, can not be completely attributed to an aesthetic imperative. Davis (1999) argues that while body-image standards and cultural ideals are important factors in explaining compulsive exercising and eating disorders, we must also consider other issues, including family dynamics and the interplay among personality, addiction, and obsessive behaviour. Sport is not always a healthy enterprise.

The above-mentioned social problems demonstrate both a connection to broader cultural values of performance, appearance, and the use of science and technology to alter human performance and a specific logic of behaviour that exists, internally, within modern sport. Athletes and coaches understand the normative codes of behaviour in sport—whether positive or negative, healthy or destructive—and generally operate within those codes to achieve success. Fighting or rough play in hockey, for example, has a long history and is generally understood and accepted as being part of the game. Yet on the street outside the arena participants in a fight would most likely be charged with assault. Norms in sport change and differ among sports. Fighting in women's hockey is no longer common. Fighting and violent behaviour is not as common in soccer as it is in hockey. Consequently, when Zinedine Zidane head butted Marco Materazzi in the 2006 World Cup, the incident generated tremendous media attention.

As studies by Young (1993) and Nixon (1996) demonstrate, athletes are aware of how they can be exploited by the media or sport owners and there appears to be a certain degree of ambivalence on the part of athletes toward bodily harm and the risks that they are willing to take (Donnelly, 2004). It is evident, however, that in some sports harm and risk are more actively promoted and celebrated by participants, coaches, and spectators.

VIOLENCE AND SPORT

On March 8, 2004, Vancouver Canucks power forward Todd Bertuzzi attacked the Colorado Avalanche's Steve Moore in retaliation for a hit on Canucks star Markus Naslund three weeks earlier. As evident in the newspaper reports, some fans understood very clearly that retaliation was in order. Bertuzzi's blindside punch crumpled Moore to the ice and left him with three broken vertebrae and a severe concussion. Moore did not return to hockey for the 2005–06 season. Bertuzzi was charged with assault, pled guilty, and received a conditional discharge, one year of probation, and 80 hours of community service. Moore followed up with a civil suit against Bertuzzi. Several months later, the Canadian Olympic Committee announced that it had approved the men's hockey roster for the Torino Olympic Games. Bertuzzi's inclusion on the roster ignited some debate in Canadian newspapers: some in support of Bertuzzi, some against him, and others arguing that his level of talent was at issue and not the incident of violence (Dalla Costa, 2006). Evidently, from a sampling of various Internet blog sites, Bertuzzi has many supporters among hockey fans. It was understood, they suggested, that there should have been retaliation for Moore's actions against Naslund and that Moore should have fought Bertuzzi. The National Hockey League (NHL) suspended Bertuzzi for 12 games and the remainder of the playoffs but reinstated him for the following season. Four years earlier, longtime enforcer Marty McSorley slashed Vancouver's Donald Brashear in the temple, causing him to lose consciousness before he struck his head on the ice. McSorley was found guilty of assault and sentenced to 18 months' probation. There is a long list of violent infractions in

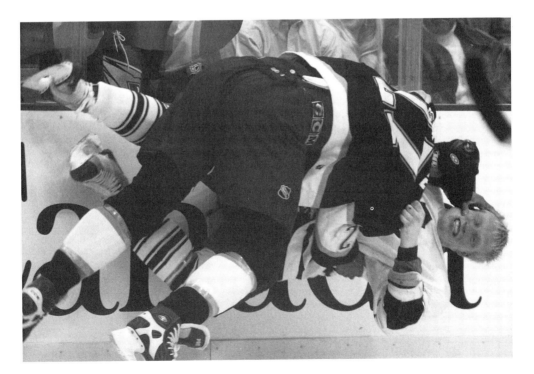

Another social problem in sport that gets media attention is violence.

KEVIN FRAYER/CP Images

professional hockey, extending back some 100 years. Recently, scholars have begun to raise questions about the legitimization of violence in sport (Atkinson, 2007; Smith, 1983; Young, 1991, 2002), attempting to explain why violence is so readily accepted in some sports—why, generally speaking, people have long thought that the courts have no place in sport, and how discourse about victimization is effectively neutralized. In short, levels of aggression and violence in sport have historically been tolerated, and these cultural attitudes toward aggressive masculinities expressed through sport help to frame our understandings of such incidents (Atkinson, 2007).

Violence has also spilled out into the stands and into arenas. In July 2001, Thomas Junta, a hockey parent, beat coach Michael Costin to death in a rink in Massachusetts. In January 2002, he was sentenced to a prison term to extend from six to ten years. Once again, the issue of violence in sport was inscribed across the news and sports pages in North America. For more than 100 years—a period coined the "modern age" of sport (Guttman, 1978)—participants, coaches, and spectators have been killed, maimed, and injured in rings, arenas, fields, and bleachers. In most instances of significant harm, whether one player sustains a catastrophic injury or several hundred fans are crushed or engaged in a brawl, journalists, academics, judicial critics, and average citizens alike ask the question Why did this happen—or, perhaps implicitly, Why is there violence in sport? Then, it seems, the question is muted until the next incident. Further, the average sports fan is likely to defend fighting in hockey, the crunching tackle in football, or the sport of boxing itself. For the entire twentieth century and now into the twenty-first, we have accepted that in sports where space is contested, where bodies are used as weapons (Messner, 1990) to gain ground or maintain control of a ball or puck, athletes can be hurt or injured (Young, White, & McTeer, 1994)—and that such physical confrontations are a necessary and exciting feature of sports. Athletes enjoy the physical contact, the violent hits and tackles; spectators seem to enjoy the body checks and fights; and television networks sometimes focus on the best hits of the week, regardless of or even particular to the physical harm experienced by the player.

With this and the historical tradition of rough sport in mind, the legitimizing functions of legal procedure generally, and the intellectual analysis of human behaviour in sport, have dichotomized such actions as violent or aggressive, unacceptable or acceptable, part of the game or not part of the game, and consensual or not consensual. As such there are different accepted norms for different sports, degrees of harm, and assertiveness—a blurring of the distinction between a measure of physical intimidation and an act of violence. Through sport, violence has been contextualized. How can we explain why violence and aggression are considered important parts of sport, often celebrated, often respected?

The popular use of "aggression" in sport suggests that it is a positive channelling of emotional and physical energy or intensity toward a legitimate goal. However, Smith (1983) and Coakley (2004) use the term aggression in reference to some behaviour designed to cause physical or psychological harm. But all forms of aggression are not harmful. Smith (1983) and Coakley (2004) categorize violence as all types of physical aggression intended to harm or injure others. It follows, then, that all violence is aggressive but some forms of aggression are used to intimidate opponents and not to cause harm.

A popular view, held by athletes and spectators alike, is that violence can be attributed strictly to human biology or *instinct*. It is argued that humans respond violently when they are confronted by particular situations, and that this type of response is programmed by evolution and the need to survive as a species. Often such a response can be labelled the "fight or flight" reaction to confrontation. Ethologists or scientists who justify human behaviour using purely biological explanations have forwarded these hypotheses, used to explain why people behave violently on or off the field. It is instinctual, they argue, for people to react violently during confrontations, such as those created through sport between opponents or between fans in the stadium and arena. Supposedly, sport provides an outlet or release for these natural tendencies toward aggression, a *catharsis* effect. In support of this theory, one would argue that tensions naturally build between two hockey players or two fans that confront one another during a game. Finally, tensions run so high that the two players or spectators decide to fight, thereby releasing these energies "safely" (Lorenz, 1966). These models purport, then, that sport becomes a *safety valve* for unhealthy aggression (Pearton, 1986). It is easy for individuals with an interest in sustaining levels of violence in sport to ensure popularity and profit, for example, to justify fighting and rough play by calling it a basic human instinct. However, there is no evidence to support this theory of aggression in human beings. Indeed, and as Dunning (1999) has concluded, sport provides the conditions for such outbursts; further, sport creates tensions.

A second theory often employed to explain violent confrontations in sport or even to provide solutions to broader social problems is the *frustration-aggression* hypothesis. It is argued that frustration in particular circumstances causes aggression. Once again, according to this model, players or fans supposedly release pent up frustration through participation in sport or through vicarious consumption from the bleachers. Sport, this theory suggests, is *cathartic* for spectators, channelling frustrations from their daily lives into harmless aggression toward opposing teams or other spectators (Dollard et al., 1939). Pearton (1986) argues that the frustration-aggression hypothesis loses much of its explanatory power because frustration is but one of a long list of factors that can lead to aggression. Sometimes aggression occurs without frustration; and, sport can cause frustration for participants, particularly if winning is equated to self-esteem or proving oneself (Coakley, 2004). Consequently, sport is not necessarily or simply an appropriate tool of emotional control, particularly when some groups and individuals find it fun and exciting (Dunning, 1999).

Advocates of the *social learning* theory (Bandura & Walters, 1963) argue that violence and aggression are behaviours people have come to understand through social relationships with others, by imitation, or learned from cultural exemplars—sport heroes, for example—or significant others. It follows, then, according to this model, that violence has a cultural history, that certain values are passed down through generations, and that various institutions, symbols, and structures of meaning reproduce or endorse aggression or aggressive tactics to achieve goals (see Box 8.1). Violence and aggression become means to attain certain ends. In some sports, according to this theory, rule-bound aggression is built in to the common cultural understandings of how they should be played and, historically, these sports leagues have been able to operate outside of the law to police themselves (Young & Wamsley, 1996). Frustration over the outcomes of games, the calls of officials, or the tactics of opposing players may lead to forms of aggression, some of which have been normalized as reasonable if not desirable behaviours— in other words, the actions of passionate athletes who care intensely about sport, the outcome of a significant championship, or standing up for a teammate. As such, the channelling of anger into ritualized confrontations, such as berating an official, has come to be naturalized within a sporting context, whereas this behaviour might not be tolerated outside of the sporting context. It is commonly asserted that certain forms of aggression on the playing field would bring criminal charges on the street.

Cultural Understandings of Violence

From the earliest eras of Aboriginal games, to the colonial period in North America, to the emerging sports of the period of the industrial revolution in the nineteenth century, violence and aggressive behaviours have always been present in various cultural forms. Physical capacity and competition were fundamental aspects of the fur trade and early agrarian economies, when

---

Box 8.1   Violence in Sport or Violence as Sport?

An alternative approach or quite different point of departure with respect to the issue of violence, distinguishing between the instrumental or goal-oriented violence commonly associated with the middle classes and their rationalized sports of the mid-nineteenth century and expressive violence or violence for pleasure, is discussed by Elias and Dunning (1986), among others (Dunning, 1999). Conley's (1999) research on fighting in nineteenth-century Ireland supports such a distinction, as does recent work on tavern culture in nineteenth-century Canada (Wamsley & Kossuth, 2001). The historical evidence in these studies suggests that understanding violence *as* sport is as important as the more frequently employed paradigm of violence *in* sport. Indeed, Conley's (1999, p. 57) citation of nineteenth-century author William Carleton (1867) is quite similar to the context frequently invoked in the current journalistic support for fighting in hockey:

> I know not however whether it was fair to expect them to give up at once the agreeable recreation of fighting. It's not easy to abolish old customs, particularly diversions; and everyone knows that this is the national amusement of the finest peasantry on the face of the earth. To be sure skulls and bones are broken, and lives lost; but they are lost in pleasant fighting—they are the consequences of the sport, the beauty of which consists in breaking as many heads and necks as you can.

men routinely tested one another for fun but more seriously while competing for labour opportunities (Wamsley, 1999). In Canada prior to the 1840s, a violent code of honour was meted out in the relationships between the self-fashioned male gentry (Morgan, 1995), and men of all classes routinely fought in the rural and urban taverns and public houses (Wamsley & Kossuth, 2001). The violence of the duel and of the public hangings, stockades, and whipping posts was reshaped in pre-Confederation Canada into institutional punishments and fines, and controlled, ritualized aggression became ensconced in organized sports by moderate political reformers who saw themselves as more civilized and rational than their predecessors in government office. In this social environment, the sons of elites were taught to be the leaders of the empire through rites of passage that often entailed measures of hardship, endurance, and violent contests (Brown, 1986). Middle-class men celebrated a public profile of physical empowerment through club sports such as lacrosse and snowshoeing, and later hockey and other sports. Through sport, masculinity was tested through an on-field, rule-bound aggression where participants and spectators came to associate the male body with power and authority, tempered by the values of Christianity and a code of fair play. Sports were viewed as rough and vigorous, a place for men.

Spectator interest in baseball and hockey piqued the interest of commercial entrepreneurs, who sought gate receipts and captivating local interest in sport for profit. Moral entrepreneurs, including instructors at YMCAs, were interested in using sport to shape the character of young Christian men; the sports promoter looked for ways to bring "respectable" citizens out to watch what were formally considered to be rough sports. Promoters and participants tended to create narratives about the modern, scientific, and highly technical aspects of their sports—boxing in particular—to attract a broader base of spectatorship (Wamsley & Whitson, 1998). By the turn of the century, organized sports such as hockey had been imbued with unique social trajectories, creating a self-contained sport subculture with norms, values, and rules that became relatively insular from legal and moral challenges registered from the "outside." Aggression and violence were accepted as being an important part of manly sports. Commenting on the issue of violence in boxing, and sport more broadly, Judge Snider in 1911 argued:

> It will be a long time before Parliament will think it wise to so hedge in young men and boys by legislation that all sports that are rough and strenuous or even dangerous must be given up. Virility in young men would soon be lessened and self-reliant manliness a thing of the past. (Wamsley & Whitson, 1998, p. 426)

Communities supported town teams and the character and tactics employed to gain victory; in order to compete with other towns, team owners and town boosters attempted to build local support by hiring the best players available from outside of the community. The enthusiasm and rivalries promoted through hockey and other sports sometimes led to fan aggression and incidents of violence during the early twentieth century (Gruneau & Whitson, 1993; Young & Wamsley, 1996).

Following both World Wars, thousands of men returned home after witnessing and surviving the horrors of war violence, killing other human beings, and trying to rationalize why people were dying painful deaths around them; it was no coincidence that the sports of boxing and wrestling were very popular in these eras, and that rough versions of masculinity were celebrated through rugby, football, and ice hockey.

During the 1930s, 40s, and 50s, radio broadcasts brought sanitized but exciting commentaries to living rooms. However, the popularization of television in the 1960s brought clear visions of aggressive and exciting play to most households in Canada. And town boosterism, capitalizing on performance and local spirit with respect to all levels of sport, was well entrenched (Gruneau & Whitson, 1993). On the margins of amateur and professional sports, professional wrestling and roller derby, theatres of violence and hyper-masculinity complete with villains and heroes, began to grow in popularity as well. After Hockey Night in Canada on Saturday nights, parents and children could tune in to All Star Wrestling to watch former Canadian Football League player, self-professed "Canada's Greatest Athlete" Gene Kiniski, as he battled make-believe villains such as "The Sheik" or "Abdullah the Butcher," supposedly from the Middle East, or "Siegfried Stanke," who sported German officer's boots and a Nazi flag. On Saturday afternoons, children could watch Paul "The Bear" Rupert and "Skinny Minny" Miller deliver punches and elbows and mock violence on the roller rink.

When second-wave feminism had made some social and political gains by the early 1970s, contends Nelson (1994), men sought solidarity and assurance through watching and admiring violent sports. Leagues such as the NFL and NHL did little to curtail aggression and violence. Indeed, the expansion hockey teams of the late 1960s and early 1970s used physical intimidation and violent tactics to offset the skill imbalance created among NHL teams as a result of league expansion. Further, this type of intimidation—and frequent fisticuffs during games—marked an era in professional hockey during which certain teams, such as the Philadelphia Flyers or "Broad Street Bullies" and "Big Bad Bruins," capitalized upon the media reputations created by them, for them, to gain respect on the ice. Specialized sport television, such as the American Broadcasting Corporation's *Wide World of Sports*, capitalized on exciting highlight packages, violent tackles, and body checks, dramatizing rough play and reinforcing the dangers and excitement of sports for men. Historical traditions, tactics, techniques, and long-accepted codes of physical manhood were punctuated in elaborate and systematic fashion by sport television. Such media representations of violent but revered masculinities were powerful endorsements of appropriate manhood. And owners, league administrators, coaches, and players were all too willing to capitalize on the popularity of aggressive sports, in spite of any risks of injury, pain, or physical and psychological impairment to the athletes involved. The athletes had to embrace these values wholeheartedly, lest

Table 8.2   Some Examples of Sport Violence*

1905–82	Sixty-six cases of assault charges in hockey
1905	Allan Loney strikes and kills Alcide Laurin with his hockey stick
1907	Charles Masson strikes Owen "Bud" McCourt over the head with his hockey stick; McCourt dies
1913	Arthur Pelkey delivers a punch to Luther McCarty in the White Heavyweight boxing championship in Calgary, killing him.
1933	Hockey player Eddie Shore hits Ace Bailey from behind, causing him to hit his head on the ice; Bailey does not play again
1955	Hockey player Maurice "Rocket" Richard suspended for hitting Hal Laycoe and the intervening linesman
1969	Hockey player Wayne Maki retaliates against Ted Green by slashing him in the head with his stick, causing brain haemorrhaging and concussion
1975	Hockey player Dan Maloney attacks Brian Glennie; Maloney charged with assault but acquitted
1977	NBA player Kermit Washington punches Rudy Tomjanovich, breaking his nose and jaw and causing a skull fracture and concussion
1982	Hockey enforcer Jimmy Mann fined $500 and given a suspended sentence after being charged with assault for hitting Paul Gardner, breaking his jaw in two places
1987	NHL enforcer Dave Brown crosschecks Tomas Sandstrom in the face and breaks his jaw
1988	Dino Cicarelli convicted of assault on Luke Richardson; spends one day in jail and is fined $1,000
1997	Boxer Mike Tyson bites off part of Evander Holyfield's ear during a heavyweight title match

* See also Young & Wamsley, 1996.
Source: Reprinted with permission of CAHPERD.

they be left in the minor leagues or forced into another line of work. Table 8.2 highlights some of the major infractions of sport violence.

The celebration of violence and intimidation in sport, endorsed through media representations and league administration, had deep ramifications for all levels from early children's participation through the junior ranks. Codes of conduct for all participants were well understood, from the "good" penalty to the "necessary" fight to stand up for a teammate or just to inspire play to gain team momentum. However, a fundamental corollary to these extensive and rather complex codes of masculine conduct has been the tendency to endure and even celebrate pain and injury as a rite of passage and part of being a man in a men's sport. Men who grew up playing sport in the 1970s and 1980s have been told to "suck it up" and "be a man," or have been accused of playing like girls or old women. Sporting goods giant Nike has featured ad campaigns to counteract the "throw like a girl" mythologies in order to expand its market in women's sport and exercise. The bipolar association of male weakness or frailty with femininity has been a feature of organized sport for more than a century. As a consequence, and as discussed above, participants in sport have tended toward positioning bodily injuries as badges of male courage at all levels. Being tough and tolerant or resistant to pain has been normalized in most sports. However, research suggests that female athletes view the pain and sport injury nexus in a similar light. Young & White (1995) found similarities in the attitudes of male and female athletes with respect to physical danger, aggression, and injury.

At the elite levels, Young (1993) concludes that sports have become hazardous work-places, where profit, socially recognized and celebrated, comes at significant cost, "in the form of compromised health and safety standards, or, in other words, injury, disablement, and human loss" (p. 390). Day to day pain and injury, disabled lists, injury-reserve lists, team doctors and physiotherapists, drugs, therapeutic medicines and techniques, massage tables, hot tubs, and ice packs are all part of the emotional or technical inventories of most sport teams. More broadly, falls, hits, and catastrophic injuries are the mainstays of highlights packages for specialized sport channels and even "news" stories on network television. Scenes of broken legs in football, such as Joe Theisman's; knockout punches at the hands of Mike Tyson or even ring deaths in boxing; hard slides and bean balls in baseball; blood-letting, lost teeth, broken bones, and concussion-causing body checks in hockey, such as those on Eric Lindros; cartwheeling, ragdoll spills in alpine skiing, such as Todd Brooker's; end-over-end or wall-smashing car crashes and deaths, such as Dale Earnhardt's in NASCAR auto-racing or Ayrton Senna's in Formula One racing; jockey and horse spills in horse racing; stomping and raking in rugby; torn muscles in sprinting and weightlifting; severe crashes in cycling; or mishaps such as heads hitting diving boards, such as Greg Louganis's did in diving—all are replayed over and over for popular consumption. Often the catastrophic damage done to human bodies is presented as news; recently, however, a market has developed for the sports "blooper," where suffering is often invoked as having comedic value. Entire videotaped volumes are dedicated to violent highlights in the context of a comedy of physical wonders, such as Don Cherry's *Rock 'em Sock 'em Hockey*, now beyond 16 editions.

In this era of widespread, edited, graphically represented violence, professional wrestling and other forms of sport entertainment, such as ultimate fighting, have captured significant market followings. Sports entertainment entrepreneur Vince McMahon has parlayed his father's business into the multimillion-dollar World Wrestling Entertainment (WWE) extravaganza, which reaches from weekly television, to pay-per-view events, to music recordings, wrestler fashions, movie character spin-offs, magazines, product lines, video games, and children's clubs and cartoons. Professional wrestling sells violent sport theatre to millions of viewers. Older gimmicks of staged, severe facial bleeding, chair throwing, and "foreign object" wielding have given way to more complex plot lines, steroid-induced hyper-muscular figures, "giants" and "little people," and elaborate technical displays of lighting and fireworks in staged matches that often have real consequences such as severe injuries—foremost the death of Calgary wrestler Owen Hart, who fell 15 metres before a match when a poorly choreographed stunt went sour.

Professional wrestling remains an extant caricature of many of the worst qualities of sport, bodybuilding, Hollywood acting, and beauty pageantry. Yet, such caricatures are a chilling reminder of some of the common features of modern sport: violent plotlines, overtraining and hyper-muscularity, anger and suffering, drug taking, and the reproduction of gender stereotypes (Atkinson, 2002). It could be easily dismissed as pure entertainment if not for its significant place in popular culture as part of a much broader constellation of actively created social meanings about human bodies utilized as weapons that are reproduced day-to-day for both spectators and participants through sport and sport theatre.

Youth Sport and Violence

Violent and aggressive altercations at children's sporting events are all too common. While coaching education programs deal explicitly with the issue of winning and the use of aggressive play and tactics of intimidation, there are few programs that deal with issues of parent aggression against officials and against one another. This ranges from berating a referee for a particular call to committing violent acts over game outcomes. The incidents of assault on referees have become so common that the National Association of Sports Officials now provides assault insurance for officials (Albom, 2000). On the heels of the Junta–Costin incident, there have been numerous examples of violence and aggressive acts by parents and coaches in North America. Fathers have struck other fathers during baseball games; full-scale brawls involving both players and parents have ensued during youth football games; Little League managers have been beaten up by irate parents; young players and young referees have been assaulted during and after baseball, hockey, football, and soccer games. The consequences of such assaults have ranged from punch abrasions to facial lacerations to broken jaws. Athletes in the highest leagues of competitive sport serve as exemplars of appropriate behaviour with respect to technique, performance, attitude, and codes of conduct. Further, the sort of behaviour tolerated by officials, league administrators, and team owners—and the media conglomerates which, in many instances, reinforce these subcultural values—serves to inform the public about normative behaviours in sport. The junior hockey leagues in Canada, for example, tend to follow rule changes and behavioural initiatives of the NHL. This is not to suggest that children view hockey fights on television and immediately fight as a direct consequence. However, it is reasonable to assert that the behaviours of well-respected players are closely watched and, from the previous evidence cited, that athlete behaviours are often defended even if they would be criminalized in other settings. Hockey Canada has attempted to deal with such incidents through a broad-based ad campaign targeting parent behaviour that outlines inappropriate conduct.

Spectator Violence

Many Canadians are familiar with the famous Maurice "Rocket" Richard riots of 1955, during which significant property was destroyed, looting occurred, and many were arrested in the streets of Montreal. Rioting and property destruction was similar in 1994 in Vancouver and most recently in 2006 in Edmonton, both during the Stanley Cup playoffs. Five people were charged in Edmonton after setting fires, destroying property, and facing off against police ("Edmonton Police, Mayor . . . ," 2006). Although these and most of the above examples are particular to the United States and Canada, fan violence is considered to be an international phenomenon. Young (1991) has analyzed several explanations for collective violence, including British soccer hooliganism. He offers examples (p. 540) of crowd violence including:

- a soccer riot in Peru, where 300 died and 500 were injured following a disallowed goal;
- a "Nickel Beer Night" in Cleveland, Ohio, when fans fired objects at players and umpires;
- a World Cup cricket match in Sydney, Australia, when 80 fans were arrested and jailed;
- a soccer match in Juventus, Italy, when 39 soccer fans were crushed to death after Liverpool, England fans charged the seating area;
- a riot in Hamilton, Ontario, when 3,000 fans destroyed significant property after a Grey Cup victory.

Young (1991) calls for a careful consideration of many factors to explain this phenomenon. He concludes,

> Collective crowd disorders at sports events are extremely complex, varied, and often highly organized rather than spontaneous phenomena, and attempts to explain their occurrence must be based on historically-grounded interpretations of, among other factors, social structure, class, politics, and gender. (p. 542)

Both Young (1991) and Dunning (1999) point to unique historical circumstances and political contexts and explicit political reactions to hooliganism and crowd violence, whether in Europe or North America, as being vital considerations to any understanding of collective behaviour, or fan aggression more specifically. The social origins of spectator violence, Dunning argues, are to be found in what he refers to as the social, political, and economic "fault-lines" or points of tension in each country, be they religious, ethnic, or related to social class or language. Young's call for historically grounded interpretations is particularly important. The Richard riots, for example, cannot be explained merely in terms of specific crowd behaviour. They were deeply rooted in extant historical tensions between French and English communities, manifested through political, economic, and religious relations between diverse populations. Some determinants such as longstanding political policies of assimilation were clearly evident, while the response of individuals during the riots was significantly different.

As Murphy et al. (1990) have suggested, there are many factors that may come to bear on spectator behaviour during sporting events, including alcohol consumption, the social significance of the event, the historical importance of rivalry between teams or towns, the type of crowd management techniques and infrastructure employed by stadium organizers, and the type of sport being played. As Coakley (2004) has argued, crowd behaviour tends to be sport-specific with respect to disruptions and emotional eruption, but watching contact sports does not necessarily lead to violent actions by spectators. North American hockey is far more violent than soccer in Europe, but this is not a good indicator of the potential for crowd violence. Indeed, the subcultural organization of soccer fans is significantly different than for hockey or American football. The outcome of important games or championships is also not a good indicator or predicting factor. Rioting or crowd violence may occur during the celebration of victory, during losses, or without respect to outcome. In this sense, sport managers and promoters must be aware of the historical and social specificity of each event, the meanings attached to the sport itself, the extant rivalries between teams, and the potential for violence when emotionally charged spectators congregate in significant numbers.

Biologically based theories do not adequately explain the problem of violence in modern sport. To suggest that human instinct is the primary factor in determining behavioural outcomes in volatile social situations is to ignore the historical context of aggression and the culturally approved and endorsed methods of dealing with confrontation both on and off the field. Research suggests that complex social and historical factors intertwine to produce a sporting culture through which ritualized aggression is normalized and psychological and physical intimidation is wielded as a strategy to achieve desired goals in sport, sometimes with violent outcomes. As a result, during and since the twentieth century, some professional sports arenas have become dangerous workplaces where pain, chronic and catastrophic injuries, and unhealthy training patterns are not only commonplace but also routinely celebrated as being appropriately masculine and team-oriented environments. A significant and disturbing corollary to the widespread spectatorship and conspicuous consumption of violence-oriented sports and sport spectacle entertainment is the prevalence of violent incidents involving youth sport in North America.

Violence has a long history in organized sport embedded in exemplary masculinities (now some femininities), and that interested parties such as owners, fans, and participants have been reluctant to seriously address issues of aggression, violence, pain, and injury. However, it appears as though there are more popular concerns about violence and aggression in youth and children's sports. Coaching education programs have been established in Canada, for example, to deal with issues of competitiveness, aggression, fair play, and appropriate conduct on and off the field. If coaches and administrators sincerely adopt an athlete-centred philosophy of coaching, one that places full emphasis on a balanced approach to athlete development, health, and well being, then at least a part of the competitive environment for youth sports will have some checks and balances. However, the issue of aggression and violence in professional and elite sports will remain until the very culture of sport changes: how it is understood, watched, and appreciated. If Dunning (1999) is correct in his assertions that organized sport is a rationalization for violence, then the changes to sport will indeed have to be significant.

CONCLUSIONS

Certainly, it must be recognized that athletes make choices in sport: whether to take drugs; to play through pain and injuries; to restrict dietary intake or ingest supplements; or to act violently against opponents. The literature suggests that spectators are ambivalent about their opposition to doping or, in the case of some aspects of violence, defend its place in some sports and enjoy the spectacle of aggression, whether ritualized or spontaneous. The way that sport has been historically constructed and how it is currently organized and celebrated has a direct bearing on values extant in the sports process. A pervasive win-at-all-costs approach to participating in and watching sport has created and sustained significant pressures on athletes. Further, the commercialization of Olympic and formerly amateur sports and the prevalence of the corporately modelled professional leagues have directly influenced the way athletes play sports, how they treat their own bodies, and how they relate to their opponents. In order to understand social problems in sport as researchers, we must continue to explore unique subcultural values, behaviours, and codes of conduct, and to beware of simple and singular causal explanations but also to recognize and study the connections of these values to broader political, economic, and social issues.

CRITICAL THINKING QUESTIONS

1. Is athlete doping any different than the day-to-day consumption of stimulants and medications?
2. Should athletes and sports leagues be permitted to police themselves or should the law intervene?
3. Anti-doping measures don't appear to be removing the urge to cheat. Should we permit medically supervised doping?
4. When should violence in sport be a concern?
5. Should Todd Bertuzzi have been considered for the Canadian Olympic team?

SUGGESTED READINGS

Coakley, J. (2004). *Sport in society: Issues and controversies*, 8th ed. St. Louis, MO: Mosby.

Dunning, E. (1999). *Sport matters: Sociological studies of sport, violence and civilization*. London: Routledge.

Gruneau, R., & Whitson, D. (1993). *Hockey Night in Canada: Sport, identities and cultural politics*. Toronto: Garamond Press.

Hoberman, J. (1992). *Mortal engines: The science of performance and the dehumanization of sport*. New York: The Free Press.

Smith, M. (1983). *Violence and sport*. Toronto: Butterworth.

Wilson, W., & Derse, E. (Eds.). *Doping in elite sport: The politics of drugs in the Olympic movement*. Champaign, IL: Human Kinetics.

Young, K. (1991). Sport and collective violence. *Exercise and Sport Science Review, 19*, 539–587.

Young, K., White, P., & McTeer, W. (1994). Body talk: Male athletes reflect on sport, injury, and pain. *Sociology of Sport Journal, 11*, 175–94.

Young, K. (Ed.). *Sporting bodies, damaged selves: Sociological studies of sports-related injury*. Amsterdam: Elsevier.

WEB LINKS

Free Reference Lists

http://playlab.uconn.edu/frl.htm

Includes a lengthy list of references on violence and aggression in sport.

The World Anti-Doping Agency

http://www.wada-ama.org/en/

Official site; includes a mission statement and educational initiatives.

Mentors in Violence Prevention Program

http://www.sportinsociety.org/mvp.html

A gender violence prevention and education program based at Northeastern University's Center for the Study of Sport in Society.

Scholarly Sport Sites

http://www.ucalgary.ca/library/ssportsite/biblio.html

The most comprehensive listing of coaching-related articles.

Sport Safe

http://www.tsa.gov.bc.ca/sport/Sportsafe.htm

A downloadable document with extensive suggestions on how to keep recreation facilities violence free.

CHAPTER 9

SPORT IN CANADIAN EDUCATIONAL INSTITUTIONS

Patricia S. Lally

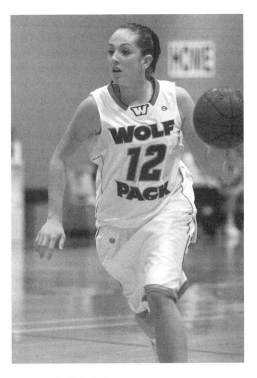

CIS varsity basketball player.

Photo by Matt Silver/TRU Athletics

Sport gives you so much unconsciously. You learn to achieve, to struggle, to fail. You learn to do a lot of things, sometimes in one game or one competition, that you can't be taught in a classroom. When you do learn from sport, you can transfer it to any other situation.
Miller, 2000. "The psychosocial development and academic achievement of Canadian intercollegiate student–athletes." Doctoral dissertation, University of Toronto

Sport and movement are visible at all levels of the Canadian educational system, from elementary through middle school, high school, college, and university. Sport is offered in different forms in the various educational settings. We will see, for example, that sport and physical activity are promoted through physical educational classes, intramural opportunities, and interschool competition in most schools across the country. Many Canadian colleges and universities offer a program of study in physical education or a closely related academic discipline, and provide participant opportunities through recreational, intramural, and intercollegiate programs.

Historically, there was strong support for the inclusion of physical activity in school settings. Functional theorists have long argued that sport has important educational benefits, that sport complements the educational mission of schools. Athletes gain from participation in sport through the exposure to significant role models and mentors, the opportunity to be physically active, and the acquisition of skills such as discipline, determination, and teamwork. This philosophy is exemplified in the opening quote. Further, along with a strong body, involvement in sport and physical activity strengthens the mind and prepares it for the rigours of academic study. Schools gain by the sense of community and loyalty sport can instill, perhaps more so than any other activity.

More recently, however, others have questioned the inclusion of sport in educational settings and this philosophy of education through sport. Some educators have demanded proof that sport directly complements the educational experience of students, rather than detracts from it. Others have wondered if sport really contributes to an inclusive sense of community for all students, teachers, and staff. Feminists have begun to critique school sport as a traditionally gendered enclave that privileges strong, male athletes while marginalizing non-athletic males, and females in general. We will examine the theme of education through sport in the public school system and later at the university and college levels and pay particular attention to these diverse perspectives throughout the chapter.

PUBLIC SCHOOL SYSTEM

The British North America Act of 1867 granted provinces individual jurisdiction over the direction and operation of their schools (Anderson, Broom, Pooley, Rhodes, Robertson, & Schrodt, 1989). As a result, there are numerous organizational and curricular differences across the country. However, sport is almost always incorporated in school curricula under physical education, and in co-instructional activities in the form of intramural and interschool sport programs.

Physical Education

We will begin by considering physical education in Canadian schools, starting with a brief history and moving forward to examine the current status of school physical education.

History of Physical Education

Physical education programs in Canadian schools date back to the middle of the eighteenth century, at which time they were heavily focused on drills and gymnastics (Anderson et al., 1989; Morrow, Keyes, Simpson, Cosentino, & Lappage, 1989). Militaristic interests dominated physical education for decades, largely due to the influence of Lord Strathcona, who developed a trust fund to support the formation of cadet corps and teacher training in physical education (Anderson et al., 1989; Morrow et al., 1989). This military influence was later championed by a warring government in need of a healthy, young population. Repetitious, rigorous calisthenics characterized physical education programs in Canada until the middle of the twentieth century.

The concern for fitness persisted, but progressive steps were taken to incorporate sports and games into physical education programs in the 1940s and 1950s (Anderson et al., 1989; Morrow et al., 1989). Until then, sports such as football, lacrosse, and baseball had been promoted outside the educational system by regional, provincial, and national groups (Morrow et al., 1989). Instruction in a broad range of activities such as those listed above, as well as dance and movement, eventually became the primary focus of physical education classes.

A major trend in elementary and secondary school physical education programs of the 1970s and 1980s was the promotion of Quality Daily Physical Education (QDPE; Canadian Association for Health, Physical Education, Recreation, and Dance, 1989). Schools across the country began to introduce mandatory physical education throughout their regular curricula, requiring students to complete a physical education course in each year of study.

Current Status of Physical Education

The status of physical education has changed dramatically in the ensuing years. Despite the continued support, at least theoretical, for health and physical activity (Chad, Humbert, & Jackson, 1999), school physical education is being devalued in new curricula across the country (Kidd, 1999; Lathrop & Murray, 1998). Elementary schools providing daily physical education are in the minority (Chad, Humbert, & Jackson, 1999). In fact, only one in four children enjoys daily physical education classes (Canadian Fitness and Lifestyle Research Institute, 2000). Only 47 percent of elementary schools across the country actually teach the required physical education curriculum (Hardman & Marshall, 2000). At the secondary level, only Quebec and Nova Scotia require students to take physical education beyond Grade 10 (Spence, Mandigo, Poon, & Mummery, 2001). Educational reform in the other provinces has significantly reduced the number of physical education credits students must fulfill before graduation, and in many cases even these abridged requirements are not met (Hardman & Marshall, 2000). The outcome, of course, has been a drastic decline in the number of students enrolled in physical education across the country. In a study of the secondary school physical education enrolment in Alberta, for example, Spence and his colleagues (Spence et al., 2001) found a significant decline in enrolment beyond Grade 10, when physical education was no longer compulsory. This displacement of physical education is occurring at the same time obesity among Canadian children is on the rise (Kidd, 1999; Limbert, Crawford, & McCargar, 1994) and more Canadian youth are leading inactive lifestyles than ever before (Cragg, Cameron, Craig, & Russell, 1999).

Barriers to Physical Education

A number of systematic barriers make it difficult for schools to provide quality, regular physical education (Humbert & Chad, 1998). First, parents and teachers place greater emphasis on academic subjects as a result of increasingly competitive university entrance requirements and an ever more uncertain job market. Second, the preferential scheduling of academic subjects discourages students from selecting physical education options. Third, schools lack the financial resources to support regular health and physical education programming as a result of drastic and repeated budget cuts. Many schools have introduced user fees for physical education and have become involved in fundraising in order to sustain curriculum and facilities—in many cases aging facilities in much need of repair. Available records indicate that 45 percent of all high school physical education programs charged user fees in 2002–03. Notably, many schools have been forced to implement fees for community use of facilities, which is having a detrimental impact on community sport and recreation (Donnelly & Kidd, 2003).

There is also a dire need for teachers trained specifically in the principles of physical education and opportunities for their professional development. In Ontario, for example, 68 percent of elementary schools have no physical education teacher at all, and only 18 percent have full-time physical education teachers (Hardman & Marshall, 2000). Providing quality physical education is difficult without adequately prepared teachers.

Enrolment records indicate the decline in physical education classes is more pronounced among females (Gibbons & Van Gyn, 1996; Gibbons, Van Gyn, Wharf-Higgins, & Gaul, 2000; Humbert, 1995; Spence et al., 2001). Only 10 percent of British Columbia female high school students take physical education when it becomes an option in Grades 11 and 12, compared to 25 percent of their male peers (Gibbons et al., 2000). Research indicates females are discouraged from pursuing physical education due to exposure to verbal, physical, and sexual harassment from male classmates (see Box 9.1), the lack of female role models, and their dissatisfaction with curriculum content and delivery (Gibbons, Wharf-Higgins, Gaul, & Van Gyn, 1999; Humbert, 1995). Some educators have recommended that co-educational physical education be eliminated altogether, and "females-only" physical education classes have been piloted in several settings (Gibbons et al., 2000).

Intramural Sport

In addition to physical education, sport and physical activity are delivered in elementary and secondary schools through intramural programs. Intramural programs include traditional games such as volleyball, basketball, and hockey, which have been on the decline in recent years. Unstructured movement opportunities such as walking, weightlifting, mountain biking, and scuba diving, as well as cooperative games and playground activities such as Ultimate Frisbee, have become more popular among intramural participants (Grossman, 2006).

Intramural programs are typically offered before and after school and at lunch-time, although they must often compete for limited space and facilities. They are usually organized by students and supervised by teachers and/or volunteers. There is a membership-based, not-for-profit national organization, the Canadian Intramural Recreation Association (CIRA), that supports intramural and recreation programming in the education system. Founded in 1977, CIRA and its 10 provincial/territorial affiliated associations provide projects, programs, and resources including volunteer and paid staff to help teachers and student leaders plan, organize, and operate intramural and recreation programs.

CIRA currently operates three national programs including the Student Leadership Development Program (SLDP), an initiative designed to empower students through the development of organizational and interpersonal skills. In the past five years, more than 1,700 elementary and secondary schools have participated in the SLDP, which means that more than 17,000 students have delivered their own intramural and recreation programs and improved their own leadership and organizational skills (CIRA, 2002).

Interschool Sport

Interschool sport programs operate in much the same manner as physical education programs in Canada; that is, on a province-by-province basis. Even more so, however, interschool sport programs also share the philosophy of education through sport that characterizes elementary and secondary physical education and intramurals.

History of Interschool Sport

The introduction of competitive interschool sport programs followed shortly after the inclusion of sports and games into the physical education curriculum in the 1940s and 1950s, due

Box 9.1   The Jock Culture in Canadian Sports

Female students report being harassed (both verbally and physically), discounted, and marginalized by male students in their physical education classes (Gibbons et al., 1999, 2000; Humbert, 1995). To make matters worse, this mistreatment is sometimes overlooked by both male and female teachers, who either wish to avoid confrontation or assume such gender dynamics are acceptable in traditionally male physical activity settings. The consequence is a critical decline in girls' participation in physical education curricula.

This sentiment of male entitlement to sport and physical activity affects not only young girls, but also boys who may not excel at traditional physical pursuits. Those who conform to the narrow male ideal are afforded elite status, and with it, remarkable power and privilege. Those who do not meet the male ideal are by definition inferior and, as such, subject to demoralization and victimization. The concept of gender issues in Canadian sport is more fully addressed in Chapter 6. The intent here is to consider the consequences of male ownership of sport in educational settings.

Male high school athletes report being able to miss classes to attend practices and prepare for competitive events without consequence, and receiving extra support from teachers and teacher/coaches, including grade inflation. Male high school athletes have also talked about enjoying special status in their schools.

The impact of this "jock culture" in North American schools, and Canadian sport, in particular, has received considerable attention of late. There have been several tragic shootings at schools both in Canada and the U.S. in recent years. Media reports suggest these shootings were linked to school culture clashes between male student–athletes, or the "jocks," and other cliques on campus, although evidence of such has not officially emerged.

This jock culture that glorifies traditional male attributes such as aggression and violence and, as a consequence, devalues feminine traits and women has also been implicated in recent exposés on sexual abuse in Canadian sport. In 1993, a Canadian television network broadcast *Crossing the Line*, a public-affairs program that examined the sexual harassment and abuse of young athletes by their male coaches. A number of segments highlighted the abuse by national team and other elite-level coaches. However, the reports of male high school and university coaches violating the trust and the bodies of the young athletes they coached was perhaps most distressing.

Educators and policymakers have tried to revise curriculum so that it would have greater appeal to both male and female students. Many health units, for example, now address such topics as disordered eating, body image, and the effects of steroids and other performance-enhancing drugs. In physical education units, there has been a shift away from traditional competitive sports like basketball and volleyball toward more fitness/leisure-based individual activities such as yoga, fitness walking, and rock climbing. These innovations have enjoyed initial successes, yet their full effect remains unclear.

The future of physical education in school settings throughout the country is in jeopardy. Physical education as a subject is not being taught in many schools today, and this is unlikely to change unless the problems outlined above can be adequately addressed. The absence of a successful lobbying group and indifferent federal and provincial governments will make this a difficult undertaking.

largely to the efforts of interested teachers. Interschool sport programs continued to expand in the following years and sports such as track and field, volleyball, and rugby grew in popularity among boys and gymnastics and field hockey among girls (Anderson et al., 1989; Morrow et al., 1989).

In the late 1970s and into the 1980s, several forces hampered the progress of interschool sport programs (Macintosh, 1990). First, Canada experienced a recession and provincial transfer payments for education were cut. School board funding for co-instructional activities including interschool sport programs were affected. Second, the aging teaching population lost enthusiasm for volunteering in extracurricular activities. Traditionally, teachers volunteered an average of 10 years to coaching, after which they were replaced by new, eager teachers. However, the climate of financial restraint that existed in the 1970s and 1980s meant new teachers were not being hired and there was a shortage of teachers interested in coaching interschool sport programs. Third, teachers who did continue to contribute to after-school activities became more aggressive in their efforts to secure compensation, and when it was not forthcoming were forced to withdraw their input. Finally, liability issues reduced participation in traditional, yet high-risk interschool sports such as football and gymnastics. In some provinces—Alberta and Nova Scotia, for example—gymnastics was eliminated altogether from interschool sport programs.

One more event occurred during this time that changed school sport programs. Several highly publicized court cases challenged policies that prohibited girls from participating on boys' teams (Macintosh, 1990). The incidents drew attention to the inequity of opportunities for male and female athletes across sport. Schools recognized that greater opportunities for female students had to be created, a considerable task given the declining financial and human resources of the period.

Current Status of Interschool Sport

Today, each province has a secondary school athletic association (for example, the Ontario Federation of School Athletic Associations, and the British Columbia School Sports Federation) that outlines eligibility and playing rules and organizes provincial playoffs. Sports are divided by gender, age, and level of competition. Seasons are purposefully kept short, about 6 to 10 weeks, to allow students to participate in multiple activities, the most popular of which are soccer, rugby, and volleyball. Unlike the U.S., which holds national championships in partnership with major corporate sponsors like McDonald's and Dr. Pepper (Eitzen & Sage, 2003), there are no national championships in Canadian high school sports. Educators fear the introduction of national championships would expose participants to the same abuses seen in the U.S., including sport specialization at a young age, greater emphasis on athletic rather than academic achievement, and greater accountability to corporate sponsors than to students, parents, and the community.

Many of the barriers that emerged in the 1970s and 1980s have yet to be fully resolved. In fact, in many provinces, they have been exacerbated by further financial constraints and educational reforms. One of the major problems facing interschool sport programs today is the escalating workload of teachers. Increasing teaching and supervision responsibilities and changing curricula have reduced the time teachers have to contribute to co-instructional programs. Labour conflicts between teachers and school boards have led to restrictions on teacher involvement in after-school activities in several provinces in recent years. Quebec and Manitoba have experimented with different incentives to encourage teachers' continued investment in extracurricular activities including time off, reduced workloads, and financial remuneration. However, most provinces continue to rely on teachers to volunteer, and many have been pressed to increase the involvement of community volunteers despite concerns about liability and educational integrity. For example, in Ontario, where the future of interschool sport programs is in crisis, approximately 10 percent of coaches are students and 15 percent are community volunteers (Ministry of Education, 2001).

Given the shrinking volunteer network, dwindling funding, limited sources of new revenue—particularly without national championships and the commercial sponsorship they would bring—why do schools labour to maintain interschool sport programs? There are two ways to answer this question. First, we can look at how schools benefit from interschool sport programs; second, we can consider how students purportedly benefit.

Schools use sport to help build a sense of community, to help school members including students, teachers, and staff feel a sense of loyalty to the school and each other. Schools hope such loyalty translates into less conflict between each of these groups and an enhanced climate of tolerance and acceptance (James, 2005). This goal of civil order through a unifying sport program may be particularly important in racially and economically diverse schools. Schools also use sport and sporting events to establish ties with their local communities and alumni, two groups schools have come to rely on more heavily for funding and support. Finally, schools use student–athletes, who must meet certain academic standards in order to be eligible to participate, as exemplary role models for other students.

Let us turn now to look at how students benefit from involvement in interschool sport programs. The bulk of the research comes from the U.S. and indicates participation in high school sports is positively associated with a range of academic and developmental benefits. Athletic participation tends to contribute to increased academic achievement for both boys and girls (Fejgin, 1994; Kerr, 1996). Athletic participation also seems to be related to higher educational aspirations and higher post-secondary obtainment (Fejgin, 1994; Kerr, 1996; Melnick, Sabo, & Vanfossen, 1992a).

Researchers in the U.S. have also found that high school athletes, particularly boys, enjoy higher self-esteem (Holland & Andre, 1994) and greater popularity among peers (McNeal, 1995; Melnick, Sabo, & Vanfossen, 1992a). Boys and girls who participate in high school sports drop out (Kerr, 1996; McNeal, 1995; Melnick, Sabo, & Vanfossen, 1992b) and engage in delinquent behaviour (Kerr, 1996; Landers & Landers, 1978; Spreitzer, 1994) less often than non-athlete peers.

Some caution is warranted. The literature on U.S. high school sport has not been entirely positive. Melnick and his colleagues cautioned that many of the advantages noted above are mediated by gender, race, and social class. For example, Sabo, Melnick, and Vanfossen (1993) reported participation in high school athletics had little effect on the educational expectations or later attainment of Black males and females. Some critics reason higher academic achievement among athletes is due to the influence of their affluent home settings where education is reinforced, and lower delinquency rates are linked to athletes' tendencies to conform to strict, oppressive sport norms. Further, there is growing concern in the U.S. that high school sport is approaching intercollegiate athletics and will succumb, if it has not already, to the same excesses seen at the university level—including the recruitment of under-prepared students, poor academic performance and low graduation rates, and the exploitation, both physical and psychological, of student–athletes (see, for example, Adler & Adler, 1991; Blinde, 1989).

Similar concerns are not widespread in the Canadian setting. In fact, the limited available research suggests Canadian high school athletes experience the same benefits, but not necessarily the same risks. There appears to be either no (Tremblay, Inman, & Willms, 2000) or a positive (Anderson et al., 1989; Okihiro, 1984) relationship between school sports and academic achievement among Canadian students. Student–athletes from the province of Ontario, for example, performed better academically than their non-athlete peers (Anderson et al., 1989). Likewise, there are suggestions participation in Canadian interschool sport is linked to higher retention. James (1995), for example, found male and female African Canadian high school athletes used sport to cope with their alienating school environments and to develop meaningful connections to peers and teachers. More recently, James (2005) found similar patterns among Canadian middle school male and female athletes. Maybe more important to the long-term health of Canadians, researchers have found participation in high school sport is a valuable predictor of sport participation among adult males and females, even for those more than 20 years beyond high school (Curtis, McTeer, & White, 1999).

The future of interschool sport programs will depend heavily on the willingness of teachers to invest their time, in many cases without compensation, and the openness of the provinces, school boards, trustees, and parents to consider creative alternatives.

UNIVERSITIES AND COLLEGES

Interuniversity Sport

Interuniversity competition dates back to before the turn of the twentieth century, although it was quite different from the highly centralized bureaucratic organization that exists today (Moriarty & Holma-Prpich, 1987). Then, student leaders at a handful of Canada's older universities—McGill, Toronto, and Queen's—put together teams and challenged each other in football, hockey, and track and field (Morrow et al., 1989). As interest in interuniversity sport grew, universities assumed a leadership role and subsumed interuniversity competition within their educational agendas.

History of Interuniversity Sport

The Canadian Intercollegiate Athletic Union–Central (CIAU) was formed in 1906 to oversee athletics in Ontario and Quebec universities (Canadian Interuniversity Sport [CIS], 2002; Morrow et al., 1989). The Maritime Inter-Collegiate Athletic Association in the east and the Western Intercollegiate Athletic Association in the west emerged in subsequent years. In the early part of the century, universities focused on competition between member institutions and did not have strong interests in national-level competition (Anderson et al., 1989). By the late 1950s, athletic unions across Canada determined national collaboration would be beneficial. A national organization could establish consistent sport regulations, help universities coordinate agreements with national sport bodies, and introduce and oversee national championships. National championships could augment the profile of interuniversity athletics across the country and bolster student interest and support. The CIAU was reconstituted in 1961 as the governing body of interuniversity sport for all provinces and operated as an autonomous organization for almost 20 years.

The CIAU experienced significant changes in the 1970s (Anderson et al., 1989; Hall, Slack, Smith, & Whitson, 1991; Morrow et al., 1989). The status of sport within the larger social context in Canada was changing. Greater numbers of sporting events were being televised and, as a result, sport became an attractive vehicle to sell goods and services, including political ideologies and platforms (Schneider, 1997; Taylor, 1986). The government saw the potential of sport to promote the Canadian culture on the international scene and national unity on the domestic scene. The Ministry of Fitness and Amateur Sport developed an agenda of high-performance sport and looked to universities to develop high-performance training centres (Department of National Health and Welfare, 1969). Additionally, federal funding was earmarked for travel equalizations, national championship travel, and involvement in international competition.

Federal government involvement in interuniversity sport was controversial (Schneider, 1997; Taylor, 1986). Some feared a focus on high-performance sport in educational settings would lead to increased costs from supporting national teams, disagreements over access to and use of space and facilities, and philosophical clashes between high-performance sport and sport as an educational experience (Jackson, 1986; Semotiuk, 1986). Yet, incorporating high-performance sport systems within institutions of higher education would also mean more qualified and experienced coaches for intercollegiate programs, improved competition, new revenues through renting of facilities and services to national teams, and research and athlete testing opportunities for sport science labs (Hall et al., 1989; Jackson, 1986).

Indeed, one of the outcomes of federal funding and greater emphasis on high-performance sport was that universities created full-time coaching positions and hired male and female coaches on non-academic routes, ending a long tradition of faculty-coaches (Schneider, 1997; Taylor, 1986). Many universities also instituted separate athletic and academic units (Schneider, 1997), despite earlier recommendations to maintain integrated athletic and physical education departments (Association of Universities and Colleges of Canada, 1966; Mathews, 1974).

The recession that hit Canada in the early 1980s reverberated throughout Canadian interuniversity athletics. Federal funding declined and funds allocated for university sport were no longer available, triggering more than a decade of fiscal restraint (Anderson et al., 1989). Athletic departments struggled to stretch existing resources and find new sources of funding, including camps and corporate sponsorship. While under serious financial limitations, athletic departments also wrestled with providing opportunities for female athletes and operating competitive interuniversity sport programs for a small population of student–athletes concurrently with broad-based sport and recreation opportunities for the wider student and local communities (Schneider, 1997; Taylor, 1986).

In June 2001, members of the CIAU agreed to the new name Canadian Interuniversity Sport (CIS), and today CIS includes all 50 major degree-granting institutions in four regional conferences: Atlantic University Sport (AUS), Quebec Student Sports Federation (QSSF), Ontario University Athletics (OUA), and Canada West (the CIS will add the Ontario Institute of Technology in 2006). The CIS is a single-tiered system that offers national championships in nine sports for men and 10 for women, a collective of more than 11,000 student–athletes and 550 coaches.

In addition to the CIS, there is a national body that governs athletic competition among colleges throughout Canada. The Canadian Colleges Athletic Association (CCAA) actually outnumbers the CIS, with 95 member institutions representing five regional conferences. Historically, colleges in one province competed against each other in a small and variable number of sports. In 1971, the provinces of British Columbia, Alberta, Saskatchewan, and Manitoba formed the Four-West Championship for interprovincial competition in seven sports. Four-West merged with the Ontario Colleges Athletic Association and the Quebec Colleges Athletic Association to form the CCAA. Today, the CCAA holds national championships in eight events: men's and women's badminton, soccer, volleyball, and basketball, and holds open championships in golf and cross-country.

Current Status of Interuniversity Sport

There are a number of challenges facing Canadian interuniversity sport today. Among the most pressing is the funding and governance of intercollegiate athletics in institutions of higher education, followed by concerns about equity, the value of intercollegiate sport for student–athlete participants, athletic scholarships, and sport initiations and hazings on Canadian campuses (see Box 9.2). Let us consider each in turn.

Box 9.2   Initiation and Hazing in Canadian Interuniversity Sport

---

Recent hazing incidents at Guelph and McMaster Universities and the University of Western Ontario triggered alarm over sport initiations on Canadian campuses. A hazing activity involving a first-year wide receiver with the University of Western Ontario and two male engineering students from the same university left one student injured, another charged with criminal negligence causing bodily harm, and a university community reeling.

Despite anti-hazing laws in all but six states, surveys of U.S. high school and university students revealed both groups were subjected to sport-related initiations in overwhelming numbers (Hoover, 1999; Hoover & Pollard, 2000). Hazing incidents included forced drinking, physical humiliation, public nudity, sexual games, being exposed to physical danger, and even performing criminal acts. Some student–athletes reported initiations were fun and exciting, made them feel closer as a group, or gave them an opportunity to prove themselves. Others, however, said they just went along with it, were scared to say no, or did not know what was happening.

A Canadian study on sport initiations warrants special mention. Johnson (2000) conducted in-depth interviews with current and former male and female student–athletes from a Canadian university with a large athletics program about the incidence, significance, and consequences of sport-related hazing practices. All of the athletes interviewed had been hazed during high school and all had been involved in some initiation activity upon arrival at university. Many later organized initiation events for incoming student–athletes, despite unpleasant and lasting memories of their own experiences. Johnson characterized initiations as acts that articulate the masculine ideals of power and hegemony, reinforce the patriarchal structure, and marginalize homosexuals and women through humiliation and objectification.

Johnson (2000) did sense student–athletes were primed to question abusive hazing practices and described them as poised for change. In collaboration with a colleague, Johnson developed a handbook for coaches and student leaders outlining alternative, welcoming orientation activities (Miller & Johnson, 1998). One of these activities, a weekend retreat at a ropes and challenge camp, was organized for athletic teams at the University of Toronto in the fall of 2000. Student–athletes from six athletic teams and their coaches participated in a low ropes course, rock climbing and belaying, canoeing, kayaking, and cooperative games. Initial feedback from first-year players, team leaders, and coaches was positive, and organizers believe such alternative activities will help break the cycle of initiations (Johnson & Miller, 2004).

The Funding and Governance of Canadian Intercollegiate Athletics. University administrators have been cutting transfer payments to athletic departments for a number of years. Likewise, students across the country have voted down requests from athletic departments for larger portions of their student fees (athletic departments across the country receive anywhere from less than 3 percent to more than 11 percent of student fees for intercollegiate programs). With decreasing funding from traditional sources, university athletic departments have had to look for alternative revenues. A number of possibilities exist, but as we will see, each presents unique challenges to who then actually controls intercollegiate athletics (Armstrong-Doherty, 1995; Inglis, 1991). Athletic departments could venture more deeply into nonuniversity contracts with commercial sponsors like food, beverage, and service companies. This would be similar to what we have seen in U.S. intercollegiate athletics, where many sporting events are sponsored by such companies as Tostitos, Fed-Ex, and Coke. However, educators fear reliance on commercial revenue sources would place greater emphasis on winning than education and compromise the academic mission of sport programs. Canadian interuniversity sport could risk the same problems seen in the U.S. including recruiting violations, exploitation of athletes,

---

Box 9.3   Drug Use in Canadian Interuniversity Sport

In collaboration with the Canadian Centre for Ethics in Sport (CCES), the CIS starting testing intercollegiate athletes for use of banned substances in 1990. Since that time, a very small number of athletes have been caught using substances prohibited by the Canadian Anti-Doping Program. CIS doping records indicate only 39 of the 5,000 tests conducted in the last 15 years have been positive for banned substances, representing a rate of fewer than 0.8 percent positive. These figures are consistent with a national survey of drug use in Canadian university athletics that included almost 800 student–athletes involved in eight different sports from eight different universities (Spence & Gauvin, 1996).

What the survey did reveal of particular interest was the high number of student–athletes who reported use of alcohol. Almost all respondents admitted consuming alcohol. These data are consistent with existing research, the bulk of which comes from the U.S. There, studies indicate athletes may drink less frequently overall, although the difference is small (Martens, Dams-O'Connor, & Beck, 2006; Martens, Watson, & Beck, 2006). More alarming is evidence student–athletes tend to binge-drink, defined as consuming five or more drinks at one time, more often than their non-athlete peers (Hildebrand, Johnson, & Bogle, 2001). In addition, athletes tend to drink more when binge-drinking (Hildebrand, Johnson, & Bogle, 2001).

A study of the consequences of alcohol consumption indicates athletes may be at greater risk of negatives outcomes including driving while under the influence, driving with someone under the influence, and date rape (Hildebrand, Johnson, & Bogle, 2001; Leichliter, Meilman, Presley, & Cashin, 1998). Alcohol consumption is an issue across campuses, but its prevalence among student–athletes, given the education missive of interuniversity sport, is disconcerting.

---

drug use (see Box 9.3), and academic failure. Another source of revenue is through more aggressive solicitation of government funding for the inclusion and support of high-performance training centres within educational institutions. The risk here is that accepting government funds for high-performance sport centres could place greater emphasis on training national and Olympic athletes than on providing an educational and developmental sport experience for university students. A third possibility, and one several universities have seriously explored, is to accommodate local community interests in sport and physical activity through university facilities. A large number of communities throughout the country are in desperate need of access to quality facilities. However, trying to accommodate the interests of an interuniversity program, an intramural program, and the local community may be too much to bear on already limited facilities.

Equity. CIS is coping with numerous issues of equity including institutional equity (member institutions across the country differ dramatically in their size, location, academic offerings, and student characteristics), program equity, and sport equity. Perhaps the most pressing, however, is the issue of gender equity.

The first conference for women's intercollegiate athletics was founded in Ontario in 1923 (Women's Intercollegiate Athletic Union, WIAU). Other provincial and regional organizations were introduced in Quebec and the Maritimes in the ensuing years. In 1969, a proposal to develop a national organization was endorsed by each of the conferences, and in 1970 the Canadian Women's Intercollegiate Athletic Union (CWIUA) sanctioned the first women's national championship in volleyball.

Many of the women's regional conferences merged with the men's during the following years, and the CWIAU itself converged with the CIAU in 1978. The last major merger took place only recently. The Ontario Women's Intercollegiate Athletic Association, after 60 years of providing competitive athletic opportunities for female students in Ontario universities, joined the Ontario Universities Athletic Association in 1997 to become Ontario University Athletics (OUA).

Numerous factors have influenced women's intercollegiate sport in Canada and the U.S. (Hums, MacLean, Richman, & Pastore, 1994). The U.S. has been largely affected by Title IX, a key provision of the Education Amendments Act of 1972 stipulating funding would be withheld from any institution that failed to provide equal access and quality of services based on gender. A 1984 Supreme Court decision that excluded athletic departments from Title IX requirements on the basis they did not receive direct federal funding was reversed by the Civil Rights Restoration Act of 1988. All athletic departments were required to provide equal access and opportunities for female students (Sage, 1998). Female athletes, coaches, and administrators in the U.S. have secured greater opportunities as universities work to meet Title IX, although there is still a long way to go before these women enjoy true equity.

Canada does not have similar legislation. Instead, under the general principles of the Charter of Rights and Freedoms, universities are compelled to provide equity with regard to athletics. The CIS conducts gender equity studies approximately every five years, with the most recent in 2005 (CIS, 2005a). Data indicate Canadian universities have made some advances toward gender equity during the last decade. Women now compete in 10 CIS sports, including the most recent additions of hockey, rugby, and wrestling, outnumbering the nine available men's programs. However, disparities persist in areas such as mode of team travel, meal money, equipment funding, and opportunities for exhibition competitions. Significantly fewer dollars are spent on recruiting, marketing, and promotion of women's programs. Member institutions report the most difficulty achieving equity in areas that rely on external funding or alumni contributions, most notably athletic financial awards. Fewer than half of our universities (47 percent) have achieved equity in this area. In 2003–04, male athletes were awarded 65 percent of athletic award dollars.

Equity figures also indicate notable differences remain in the opportunities for women in coaching and administrative positions within the CIS. While there were slight increases

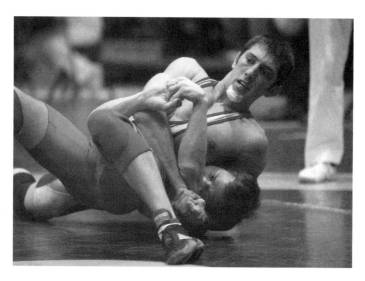

CIS varsity wrestler.
ROB LINKE/CP Images

in female university coaches in the early 1990s, these were primarily assistant or part-time head coaching positions. Few head coaching opportunities exist for female coaches in university sport. As of January 2005, only 86 of the 348 or 20 percent of CIS coaches were female (CIS, 2005b). Although many coaches are members of university collective labour agreements and perceive equitable compensation, available data reveal that both women and men coaching women's programs often earn less than men coaching men's programs. Notably, this pattern parallels the distribution of coaches for our Olympic teams, where women have made up only approximately 20 percent of head coaches for the 1998, 2000, 2002, 2004, and 2006 Games.

The dearth of women in coaching and administrative positions exists in a post–Title IX NCAA, as well. More coaching and administrative positions for women were anticipated following Title IX. Yet, as women's programs received intercollegiate status and improved funding, coaching and administrative openings became more attractive to men (Carpenter & Acosta, 1985).

Some argue the lack of women in these positions persists today because women are not qualified for or interested in coaching or management positions, are deterred by the long and/or weekend hours such positions typically demand, or are restricted by their domestic responsibilities, primarily childcare. Conversely, women argue they are both interested in and qualified for high-level coaching and administrative positions, but never learn about open postings, are not interviewed for them despite ample qualifications, or are not seriously considered for them simply because they are women. They also contend that, in many cases, positions have already been passed down to former male athletes or assistant coaches by an "old boys' network" of male coaches and administrators (Inglis, Danylchuk, & Pastore, 2000, 1996).

Clearly, close examination of announcement, interviewing, and hiring practices in Canadian sport is warranted. In the meantime, however, the lack of female coaches and administrators means fewer role models for young girls, unfortunately at a time when such role models are of critical need.

Value of Interuniversity Sport for Student–Athlete Participants. Dominant ideology contends sport contributes to students' overall development in two ways. First, university sport promotes the academic achievement of student–athletes. Second, it encourages the acquisition of valuable life skills and the successful negotiation of age-appropriate developmental tasks, notably identity formation. Although closely held, research suggests these ideals are not always met.

Academic achievement of student–athletes. As noted earlier, the escalating emphasis on high-performance sport, growing autonomy of athletic departments, and increasing number of coaches accountable to athletic and not academic mandates, caused concern that the integrity of educational institutions was being compromised. Prompted by these changes, and in part by the research coming out of the U.S. (see, for example, Adler & Adler, 1991; Thelin, 1994), several Canadian researchers examined the academic performance of Canadian student–athletes (Curtis & McTeer, 1990; Danylchuk, 1995; Martens, 1985; McTeer & Curtis, 1999).

Two early studies suggested Canadian student–athletes were doing as well if not better than their non-athlete peers. Martens (1985) found the annual and overall GPA of male student–athletes from 10 different sports did not significantly differ from non-athletes, and athletes graduated significantly more often than their non-athlete peers, although they took longer to do so. Curtis and McTeer (1990) reported athletes and non-athletes took about the same amount of time to graduate, and athletes achieved GPAs equivalent to their non-athlete peers. Athletes in honours programs actually achieved significantly higher cumulative GPAs.

In the most recent Canadian study, however, Danylchuk (1995) found student–athletes were struggling academically. The high school grades of the athletes and non-athletes did not significantly differ, yet non-athletes consistently outperformed both male and female athletes while at university.

Although only several studies of the Canadian case exist and the latest is already more than 10 years old, the findings are sobering. Less than a decade after student–athletes achieved grades and graduation rates equivalent to, if not better than, non-athletes, they were earning lower grades and graduating less often.

McTeer and Curtis (1999) suggested a number of factors may be to blame. The demands placed on student–athletes by coaches and administrators may be on the rise as universities use interuniversity sport to increase student and community interest. Student–athletes' time may be stretched even thinner than in the past as greater emphasis is placed on academic performance and graduate studies. Finally, tuition increases mean most students must now work throughout the school year and may have less time and energy to devote to academics.

The NCAA closely tracks and reports the academic performance of its athletes across all three divisions. Clearly, more contemporary research of the Canadian setting is needed to determine why the academic performance of student–athletes has declined in recent years and if this pattern persists today. The CIS is considering tracking the academic performance of its student–athlete members, but no information was available at the time of publication.

Acquisition of life skills. Athletic administrators across the country were surveyed about the goals of intercollegiate athletics (Chelladurai & Danylchuk, 1984). In addition to athletes' physical growth, intercollegiate athletics were intended to promote psychological and emotional development. The athletic administrators believed the acquisition of skills relevant to future employment, including leadership, responsibility, and respect for authority, and increasing student–athletes' future career opportunities were fundamental goals of Canadian interuniversity sport. Indeed, when athletic departments are criticized for placing too much emphasis on sport or for expecting too much from student–athletes, they often assert that interuniversity sport encourages not only physical but also overall development, and not only for those students directly involved, but also for those who act as coaches, team managers, officials, sports information officers, and even fans.

Despite the developmental goals of interuniversity sport programs, there is little empirical evidence student–athletes benefit directly from participation in university sport. For the most part, the acquisition of skills such as those listed above is assumed or inferred. Furthermore, there is little proof that skills learned in sport are transferred to and facilitate success in other settings, particularly the classroom.

One of the major problems with examining the developmental outcomes of involvement in university sport is the difficulty in teasing benefits related specifically to sport from general maturation effects. Miller and Kerr (2002) attempted to address this by asking male and female student–athletes from a large Canadian university what developmental benefits, if any, they experienced as a result of participating in university athletics. The researchers also asked student–athletes to what degree they were able to transfer skills learned in university sport to other settings. The student–athletes asserted they acquired valuable life skills through sport including leadership, communication, independence, and self-confidence. However, the student–athletes had difficulty recalling how and in what context they had acquired these strengths, as well as how they might be useful in future pursuits, conditions developmental theorists argue are necessary for successful skills transfer (Danish & Nellen, 1997). Research documenting the developmental outcomes of participating in Canadian interuniversity sport is needed if we are to advocate these as educational experiences of lifelong value.

Identity formation. Identity formation is of particular significance to our discussion of the overall development of university student–athletes. It is during the college and university years that we wrestle with such questions as, "Who am I?", "What do I want to do with the rest of my life?", and "Where am I going?"

Marcia (1993) isolated four identity statuses; two suggest the individual is working toward establishing a stable and multidimensional sense of self, while the remaining two denote negative outcomes. Identity foreclosure occurs when an individual prematurely commits him or herself to a particular role, often a socially prescribed or accepted role, without adequate exploration of the role and his or her likes, dislikes, ambitions, and goals (Marcia, 1993).

Evidence suggests student–athletes may be at risk of developing identity foreclosure because the demands of being both a student and an athlete prohibit the exploration of self within a broad range of roles. Murphy, Petitpas, and Brewer (1996), for example, found both male and female student–athletes had higher identity foreclosure scores than non-athletes. However, much of the research published to date considers student–athletes from the U.S. (Brewer, 1993; Chartrand & Lent, 1987; Grant & Darley, 1993; Pearson & Petitpas, 1990). Miller and Kerr (2003) investigated the identity formation of Canadian student–athletes in particular. Canadian male and female athletes from volleyball, basketball, track and field, and swimming over-identified with the athlete role during their early university careers at the expense of meaningful investment in their academic and social selves, consistent with the experiences of their U.S. peers. However, the Canadian student–athletes shifted their investment from athletics to academics as they progressed through university and demonstrated deferred role experimentation in their academic and social lives in their upper years. These findings suggest that Canadian student–athletes may over-identify with the athlete role in their early university careers, yet they are able to avoid identity foreclosure through the exploration of other roles during their senior years. It may be that Canadian student–athletes falter initially, but eventually recover and successfully progress through the developmental task of identity formation.

Athletic Scholarships. Athletic scholarships have been a very contentious issue in the CIS, at times threatening to divide the organization (Hall et al., 1991). Financial aid for returning student–athletes was sanctioned by the CIAU in 1981 provided the value of the scholarship did not exceed $1,500 and the recipient met certain criteria. Athletic awards for first-year students were prohibited. Frustrated by losing talented athletes to U.S. colleges, some universities, notably those in western Canada, aggressively contested CIAU scholarship regulations. They argued larger athletic scholarships and scholarships for first-year students would entice Canadian student–athletes to stay home and enrich Canadian interuniversity competition. Other schools, however, were philosophically opposed to scholarships based on athletic ability alone. Many of the Ontario universities argued athletic scholarships would threaten the academic integrity of athletic programs and their schools and lead to exploitation and corruption similar to that seen on U.S. campuses.

The issue of athletic scholarships was revisited at the CIS annual meeting in June 2000. Ontario universities, which make up two-thirds of available votes in the CIS General Assembly, were expected to block-vote against proposed changes, including a revision allowing scholarships for entering student–athletes. In spite of anticipated and, indeed, initial disagreements, member institutions agreed to a number of changes. Most notably, the CIS moved to allow athletic scholarships equivalent to tuition and compulsory fees for entering students provided they had a minimum average of 80 percent and for continuing students provided they completed two semesters of full-time study in the preceding academic year and achieved a 70-percent average.

While the CIS provides overriding principles, individual institutions can agree within their conference to operate under different policies provided they meet the CIS minimum requirements. OUA member institutions voted not to provide athletic scholarships to entering student–athletes (OUA, 2001). This decision reflected their continued concern that athletic scholarships for incoming student–athletes would preference athletic over academic perform-ance, as well as fears about the impact of CIS policy changes on recruiting practices and the policing thereof. Some observers predicted the OUA's position would eventually make it difficult for Ontario universities to recruit talented athletes and result in a two-tiered system in Canadian interuniversity sport, reminiscent of the NCAA (Rayner, 1998). The impact of these developments remains to be seen. However, the University of Ottawa and Carleton University recently threatened to move from the OUA to the Quebec Student Sport Federation if the OUA did not loosen its scholarship restrictions.

In June 2000, members also agreed to a new gender-equity policy mandating financial sup-port for male and female student–athletes must be proportional to the number of CIS male and female student–athletes at issuing institutions (CIS, 2000a). Scholarship data from 2000–01 revealed male athletes, who make up 53 percent of CIS student–athletes, received an unequal 66 percent of athletic scholarships (CIS, 2000b). CIS expects universities to eliminate this discrepancy, and were to assess their progress in 2003 and their compliance by 2005–06 (Charbonneau, 2002). No data were available at the time of publication to determine the status of scholarships in the CIS today.

CONCLUSIONS

The purpose of this chapter was to consider the relationship between sport and educational insti-tutions in Canada, while paying particular attention to the theme of education through sport. The material presented suggests that while this is a noble goal, it is not being fully realized.

In the school system, students enjoy participation in recreational activities in physical education classes and competitive opportunities through intramural and interschool programs. These are being threatened by sweeping educational reforms that devalue physical education and shrinking financial and human resources critical to co-instructional activities. Physical educators across the country are faced with the daunting task of rallying public and official sup-port for physical education and interschool sport programs. Promoting education through sport will be difficult if both physical education and interschool programs continue to be displaced.

At the university level, interuniversity programs continue to enjoy support among sport enthusiasts and those who believe in the philosophy of education through sport. Yet, diverse interest groups including Canada's high-performance contingent, the general student popula-tion, and the broader communities in which universities exist are challenging varsity programs for increasingly limited space and resources. Further, research suggests university student–athletes' education, both academic and personal, may not be directly enhanced as a result of participation in interuniversity athletics.

These trends should not be disheartening. Sport has the potential to contribute to the development of our youth, and our education system is the best way to help children and youth develop healthy, active lifestyles. The challenge is to provide sport opportunities that truly embody the philosophy of education through sport.

CRITICAL THINKING QUESTIONS

1. Physical education is being devalued in curricula nationwide. Explain why this is taking place and the efforts being made to reverse this trend.

2. Interschool sport programs face a number of significant challenges. Identify these challenges and discuss how you would address them if you were a member of a local school board and supporter of the inclusion of sport within educational institutions.
3. The governance of interuniversity sport programs is being threatened from multiple directions. Explain the changes that made this possible, the perspectives of the different interest groups vying for control of interuniversity sport, and how athletic departments across the country are responding.
4. Research suggests the academic achievement of Canadian student–athletes has changed over the last three decades. Describe these changes and why they have taken place.
5. Why are athletes at risk of developing identity foreclosure? What are the consequences of doing so?
6. Considerable debate has surrounded the issue of athletic scholarships. Summarize the arguments for and against athletic scholarships and predict the impact of recent CIS policy changes on interuniversity sport in Canada.

SUGGESTED READINGS

Adler, P., & Adler, P. (1991). *Backboards and blackboards: College athletes and role engulfment.* New York: Columbia University Press.

James, C. (2005). *Race in play: Understanding the socio-cultural worlds of student–athletes.* Toronto: Canadian Scholars' Press Inc.

Johnson, J., & Holman, M. (2004). (Eds.). *Making the team: Inside the world of sport initiations and hazing.* Toronto: Canadian Scholars' Press Inc.

Kerr, G. (1996). The role of sport in preparing youth for adulthood. In B. Galway and J. Hudson (Eds.), *Youth in transition: Perspectives on research and policy.* Toronto: Thompson Educational Publishing.

Lally, P. S., & Kerr, G. (2005). The career planning, athletic identity and student role identity of intercollegiate student–athletes. *Research Quarterly for Exercise and Sport, 76,* 275–285.

McTeer, W., & Curtis, J. (1999). Intercollegiate sport involvement and academic achievement: A follow-up study. *Avante, 5,* 39–55.

Miller, P. S., & Kerr, G. (2003). The role experimentation of intercollegiate student–athletes. *The Sport Psychologist, 17,* 197–220.

Thelin, J. R. (1994). *Games colleges play: Scandal and reform in intercollegiate athletics.* Baltimore: Johns Hopkins Press.

WEB LINKS

Atlantic University Sport

www.atlanticuniversitysport.com
Regional CIS association for eastern provinces.

Ontario Physical and Health Education Association

www.ophea.net
Online community of organizations and individuals committed to promoting physical activity among children and youth.

The Ontario Federation of School Athletic Associations

www.ofsaa.on.ca
Interschool sport programs in Ontario.

Canadian Interuniversity Sport

www.universitysport.ca
Interuniversity sport programs in Canada, including media and corporate information about the CIS.

Canada West Universities Athletic Association

www.canadawest.org

Information about interuniversity sport in British Columbia, Alberta, Saskatchewan, and Manitoba.

Ontario University Athletics

www.oua.ca

Information about interuniversity sport in Ontario.

Fédération Québécoise du Sport Étudiant

www.fqse.qc.ca

Information about high school, college, and university sport in Quebec.

Canadian Colleges Athletic Association

www.ccaa.ca

Information about intercollegiate competition across Canada.

National Collegiate Athletic Association

www.ncaa.org

The governing body of intercollegiate sport in the U.S.

CHAPTER 10

SPORT AND THE MEDIA

Steve Jackson, Jay Scherer, and Scott G. Martyn

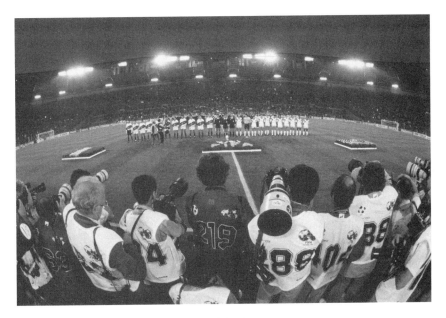

There is more than meets the eye in producing televised sport.

Bob Thomas/Stone/Getty Images

Television won't be able to hold on to any market it captures after the first six months. People will soon get tired of staring at a plywood box every night.

Darryl F. Zanuck, President, 20th Century Fox, 1946

Despite the prognostications of Darryl Zanuck and others within the print and broadcast industry, television audiences have continued to grow both nationally and globally. For example, audiences for televised sport remain among the largest and most dedicated of all tele-visual spectators, leading one commentator to describe the sport–television relationship as a "global love-match" (Rowe, 1996). While care needs to be taken in how data for television rat-ings are both collected and interpreted, we are regularly informed that audiences for major sporting spectacles, such as the Summer Olympics, are now in the billions. One indication of the immense power and reach of what has been referred to as the *sports-media complex* (Jhally, 1989) is evident in the *Athens 2004 Olympic Broadcast Report* (2004), which states that:

> dedicated coverage reached an unprecedented global audience. More than 300 channels pro-vided 35,000 hours of dedicated Olympic Games coverage over 17 days, delivering images from Athens 2004 to an unduplicated 3.9 billion people in 220 countries and territories. (p. 77)

Similarly, it is estimated that there were a half-billion television viewers for each of the 2006 FIFA World Cup soccer games in Germany, for a cumulative audience of nearly 30 bil-lion for the month-long tournament ("FIFA World Cup . . . ," 2006). The television audiences for North American professional sports are equally impressive. It is estimated that the 2006 Super Bowl was watched by 90.7 million people. Moreover, consider that of the top 15 rated television shows in U.S. history, nine have been Super Bowls. North of the 49th parallel, one of the longest-running television shows in world history, *Hockey Night in Canada* (HNIC), has consistently achieved some of the highest ratings of any Canadian television broadcast. Such facts are cited so regularly that we often forget some of the other epic moments in the history of television, including the first human landing on the moon. Thus, even a cursory view of con-temporary sport reveals its intimate relationship with the media. "Indeed, it is difficult to imagine the cultural form of sport before television became its defining medium" (Whannel, 2005, p. 405). Furthermore, the previous examples and statistics confirm something that we all seem to know but tend to take for granted; that is, that sport is an important and pervasive part of Canadian culture and society. Rod Brookes (2002), for example, highlights the significance of sport in society generally and the role of the sports-media complex in particular:

> Sport appears to be ever more visible within the media. Live sports events have been crucial to the introduction of new pay television services. Sport stars provide a rich source of human interest for a news and entertainment industry in which celebrity and scandal stories in gen-eral are particularly newsworthy. Sports journalism has become a staple of rolling news chan-nels on television and radio, and is already central to the business strategies of Internet content providers. (p. 1)

Even a brief glance at a daily newspaper or local news broadcast reveals the extent to which the media regularly devote substantial segments of their productions to sport. Indeed, as a popular and powerful social institution, sport is an important conduit for the transmission of images, symbols, and meanings that are central to our society. The latter point is extremely important when we consider the media's role in producing, representing, and circulating ideo-logical images of national, gender, racial, sexual, and other identities. Increasingly, it is through the media that we learn about dominant and stereotypical as well as subordinate and alterna-tive identities that are socially constructed for our consumption and often become a part of our everyday common sense. As Harvey and Law (2005) note, the

> mass media and cultural industries. . . . do not sell an innocent product. Rather, they produce cultural texts that affect society's values, beliefs, the way citizens see themselves and debate about society, culture, politics and sport. (p. 200)

Thus, in light of the media's central role in defining and shaping much of our contemporary existence, including our sporting practices and identities, the purpose of this chapter is to outline and explain the relationship(s) between sport and the media. First, the terms "media" and "mediamaking" will be defined and conceptualized. Next, we discuss the value of sport as a commodity, not only in terms of an entertainment sporting spectacle, but also as a vehicle through which advertisers reach targeted audiences/consumers. Here we are referring to the overall significance of the sport-media complex. In turn, we provide a brief historical outline of the relationship between sport and the media in Canada, with a particular focus on Canada's national network, the Canadian Broadcasting Corporation (CBC). Finally, we offer some perspective on the future of sport and the "new media."

DEFINING MEDIA AND MEDIAMAKING

Communication has always been central to human life. Within contemporary society, however, the media have become so intertwined with all aspects of reality that the boundaries between media and reality have become increasingly blurred. We receive mediated information, entertainment, and imagery from around the world that shapes the lived realities of our day-to-day lives and our understandings of important historical moments and events. In other words, to discuss the media as a separate entity or in isolation from other aspects of our lives and culture (i.e., media and politics, media and society, media and sport) is an oversimplification: the media are already actively implicated in socially constructing/producing these realms even as these realms are in turn involved in shaping the media.

Most people are familiar with and use the term media commonly. But what exactly do we mean by *media*? Media is plural for medium, which is related to the process of circulation of information by some channel of communication. Central to this process is the distribution of signs or symbols by means of an ordered system that constitutes the medium for their transmission. According to Grossberg et al. (2006), every medium is comprised of and shaped by technology (the physical means of producing and distributing signs and symbols), institutions (a large-scale entity, embodying a range of social relations/functions created to perform a function for society), and cultural forms (how the products of media organizations are structured).

In contemporary society the term media is generally understood to refer to the institutions of electronic broadcasting (television, radio, film, the Internet) and various forms of print media (newspapers, magazines, books) that address mass audiences. As David Morley (2005) explains, "by contrast to interpersonal or two-way forms of communication, the emphasis is usually on the sense in which mass media constitute powerful one-way systems for communication from the few to the many" (p. 212). Most people are dependent on some form of media for information, entertainment, and interpretation of events outside their direct or immediate experiences. In this sense, much of our social existence is heavily mediated, and it has been claimed that we live in a "society of the spectacle" (Debord, 1967) constituted by "media culture" (Kellner, 1995).

Consequently, it is important to note that the media act as mediators that occupy the space of interpretation between the subject and reality, actively shaping and re-presenting selected content and experiences. In this chapter we use the term *mediamaking* to suggest that "we see the media and all of the relationships that the media are involved in as active relationships, producing the world at the same time that the world is producing the media" (Grossberg et al., 2006, p. 7). Thus, we cannot study the media and their products separately from the context of their economic, political, historical, and cultural relationships.

Most of the media operating in the global economy, for example, are privately owned and concerned primarily with profit-making through advertising revenues; no more than 12 giant corporations dominate the global media market, including AOL-Time Warner, Disney, Viacom, General Electric, and Sony. In Canada, a very small number of corporations including Bell Globemedia, CanWest Global, Rogers, and Quebecor control most of the media landscape (Harvey & Law, 2005). Although the concentration of media ownership runs parallel to other sectors of the economy, the media warrant special consideration and critical attention because of their role in setting public agendas and framing social issues. The importance of this cannot be overemphasized, particularly in relation to concerns surrounding the effects of concentrated ownership of democracy. While often assumed to be objective, unbiased, and politically neutral, most media are controlled and operated by owners, managers, and editors who are subject to a range of market-oriented constraints and are directly accountable to shareholders and "the bottom line." It is not surprising, then, that the direction editors and owners steer media content is remarkably consistent with business values and business interests in general. As Ralph Miliband noted more than 25 years ago, "those who won and control the capitalist mass media are most likely to be men whose ideological dispositions run from soundly conservative to utterly reactionary" (1969, p. 204). Indeed, in Canada there has been no shortage of cases where the intervention of owners with respect to editorial policy and media content has been direct and remarkably heavy handed (Hackett & Gruneau, 2000; Winter, 1997).

In the case of sport, the media have a major impact on the meanings and values assigned to sporting events, while at the same time trivializing or ignoring others. According to Michael Real, no force has played a more substantial role in socially constructing mediated sporting texts than "commercial television and its institutionalized value system—profit, sponsorship, expanded markets, commodification, and competition" (1998, p. 17). Those in positions of power within the media select and determine not only the sports we see, but also what sort of images, commentary, and ideologies will be emphasized. Often we simply take for granted the fact that our mediated sporting experiences are in fact carefully produced and manufactured for our consumption and naturalized as common sense. That is, we are shown selected versions of sporting events that are determined by those who control the media in relation to cultural, political, economic, and technological contexts, including dominant ideologies. Indeed, Rowe (1999) outlines three forms of cultural power that are manifest in the sport-media complex: institutional power, symbolic power, and relational power. He suggests that

> by gaining a better knowledge and understanding of how media sport texts are produced and what they might mean, it is possible to learn more about societies in which "grounded" and "mediated" experience intermesh in ever more insidious and seemingly seamless ways. (p. 34)

Within the sociology of sport community there have been a number of excellent ethnographic case studies that have provided insights into the nature and politics of how televised sport is produced for audiences in relation to a range of enabling and constraining features. Gruneau's (1989) case study of the CBC's production of a World Cup Downhill ski race, MacNeill's (1996) analysis of CTV's production of the 1988 Calgary Olympics, Stoddart's (1994) analysis of an Australian network's coverage of professional golf, and Silk's (2001) ethnographic analysis of the production of the Kuala Lumpur Commonwealth Games confirm that sporting texts are the result of complex processes associated with making live sport. Meanwhile, Lowes (1999), Rowe (1999), and Theberge and Cronk (1986) have examined a range of aspects associated with the politics and day-to-day operations surrounding the production of sports news for daily newspapers. Of course, production is only one part of the overall process by which sport is produced, represented, consumed, and regulated. It is important that we gain an understanding of each of these particular elements along with their relationships, because as previously noted, sport circulates more than just the event itself; rather, it makes available a whole range of ideologies and meanings about the value of sport in society. Notably, a wide range of research has been conducted in the area of media representation, including both television and print, and the politics of identity within sport.

It is worth highlighting the significance of the print media because it offers some interesting insights into the complex and often contradictory position of sport. Indeed, newspaper sports departments have been described as leading a schizophrenic life (Wanta, 2006). This is due to the fact that sports sections often feature some of the best writing and are among the most read sections of a newspaper, but at the same time are given very little respect (Miller, 1989). As a consequence, there has been very little research concerning sports journalism per se (Lowes, 1999; Rowe, 1999; Theberge & Cronk, 1986); but, as previously noted, there has been fairly extensive research conducted on the media's role in identity politics.

Consider the symbolic annihilation of women's sport through the persistent lack of coverage and the hyper-feminized representations of female athletes deployed in the commercial mass media targeting a primarily male audience (Adams, 2006; Crossman, Hyslop, & Guthrie, 1994; Crossman, Vincent, & Speed, forthcoming; Duncan & Hasbrook, 1988; Duncan &

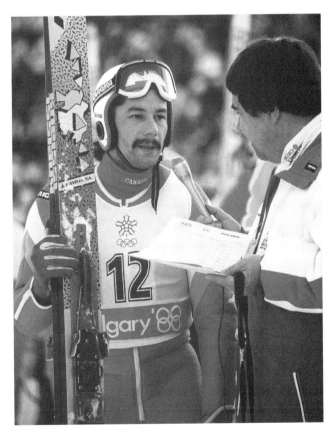

Canada's Steve Collins gives an interview during the ski jumping event at the 1988 Winter Olympics in Calgary.

CP PHOTO/STRCOC/J. Gibson

Messner, 1998; Robinson, 2002). For example, the Canadian Association for the Advancement of Women in Sport (CAAWS) used to do an annual report that examined the amount of newspaper space given to women's sport and consistently found that coverage ranged from a low of 2 percent to a high of 8 percent depending on the newspaper (Robinson, 2002). According to Laura Robinson (2002), the CAAWS ceased to measure these numbers simply because they never changed. Although the power of omission is a sizeable ideological weapon, other strategies of marginalization include "the application of condescending descriptors, the use of compensatory rhetoric, the construction of female athletes according to an adolescent ideal, and the presentation of female athletes as driven by cooperation rather than competition" (Burstyn, 1999, p. 154). However, the issue of how particular sporting identities or issues are represented in the media is not limited to gender. Indeed, this type of research addresses a wide range of issues including how the media represent a range of political issues (cf. Scherer, 2001; Scherer & Jackson, 2004; Whitson & Macintosh, 1993; Wilson & White, 2002); racial/ethnic identity politics (Andrews, 1996; Jackson, 1998a, 1998b; King & Springwood, 2001; Wilson, 1997); sexuality (Jones & LeBlanc, 2005; Lenskyj, 1990; Wright & Clarke, 1999), and national identity (Bairner, 2001; Darnell & Sparks, 2005; Gruneau & Whitson, 1993; Jackson, 1994, 1998c; Whitson & Gruneau, 2006). Although these studies vary with respect to their specific theoretical and methodological framework, central to all of them is a focus on how the media represent particular identities and how this reproduces existing power relations.

THE SPORTS-MEDIA COMPLEX

The foundation of today's sports-media complex was laid in the 1890s with the development and proliferation of the daily sports section of commercial daily newspapers (Burstyn, 1999). This was, in fact, a sizeable acknowledgment of the powerful draw of sports for readers: "the growth of the advertising-dependent mass press and the consolidation of men's sports— especially team sports—went hand in hand in the latter decades of the nineteenth century and the early decades of the twentieth" (Burstyn, 1999, p. 105). As Burstyn (1999) astutely notes:

> Because sport sold newspapers and newspapers sold sport, many newspaper owners in the early years of this century began investing in athletes, sports teams, and sporting facilities, and then in the advertising that promoted them. This marked an early stage in the trend to the corporate integration of ownership of athletes, teams, parks, arenas, stadiums, and newspapers. (pp. 105–6)

Yet, this was clearly just the beginning. Today, one can examine any major commercial sporting event and find an intricate and complex web of interdependent key groups at work, including sports teams/organizations, media/marketing organizations, and transnational corporations (Maguire, 1999). The complex relationships among such groups have been conceptualized in various ways, including the "sports/media complex" (Jhally, 1989), the "media/sport production complex" (Maguire, 1993), the "media sports cultural complex" (Rowe, 1999), and simply "mediasport" (Wenner, 1998). Although there are subtle differences among these views, central to all of them is the recognition of the essential, multifaceted, and powerful relationship embodied by many, but not all, sports, media, and a range of other cultural practices and institutions. Consider the fact that most major sporting spectacles (the Olympics, various World Cups, and many professional sporting leagues) require the cooperation of nation-states, the large global corporations (AOL-Time Warner, ABC/ESPN, Viacom, Rogers, etc.) that own the network and satellite television services (and sometimes the teams and athletes themselves), along with the allied print, radio, and Internet media outlets that circulate information. Jean Harvey and Alan Law (2005), for example, map what they refer to as the "oligopoly" of global sport media ownership that illuminates a shift toward corporate integration of content and distribution with respect to the media and entertainment industries, including the ownership of professional teams and the acquisition of broadcasting rights.[1] As Harvey and Law (2005) note, it is through the ownership of distribution platforms and content-production capacities that corporate convergence and synergy are achieved. It is in this sense that professional sport teams and entire leagues exist as mediated sporting products within "circuits of promotion" that promote other media content and commodities, which in turn also promote sport (Whitson, 1998). Indeed, such a corporate media philosophy has been unquestionably embraced by News Corporation and its longtime chairman and CEO Rupert Murdoch, who regards sports as a "battering ram" to initially penetrate media markets while developing consumer loyalty to a range of entertainment products (Andrews, 2004).

These trends explain in part the continued interest in media corporation ownership of sport teams, but also speak to the exponential growth of broadcasting rights fees. Although initially small, broadcasting rights fees have, in recent years, mushroomed with the increased competition and complexity in the television marketplace. The television rights paid for the Olympic Games by television networks in the United States, for example, have increased exponentially for almost every Olympiad since 1960, as shown in Table 10.1.

A similar pattern of rising broadcast rights fees has occurred in Canada, where the "broadcasting system is a mixed system of public and private corporations in which wars are constantly fought for their respective interests" (Harvey & Law, 2005, p. 201). In 1988, CTV paid US$4.3 million for rights to the Calgary Winter Olympic Games. Recently, a consortium led by Bell Globemedia, incorporating CTV and Rogers Communications, secured Canadian television rights for the 2010 Winter Games (Vancouver) and the 2012 Summer Games (London) with a winning bid of US$153 million, an increase of 110 percent on the $73 million spent for the 2006 and 2008 Games. Of that, US$90 million is for the 2010 Games—a 221-percent increase from the $28 million spent for Torino in 2006—and $63 million for the 2012 Games.

The television rights for other major sporting events have also risen dramatically over the past few decades, with multi-year billion-dollar deals quite commonplace (see Table 10.2).

Table 10.1   United States Summer Olympic Television Rights (in US$)

Games	Country	Broadcaster	Amount
1960	Rome	USA CBS	$394,940
1964	Tokyo	USA NBC	$1,500,000
1968	Mexico	USA ABC	$4,500,000
1972	Munich	USA ABC	$13,500,000
1976	Montreal	USA ABC	$25,000,000
1980	Moscow	USA NBC	$85,000,000
1984	Los Angeles	USA ABC	$225,000,000
1988	Seoul	USA NBC	$300,000,000
1992	Barcelona	USA NBC	$401,000,000
1996	Atlanta	USA NBC	$456,000,000
2000	Sydney	USA NBC	$715,000,000
2004	Athens	USA NBC	$793,000,000
2008	Beijing	USA NBC	$894,000,000
2012	London	USA NBC	$1,800,000,000

Table 10.2   TV Rights for Major Sports and Events

Sport	Network	Cost (US$)
World Cup Soccer	TV rights acquired by international sports marketing agency Infront Sports & Media	$1.97 billion, 2002 & 2006*
Premier League Soccer (UK)	BSKYB	$1.8 billion, 2004–07
NASCAR	FOX, TBS, NBC	$2.4 billion, 2001–07
NFL	ABC, CBS, ESPN, FOX	1998–2005, $18 billion; $2 billion per year
NBA	ABC, ESPN, TNT	$4.6 billion, 2002–08
MLB	FOX, ESPN	$3.3 billion, 2000–06
NHL	ESPN**; OLN/Comcast	2000–05: 120 m/year; $65 million (2006); $70 million (2007) with options for 2008–11

* Horne, J., & Manzenreiter, W. (2002). The World Cup and television football. In J. Horne & W. Manzenreiter (Eds.), *Japan, Korea and the 2002 World Cup.* London: Routledge, p. 197. ISBN: 9780415275620/ISBN-10: 0415275628
** ESPN rejected 2005 optional year at $60 million, which provided an opportunity for an Outdoor Life Network (OLN)/Comcast deal.

This trend demonstrates both the dependency that has emerged between sport-governing bodies and television revenues, and, furthermore, that sport will "go to any lengths to accommodate television" (Boyle & Haynes, 2000, p. 49).

Professional leagues are similarly dependent on the revenue generated from their television rights agreements as predictable sources of income, but also for publicity without which the popularity of commercial sport would be very limited in an increasingly cluttered promotional/media culture. This is a crucial difference compared to the coverage given to other cultural events; that is, sports coverage is frequent, ongoing, and incredibly detailed. As television assumed a different, more dominant role in the mediation of sport, it was no longer willing to simply televise the event. Seeking to package sport into a pattern that ensured the maximum exposure and revenue, sport governing bodies were often lobbied to make both major and minor rule changes and alterations to meet the ongoing needs of the broadcaster. Networks sought to dictate when, where, and in what form sport could take place. For example, major sporting spectacles tend to be scheduled in relation to the largest and most lucrative markets—which in North America tend to be in the American northeast. Other, perhaps more peripheral, changes included the introduction of television time-outs and teams/leagues accommodating reporters by constructing press boxes and providing access to players, particularly during breaks in games. Another example of the media's influence on sport was the Fox network's attempt to introduce the FoxTrax glow puck beginning with the 1996 NHL All Star game. The technology was intended to help prospective new fans follow the puck, but was met with severe criticism from traditional spectators, particularly Canadians (see Mason, 2002). Yet, despite the demands of television, the relationship is symbiotic, as the partners need each other to maintain and extend their influence. The relationship is best exemplified, for instance, by the "area black-out rule" whereby television broadcasts are often restricted within a specified geographic territory in order to encourage local fans to purchase tickets to the actual event.

There have been exceptions and some observers have suggested that we may have reached the point whereby the costs of broadcasting rights are becoming prohibitive for networks and sponsors. Moreover, the media value of some sports has diminished as a consequence of low ratings caused by a combination of factors including increased competition, image problems associated with violence, scandals related to corruption or drugs, strikes or lockouts that interrupt or cancel seasons, and arguably a range of cultural barriers. Consider the NHL's precarious position in the United States. Generally speaking, the NHL has always been relatively popular in Canada whether its games were broadcast by the CBC, CTV, or TSN. However, despite successive expansions to new U.S. markets, substantive marketing campaigns, and strong regional television ratings in several major markets, the NHL remains a marginal television product in U.S. sports culture. Golf, college football, basketball, and a range of "minor" sports routinely draw larger television audiences than does the NHL (Bellamy & Shultz, 2006). In fact, almost every major national network has broadcast the NHL but, for a range of reasons, has not renegotiated their television rights. The most recent example of the difficulties facing the NHL in the U.S. occurred following the 2004–05 NHL lockout, when ESPN opted to forgo an option for 2005 that would have cost only $60 million in contrast to its regular $120-million fee for several years prior. Consequently, the Outdoor Life Network (OLN) in partnership with Comcast signed a national broadcasting deal with the NHL that offered them the 2006 season for $65 million and 2007 for $70 million, with further options until 2011. The television rights for the NHL have become much more complicated, with a range of deals signed on both sides of the Canada–U.S. border, including regional deals that have heightened disparities in income generated by large-market U.S. teams such as the New York Rangers and small-market Canadian teams. Of course, the sport-media complex in Canada today has been shaped by a range of historical factors; we now turn to a brief chronological overview of how some key events have shaped it.

THE HISTORICAL DEVELOPMENT OF THE TELEVISION–SPORT RELATIONSHIP IN CANADA

> Sport in Canada rarely generates its own change, but tends to be shaped by other forces in the society. Until more Canadians become concerned about the effects of unregulated commercialism upon other aspects of Canadian society, it is unlikely they will ever be concerned about the effects of commercialism in sport. (Kidd, 1970, p. 272)

This section outlines the historical development of the television–sport relationship in Canada. Our intention here is twofold. First, we endeavour to illuminate the sheer volume of changes in the Canadian televisual sporting landscape that have occurred over a relatively short period of time. Second, we discuss these changes in relation to a historical struggle between nationalists, who have advocated for a state-controlled broadcasting system to promote and protect Canadian culture, and the pressures of private interests to develop "media empires modeled on the U.S. entertainment media entertainment enterprises" (Harvey & Law, 2005, p. 200). The remnants and effects of these struggles are still visible today in Canada's telecommunications and broadcasting system, which features a mix, albeit an uneven one, of public and corporate corporations. For example, Canadians today have access to a number of privately owned national networks (CTV, Global) and regional networks (CityTV, A-Channel) in addition to Canada's national broadcaster, the CBC/SRC. While the CBC/SRC is a Crown corporation (i.e., it relies on support from Parliament through the Ministry of Canadian Heritage), it also derives substantial revenue from selling commercial time. Most Canadians have access to a range of U.S. networks in addition to a number of specialty channels, including dedicated sports channels TSN/RDS, Rogers Sportsnet, and

The Score. Canadians also have access to a range of digital and pay television sporting options, including Leafs TV (owned by Maple Leaf Sports & Entertainment), Raptors NBA TV (owned by Maple Leaf Sports & Entertainment in limited partnership with the NBA), and the NHL Network (owned by the NHL and Bell Globemedia), among others. Access to the diverse range of predominantly privately owned televisual sports content, however, was clearly not always the case.

The CBC was established 1936 in part as a response to concerns over the penetration of commercialized radio content by U.S. radio networks. The significance of this initial radio network cannot be overstated. Modelled after the BBC, the CBC emerged as the

> central electronic institution of cultural *reproduction*, where broadcasters could create programming, and as well a *distribution* network for delivering to the public its made-in-Canada-by Canadians-for Canadians news, public affairs, music, drama, sports, and entertainment programs. In its halcyon days through the 1940s and 1950s, the CBC helped consolidate a national consciousness among Anglophones as its French-Canadian arm, Radio Canada, did for Francophones. (Clarkson, 2002, p. 365)

Corporate sport, and more specifically professional hockey, emerged as a key element in the programming activities of Canada's new radio broadcaster. Through *HNIC*, the CBC simultaneously raised NHL hockey to the level of national passion while creating a Saturday-night ritual for many Canadians. However, as Bruce Kidd (1996b) argues, the CBC's partnership with the NHL distorted the development of Canadian sport and culture and contributed to the systematic annihilation of the coverage of women's sport in the media, a trend that is visible to this day. As Gruneau and Whitson (1993) note: "By 1934 the national General Motors broadcasts were reaching over a million listeners. By the end of the 1930s, the audience for *Hockey Night in Canada*—now sponsored by Imperial Oil—had doubled to two million listeners" (p. 101). The case of *HNIC* underscores the importance of understanding media-making processes in relation to broader social and historical contexts. Thus, while it is often argued that ice hockey is one of the most—if not *the*—defining features of Canadian identity, we need to understand that it is not something natural, essential, or inevitable. Rather, a vast range of state, corporate, and media agencies have combined to ensure ice hockey's central position in both Canadian culture and the Canadian marketplace, often at a cost to others. As Kidd (1996b) notes, *HNIC* was literally designed as an all-male affair that in turn "helped keep women's sports off the air" (p. 260).

By the 1950s, all previously existing forms of mass media, including books, newspapers, magazines, films, and radio, were being challenged by the sports–television "revolution." Television was the pre-eminent mass medium of the last half of the twentieth century and, as noted above, remains central to the delivery of sport product to Canadians. Historically, experiments with television started in the early 1920s in both Europe and the United States. Having made rapid advancements in the technology at a number of centres throughout the world, pioneering German scientists successfully transmitted the first live television images of the Opening Ceremonies of the Games of the Eleventh Olympiad in 1936 to receiving screens in viewing halls located within a two-mile radius of the stadium. At different times during the Games, four competition venues, including the Olympic Stadium and the swimming facility, housed television equipment. During 138 hours of coverage, a total of 162,228 people watched the transmitted blurred images of athletes performing (Barney, 1993, p. 17). Yet, despite the success experienced in Berlin, television was considered only an extension of the stadium, rather than an important medium in its own right.

Notwithstanding the early success with television, broadcasting was halted in Britain and the U.S. with the onset of World War II. However, when work on the commercial application of television resumed following the cessation of hostilities, progress came quickly. Twenty-four stations were licensed in the U.S. in 1946, and more than one hundred by 1948. By August 1949, an estimated two million Americans owned television sets; that number jumped to 13 million by June 1951. Sport has been credited with some of this dramatic growth. Indeed, such was the influence of the media that it "has even been suggested that the televising of major league baseball, boxing and college football in the 1940's was a key element in launching the television industry" (Goldlust, 1987, p. 81). In Canada, despite the lack of a Canadian television station, an estimated 3,600 television sets were owned in 1949 by those able to afford the costly units and those geographically positioned to receive signals from American broadcasters. As Clarkson (2002) notes, "the technology enabling the broadcast of images and the arrival of U.S. commercial television in the early 1950s revived the national debate over Canada's cultural survival" (p. 365). After three years of hurried labour by CBC's Board of Governors, television officially came to Canada on September 6, 1952, when CBFT in Montreal began telecasting, followed two days later by CBLT in Toronto.

Although the early experiments with television focused on Maple Leaf Gardens in Toronto, the first NHL game to be televised on CBC was actually a game in Montreal on October 11, 1952, three weeks before Toronto's television debut. The debut saw Imperial Oil purchase the television rights for that first season at just $100 per Maple Leafs game, as team owner Conn Smythe wanted to make sure that hockey was as appealing on television as it was on radio before asking for an appropriate fee. The following season, Imperial Oil purchased the rights to the games for $150,000 a year in a three-year contract. By the early 1960s, after Stafford Smythe had bought out his father's controlling stock in the Gardens, the rights sold for $9 million over six years, or approximately $21,000 per game. Undoubtedly a success,

> Television revenues rose steadily through the 1950s and 1960s as the size of audiences grew in North America. Less than 10% of Canadian homes had televisions in 1953, but by 1960 the number had jumped to 80%. Almost immediately, *Hockey Night in Canada* became the CBC's most popular television show, drawing audiences as large as 3.5 million English Canadians and 2 million French Canadians by the early 1960s. (Gruneau & Whitson, 1993, p. 105)

Thus, it did not take long for *HNIC* to become a valuable media commodity that could reach a large, national, and predominantly male audience. In turn, the success of *HNIC*, as opposed to other televised sports, contributed to ice hockey serving as a key site for the confirmation of a dominant masculinity predicated on physical violence (Kidd, 1996b).

The new medium developed rapidly, and its growth brought new ownership to the media industry. At the same time, many private companies in Canada that already owned and operated newspaper or radio outlets were among those granted television licences on the condition that their stations operate as CBC affiliates. By 1960 there were 47 stations in Canada: 9 wholly owned CBC stations, and 38 privately owned CBC affiliates. Each of the stations was linked to the others by a coast-to-coast microwave relay system that enabled everyone but those living in the most remote areas of Canada to receive a Canadian television station. In less than a decade, three-quarters of all Canadian households possessed a television set. With the quality of telecasts steadily improving, watching television soon became the number one in-house leisure activity of Canadians, who were increasingly viewing professional hockey and football, but also boxing, wrestling, and a range of international sporting competitions. This is but one clear example of how media technologies changed Canadian lifestyles.

Many Canadians were, however, dissatisfied with the CBC's dominant position as the country's sole broadcaster. In 1958, responding, in part, to the growing dissatisfaction of a system that saw the private broadcasters regulated by the CBC, the Conservative government of John

Diefenbaker announced it would allow competitor stations. By 1960, under the independent regulatory authority of the Board of Broadcast Governors (BBG) established two years earlier, eight privately owned "second" television stations were licensed in Canada's largest municipal centres. Shortly after, on October 1, 1961, these stations formed Canada's second television network, CTV, thus providing an alternative to the programming offered by CBC stations. In 1963, CTV established its own microwave relay system linking its affiliates from coast to coast.

Regardless of the federal government's intentions, the statute bringing these changes into effect did not clearly specify the relationship of authority between the CBC and the BBG. Given the confusion, and unwilling to relinquish its control over Canada's private broadcasters, the "CBC tried to continue its operations just as it had done in the past" (Lorimer & McNulty, 1996, p. 181). However, under the 1968 Broadcasting Act a new agency, the Canadian Radio and Television Commission (CRTC), was given full regulatory authority over all aspects of the Canadian broadcasting system, including the CBC networks and stations.[2] One of the CRTC's substantial regulatory powers included the authority to limit foreign ownership of Canadian broadcasters. More specifically, the CRTC restricted broadcast licences to those firms with at least 80 percent Canadian ownership and/or board membership.

In their struggle to compete, television broadcasters used sport as an important component of their weekly programming mix. Historically, sports programming proved to be inexpensive, popular, and easy to schedule; once sizeable audiences had been confirmed, the competing networks expanded their coverage to include other sports including golf, figure skating, and curling.

In the Canadian context, sport also helped to satisfy the networks' government-stipulated mandate to ensure that they conformed to Canadian-content requirements. First introduced by the BBG in 1959, Canadian-content requirements have risen from 45 percent of broadcast hours to be devoted to programs of Canadian origin, to the present-day regulations requiring 60 percent Canadian content and 50 percent in prime time for conventional private stations. Although somewhat restricting, the definition of "Canadian" has been generously defined to include any program produced by a licensee, all productions made in Canada, and broadcasts of events taking place outside Canada in which Canadians were participating, such as NHL hockey. It also includes events that are deemed to be of special interest to Canadians, including sporting events such as the World Series.

In an effort to achieve its Canadian-content goals, the CBC began securing the rights for, and televising, international sporting events such as the 1972 Canada–Russia Summit Series (which drew massive audiences for the network), the Commonwealth and Olympic Games, as well as those games played by professional sports teams headquartered in Canada—including the two Canadian Major League Baseball teams, the Toronto Blue Jays and the Montreal Expos.

By the 1970s, the Canadian media landscape had further evolved, with Canadians increasingly interacting with U.S.-network sporting products shown on the three major U.S. networks (ABC, CBS, and NBC), leading to nationalists' concerns over the Americanization of Canada. By the 1990s the entire Canadian media system was being increasingly challenged by a number of economic pressures resulting from globalization. On one hand, increased calls to completely privatize the CBC, as well as funding cuts by the Mulroney and Chrétien governments, resulted in declining programming quality and equally declining audiences for the CBC (Hurtig, 2002). Conversely, economic and cultural deregulation (through the FTA and NAFTA), and substantive technological developments including the establishment of digital and satellite television, have increased the variety of sports content available to Canadians.

What is at stake here is the kind of sport programming to be broadcast by particular types of corporations following particular kinds of objectives. For example, in 2002 the broadcasting of the legendary *La soirée du hockey*, a cultural institution for Quebeckers for more than 50 years, was threatened after talks between Radio-Canada and Réseau des Sports (RDS) collapsed; RDS had already negotiated with the NHL, the Montreal Canadiens, and the Ottawa Senators for the broadcasting rights for a package of regular-season and playoff games (Harvey & Law, 2005). Radio-Canada's withdrawal, however, generated criticism among fans but also from politicos, because "French-speaking fans, inside and outside of Quebec, would either have to watch *Hockey Night in Canada* (in English) or subscribe to cable or satellite television" (Harvey, 2006, p. 47). More specifically, after concern was expressed by federal Heritage Minister Sheila Copps—and the formation of a House of Commons Standing Joint Committee on Official Languages to examine the issue—RDS and the Canadiens began new negotiations with Radio-Canada, resulting in a three-year deal allowing the Crown corporation to broadcast a number of Canadiens hockey matches on Saturday nights, as well as off-season games. This is one of many examples of how market imperatives can conflict with cultural institutions, in this case a very specific francophone cultural institution, and, in turn, influence what Canadians can watch.

It is likely that debates surrounding the role of the nation's public broadcaster and its provision of sport will be ongoing and contentious. In June 2006, the Canadian Curling Association (CCA) signed an exclusive six-year broadcasting and multimedia deal with TSN, ending a 40-year association with the CBC. The deal gives TSN exclusive rights to major curling events. Concern, however, has been expressed over the fact that curling matches will be unavailable on a national network. TSN has indicated that select matches may also be shown on CTV. Notably, in June 2006, a Senate report recommended the gradual phasing out of commercials on the CBC and that Canada's public broadcaster cease coverage of professional sports and the Olympics. Meanwhile, the CBC's broadcasting agreement with the NHL,

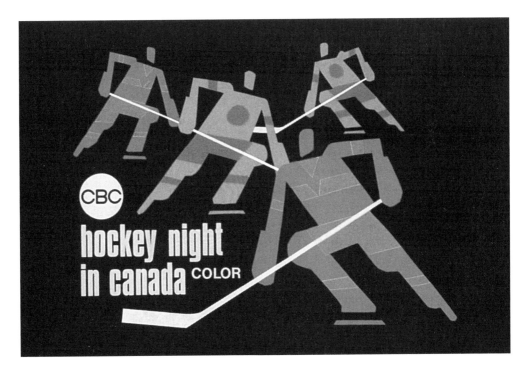

How and why has *Hockey Night in Canada* remained a "Canadian institution"?

CBC Still Photo Collection

which is estimated at CDN$65 million per year, is set to expire at the end of the 2007–8 NHL season. However, the CBC will likely be competing against an aggressive and sizeable bid from CTV-TSN for exclusive broadcasting rights, potentially marking the end of the public broadcasting of *Hockey Night in Canada* (a brand name owned by the CBC). There are several levels of irony here, most notably given the substantive role the publicly owned broadcaster has played in establishing the mass popularity of hockey since 1952.

The historical development and current operations of the CBC illustrate the processes of mediamaking that have played a large part in structuring the lives and sporting experiences of many Canadians. Other developments have seen Canadians increasingly engage sports content through a range of new media technologies and new interactive forms of mediamaking. It is to a brief discussion of these issues that we now turn.

SPORT AND NEW MEDIA TECHNOLOGIES

With the rapid advancements in communications technologies, it is easy to forget that technological changes have been a constant feature of the historical development of the sports-media complex. Advancements in photography (1830s), the typewriter (1860s), transatlantic cable (1866), telephone (1876), motion pictures (1894), wireless telegraphy (1895), magnetic tape recording (1899), radio (1906), and television (1923) have each played a significant role in the development of mediated sport. However, as we move into an increasingly networked global arena, a range of new media technologies are expanding "the possibilities of cultural production into areas normally associated with consumption, enabling fans to produce their own custom-made texts out of the 'raw' material supplied" (Rowe, 1999, p. 168). The expanding multimedia marketplace, which includes broadband, digital, and high-definition television, cable multipoint multi-channel distribution service (MMDS), and a range of new wireless/mobile technologies, is rapidly transforming the processes of mediamaking and the consumption experiences of an increasing number of Canadians. For example, according to a recent Ipsos-Reid poll, Canadians between the ages of 18 and 34 (a demographic considered to have a sizeable disposable income) are spending more time on the Internet than any other medium. Not surprisingly, the Internet and other digital distribution techniques have provided a unique avenue for existing media corporations to extend their influence and power in the aggressive competition to attract increasingly fragmented and discerning audiences.

The CBC, for example, attempts to ensure the coordinated development of its Internet products—media content, wireless products, database information, software—for the entire country. CBC websites have received repeated recognition for their effectiveness and the interest generated among audiences both at home and abroad. The main CBC website (www.cbc.ca) now receives more than 3.5 million page views each week. Using various Internet and data technologies, CBC Radio and CBC Newsworld have extended the availability of content by providing on-demand access to their hourly newscasts in Real Audio and Real Video formats. Cyber audiences are able to download news segments or the most recent diatribe by Don Cherry on *Coach's Corner*. Unlike television, which offers a restricted schedule determined by networks, audiences are able to consume media content on the Internet at their convenience, drastically altering viewing/consumption experiences. For example, in 2006 Walt Disney Co.'s ABC network made episodes of *Lost*, *Desperate Housewives*, *Commander in Chief*, and *Alias* available free for flexible viewing (but not downloading) online for a U.S. audience over a two-month trial period. Interestingly, while viewers will be able to pause, fast-forward, and rewind episodes, they will not be able to skip over the commercials of the programs' sponsors including AT&T Corp., Ford Motor Co., Procter & Gamble Co., Toyota

Motor Corp., and Walt Disney Pictures—a reminder that the Internet is an increasingly commodified medium.

Given the global visibility and cultural centrality of sport, it is not surprising that "the greatest war for market share is with regard to sports websites" (McChesney, 1999, p. 174). These electronic sporting spaces have emerged as significant battlegrounds for networks and other corporations to locate and interact with premium consumers and sports fans who are regarded as the most "rabid of Internet users" (Grover, 1998, p. 188). Other broadcasters, such as TSN-RDS and Rogers Sportsnet, have extensive websites while all the major professional leagues, franchises, and even individual athletes such as Sidney Crosby are utilizing a range of interactive and increasingly mobile media technologies as part of their global branding strategies. For example, Manchester United's website receives eight million hits per month, most of which are from overseas, enabling new fans as well as expatriates to keep up to date with the team and players (Boyle & Haynes, 2003). Of course, such a global marketing opportunity was not lost on the club's sponsor, telecommunications company Vodafone, which "intends to use the Manchester United brand to sell new products—including co-branded phones—and introduce new media services such as club-specific content across a range of platforms" (Boyle & Haynes, 2003, p. 107).

One of the main issues and debates surrounding the use of new media technologies relates to the ownership of rights to electronic images and content. While players are increasingly attempting to negotiate control over their online image rights, new media technologies are providing international sport organizations, such as the IOC, with leverage in their negotiations with broadcasters for the 2010 Winter Olympics in Vancouver and the 2012 London Summer Games. More specifically, as part of its current negotiating strategy, the IOC is "bundling" traditional broadcasting rights with those for cable television and the Internet, mobile phones, and other new media technologies. Meanwhile, other professional clubs, such as Celtic of the Scottish Premier League, have been at the forefront of the development and ownership of online content. Celtic created its own in-house multimedia production company, which enabled the club to screen live video coverage of a UEFA Cup match through its website in 1999 (Boyle & Haynes, 2003). In a similar vein, the New Zealand Rugby Union (NZRU) has recently invested in the in-house production of Allblacks.com to communicate with a global audience of rugby fans. However, the NZRU cannot display live rugby matches featuring the All Blacks on its website because those images are owned by News Corporation as per its broader broadcasting agreement with SANZAR (South African, New Zealand and Australian Rugby Unions) (Scherer & Jackson, 2005).

Beyond sponsoring individual teams and athletes, transnational sporting corporations including Nike, Reebok, and Adidas, among others, have also developed their own comprehensive websites and a number of online games complete with e-commerce capabilities to communicate and interact with a global audience of consumers and sports fans (Scherer, forthcoming). Indeed, as Schiller (1999) explains:

> For this purpose, the advertising community had already begun to fix on one of a handful of "old-standby" program genres with a demonstrated global popularity: sports and games, in a plethora of formats and business models. Games in turn engaged the potential implicit in the first of cyberspace's critical typifying features: its interactivity. (p. 130)

In a similar vein, other networks and leagues have invested in the production of branded fantasy sporting leagues that allow cyber sporting fans to select and follow their "own" teams throughout the season in a broader competition with other subscribers. Such fantasy leagues often involve an extensive commitment of time and energy on the part of the cyber fan to follow the ebb and flow of the fantasy sporting season. Indeed, the appeal of interactive websites, online games, and fantasy sports for corporations is that they are relatively cheap to produce/maintain and allow corporations to reach and communicate with premium cyber audiences on a consistent and often lengthy basis in a relatively secure and extensively branded cyber environment.[3] Here it is important to note that many of these electronic initiatives increasingly target a new demographic referred to as the "jeeks": an audience of sports-loving and computer-literate boys and men who possess a level of technological and cultural capital required to engage such electronic sporting spaces (Scherer, forthcoming).

The relatively inclusive nature of Internet communication technologies not only has enabled the mass media to extend their delivery of sport, but also has provided an opportunity for computer-equipped sport fans to communicate with each other through a number of online discussion forums. For example, new virtual communities of sports fans are created when professional sports teams allow fans to post comments on their websites. Even traditional print media have recognized the value in producing interactive online forums; for example, *The Globe and Mail* allows its online readers to post comments pertaining to particular stories or other postings, while its columnists are often available online to answer questions during virtual forums at designated times. During the NBA playoffs, *Sports Illustrated*'s website features blogs by its writers that are frequently updated after games; in a form of real-time commentary, fans are able to respond by posting comments related to particular blogs. However, it is important to note that many sites require the payment of registration or subscription fees to access unique electronic content. Beyond corporate-controlled websites, an increasing number of cyber sporting fans have created their own blogs, which allow them to post their views and opinions while interacting and debating with other bloggers over a range of sporting issues. These electronic consumption and communication experiences arguably foster a complex form of virtual togetherness (Bakardjieva, 2005) that may allow communication and interaction beyond the constraints of private interests and capital.

Beyond interactivity, a range of new media technologies are also extending the flexibility of consumption experiences by enabling consumers to engage the media–sport landscape on their mobile phones and handsets. For example, fans can receive real-time sporting updates, statistics, and stories/highlights from a range of television networks on phones equipped with video and high-bandwidth capabilities. Cellphone carriers are increasingly capable of delivering full television and music services and moving beyond the boundaries of traditional television. More specifically, the CRTC recently upheld its new media exemption order (created in 1999), setting a precedent that the regulatory agency would not set rules for broadcasting services over the Internet. As such, mobile television services won't be required to carry specific channels and will have greater content control compared to traditional broadcasters. One of the latest developments with respect to mobile technologies and media sport is "podcasts," which allow fans to receive audio and video files over the Internet via mobile devices including MP3 players and personal computers. Podcasting effectively allows consumers to download and create their own mediated and mobile sporting experiences. In this sense, consumers and sports fans are increasingly becoming an integral part of the social construction of their sporting and consumption experiences. It is unlikely that the rapid evolution of new media technologies will dissipate any time soon. For example, there is another Internet—already operational—where the minimum connection speed is almost 3,000 times faster than a dial-up modem. On average, users receive connections up to one hundred times faster than home users experience with a broadband connection. It is a network so swift and so powerful that its advocates are claiming it has already changed the way we will interact with the Internet in the future. This new Internet, called Internet2, is under development in more than 190 universities and research laboratories across the globe. Although its usage is currently limited to the research and education communities, its benefits could spill over into the mainstream in only a few years. Various media corporations, as well as companies such as McDonald's, Johnson & Johnson, and Ford, are keenly watching developments on the new network. The fast-food chain has already shown interest in the tele-immersion experiments run on Internet2, envisioning tele-immersion cubicles in its restaurants so those away from home could have dinner with their family.

With the increased bandwidth capabilities of Internet2, the development and implementation of software applications that enable such things as the broadcasting of high-definition television (HDTV) over the Internet have already become a reality. Multicasting, or broadcasting from one server to many recipients with one data stream, could enable a single Web server site to supply thousands of users with a continuous, uninterrupted feed. These developments create new possibilities not only for those involved in the distribution of media, but also for those who produce its content. In general, the discoveries made on Internet2 are poised to speed up the technological and corporate convergence of the "traditional" mass media.

CONCLUSIONS: SPORT, MEDIA, AND CULTURAL POWER

Whoever controls the media—the images—controls the culture.

Allen Ginsberg, poet and author

Sport has played a critical role in globalization processes, regularly providing audiences from different cultures, languages, religions, and political ideologies with some of the largest global spectacles of our time. The Olympic Games, the World Cup of soccer, and the Super Bowl are among those sporting events that repeatedly attract audiences in excess of 100 million. With the continued proliferation of specialty sport newspapers and magazines, sport talk radio, sport channels, and sport websites, the media have become increasingly interlinked with these and other sport spectacles. In contemporary society, the mass media are the primary vehicle through which sports texts are produced and disseminated. This is a key point fundamental to understanding the role of the media in creating our common-sense view of the world, particularly in relation to identity politics related to nationhood, race/ethnicity, gender and sexuality, and ability/disability. As such we hope that students will strive to make links between our chapter and others within this text.

Throughout this chapter we have highlighted the role of sport within what Grossberg et al. (2006) refer to as mediamaking; that is, the active role of the media in "producing the world at the same time that the world is producing the media" (p. 7). After describing the nature and meaning of mediamaking we outlined the relationship between sport and the media. In particular we explored the increasingly complex relationship that has emerged among sport, media, and transnational corporations, or what is referred to as the sport-media complex. Clearly, sport is a valuable commodity for the media given that it embodies human drama, offers up heroes and celebrities, is relatively cheap to produce, and attracts large global audiences. Arguably, in order to understand contemporary sport we need to locate it as a cultural commodity in late capitalism (Andrews, 2004), which is both transforming and transformative through new synergistic global media technologies as well the shifting nature of contemporary culture itself. The emergence of sport-related programs such as *Survivor*, *The Amazing Race*, and *Dancing With the Stars* signifies a convergence of celebrity culture, hypercommercialism, sex, commodified identity politics, and a contemporary obsession with "reality" even if its temporal and spatial composition is both compressed and highly mediated. In turn, we traced the historical development of the sport-media relationship in Canada, noting the ways in which public and private interests converge and sometimes compete.

Finally, we concluded this chapter with a brief discussion of sport and the new media, revealing that technological change has been a constant feature of the sport-media complex.

As part of this discussion we explained how it is positioned to merge the traditional media forms, as well as the roles played by spectators and participants.

The capacity of each student of sport "to decode media sports texts and to detect the forms of ideological deployment of sport in the media is, irrespective of cultural taste, a crucial skill" (Rowe, 1999, p. 8). Given the position occupied by the mass media in today's society, along with the significant impact the media have on the meanings and values assigned to sporting events, it is also essential that we understand the relationship between sport and the media. With the ability to interpret mediated sport texts, students of sport are able to embark on a journey that will illuminate the process by which media sports are presented, created, and assigned various meanings within the wider political, economic, and cultural contours of our society.

NOTES

1. An oligopoly denotes a situation where a few powerful corporations collectively own and influence a significant segment of the marketplace. Using the top five global media corporations, including NewsCorp (Rupert Murdoch), Disney, and Time-Warner, along with the two major Canadian players BCE (Bell Canada) and CanWest Global, they chart the structural and functional relationships among the various media companies within each of these major corporations. Notably, sport figures prominently within all of the media holdings of these major media corporations.
2. The name was changed to the Canadian Radio-television and Telecommunications Commission in 1976, when telecommunications was added to the commission's list of responsibilities. Today, the CRTC's responsibilities continue under the updated Act of 1991, and the Telecommunications Act of 1993.
3. Unlike traditional media, websites and online games are vulnerable to hacking (Scherer, in press).

CRITICAL THINKING QUESTIONS

1. Why are media corporations prepared to spend huge sums of money on securing the television rights to sporting events?
2. Has the integration of sports and media into a combined totality moved sports away from the classical values of fair play and toward commercialization and profit? Are the two mutually exclusive?
3. How do the powerful allegiances being forged between television and sponsors present a challenge to those bodies that have traditionally run sport at either a national or international level?
4. Considering the rapid development of new media technologies, will the increasing capacity for international communications stifle Canadian cultural production or will it expand its possibilities?

SUGGESTED READINGS

Barney, R., Wenn, S., & Martyn, S. (2002). *Selling the five rings: The International Olympic Committee and the rise of Olympic commercialism.* Salt Lake City: The University of Utah Press.

McLuhan, M., & Fiore, Q. (2001). *The medium is the massage: An inventory of effects.* Corte Madera, CA: Gingko Press.

McQuail, D. (1994). *Mass communication theory: An introduction,* 3rd ed. Thousand Oaks, CA: Sage.

Scherer, J., & Jackson, S. (2004). From corporate welfare to national interest: Newspaper analysis of the public subsidization of NHL hockey debate in Canada. *Sociology of Sport Journal, 21,* 36–60.

Simpson, V., & Jennings, A. (1992). *The lords of the rings: Power, money and drugs in the modern Olympics.* London: Simon and Schuster.

Whitson, D., & Gruneau, R. (Eds.). (2006). *Artificial ice: Hockey, commerce, and cultural identity.* Peterborough, ON: Broadview Press.

WEB LINKS

The Canadian Association of Journalists (CAJ)

http://www.eagle.ca/caj/

Contains a directory of Canadian journalists, an online archive of *Media Magazine,* and Internet resources for those interested in various aspects of journalism.

Canadian Newspaper Association (CNA)

http://www.cna-acj.ca/

For the people who publish and work for newspapers in Canada, as well as those who read newspapers, including an online resource of Canadian newspapers and media sources.

Canadian Radio-television and Telecommunications Commission (CRTC)

http://www.crtc.gc.ca/eng/welcome.htm

Provides information about the history and organization of Canada's broadcasting and telecommunication systems, as well as the relevant documents and speeches involving the Canadian agency responsible for regulating the system.

Official Olympic Website

http://www.olympic.org/uk/index_uk.asp

Provides a range of information including details of television rights contracts.

Ipsos Canada

http://www.angusreid.com/

Devoted to the collection and analysis of marketing data, providing both the public and private sector with insight into the thoughts, feelings, and intentions of people throughout the world.

Journal of Mass Media Ethics

http://jmme.byu.edu/

Devoted to explorations of ethics problems and issues in the various fields of mass communication.

Media Awareness Network

http://www.media-awareness.ca/

Provides resources for media education across the curriculum, focusing primarily on K–12, while providing the user with information and "food for thought" on the evolving media culture.

Nielsen Media Research

http://www.nielsenmedia.com/

Primarily provides information about the media measurement services available at Nielsen Media Research and the various means used to collect the data. Audience estimates for broadcast and cable networks, nationally distributed syndicated programs, and satellite distributors for various populations are made available on the website.

Scholarly Sport Sites

http://www.ucalgary.ca/library/ssportsite/

Subject directory that brings together websites that will assist the serious sports researcher on a broad range of topics.

CHAPTER 11

THE ECONOMICS OF SPORT AND THE NHL LOCKOUT

Marc Lavoie

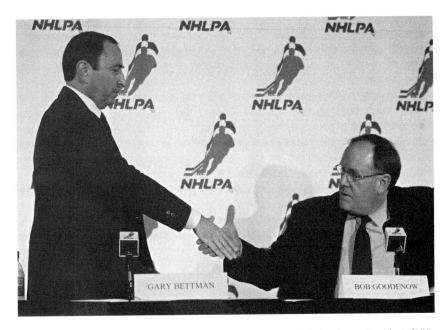

Collective bargaining at work: Gary Bettman (NHL Commissioner) and Bob Goodenow (President of NHL Players' Association) shaking hands.

ADRIAN WYLD/CP Images

. . . and a weak and desperate Goodenow was compelled to make major concessions in the new CBA in order to salvage what was left . . . Bettman took his pants.

Gil Stein, NHL president 1992–1993, *Power Plays: An Inside Look at the Big Business of the National Hockey League* (1997, p. 115)

While both sides lost heavily from the lockout, however, the owners clearly won the overall war.

Paul D. Staudohar, *Playing for Dollars: Labor Relations and the Sports Business* (1996, p. 152)

The owners were worried that the players' share of league revenues had reached 61 percent.... It looks like owners won this round.

Rodney Fort, *Sports Economics* (2003, p. 294)

The economics of sport is a rather wide field. It spreads across analyses of the demand for sport, cost–benefit analyses of sporting events and sporting venues, the local public finance implications of these same events and venues, sporting governance (meaning labour–management relations, organizational models of team or individual sports events, as well as professional leagues), the business and finance of professional leagues, wage determination, labour-market discrimination, trade in the sporting goods industry, media coverage, sponsoring, endorsements, and numerous related issues such as the economics of performance-enhancing drugs. Broadly speaking these themes have developed from two traditions in sports economics, a North American one and a Continental European one, although there is now a trend for both traditions to merge. North Americans and their colleagues from Britain and Australia have applied the standard tools of supply and demand analysis to model the behaviour of the various participants to the world of sport. They have focused most of their attention to professional sport, more specifically men's team sports, using advanced statistical methods such as regression analysis. On the other hand, Continental European sports economics is more of the institutionalist sort, relying more on descriptive statistics, with tables of numbers and the computation of various ratios, while some- times applying economic theories alternative to the standard supply and demand analysis. Continental Europeans are also concerned with professional teams, but they devote more atten- tion to the sporting goods industry (manufacturing and world trade patterns) and to the eco- nomics of amateur and recreational sport, in particular the Olympic Games.

An attempt to deal with all these issues within a single chapter would yield a rather super- ficial analysis. The agenda of this chapter is driven by the fact that most of the academic research on the economics of sport in North America, both at the theoretical level and in data gathering, actually deals with team sports, in large part precisely because of data availability. Within the Canadian context, it seems best to focus on one sport, ice hockey, and more specif- ically the economics of the National Hockey League. As much as we would like to deal with other Canadian sporting traditions—the Canadian Football League (CFL), lacrosse indoor leagues, or all sorts of minor leagues—very little can be said due to an absence of data (but see Box 11.1 about the CFL). As to Olympic sports, while the funding of amateur athletes raises important questions of public policy, these are not questions that readily lend themselves to economic analysis. The Olympic Games today clearly involve big money and invite questions about the costs and benefits of staging them, but estimates related to their net economic impact are mired in fantasies and hard to assess. The interested reader is referred to an easy-to-read introduction to the economic issues arising from holding the Vancouver 2010 Winter Olympics, such as transportation costs, speculation in the real estate market and the impact on low-income housing, high-skill labour demand and possible inflationary repercussions, and the possible cost underestimation and net impact overestimation (Fromm, 2005); these topics are examined in more detail by Preuss (2004), for all the Olympic Games staged since 1972.

The substantial transformation of the (team) sports business over the last decades is most obvious in the way sports news is being reported since the early 1990s. In the past, sports reporters and columnists were primarily concerned with players' performances, statistics, team gossip, and human-interest stories. Today, good sports journalists need to understand the eco- nomics of professional sports *as a business*. If they are to explain to their readers the intricacies of trades and the manager's likely motivations, reporters must have knowledge of team budgets, the length and structure of individual players' contracts, and the collective agreement. This knowledge is ever more important in today's NHL hockey with the advent of payroll ceilings, as players are traded or offered on waivers (and then sent back to the minors) to keep the team payroll below the ceiling, and only incidentally because of their poor playmaking performance.

When sports journalists are not discussing players' salaries, moreover, they are often trying to explain the implications for sports teams of a variety of other financial and fiscal issues. They

Box 11.1   The Economics of the Canadian Football League

While Canadian football is most popular in the western part of Canada, as attendance numbers and the greater financial stability of the western franchises demonstrate, the game itself has an increasing number of participants in Quebec high schools and colleges, leading to an influx of French Canadian players into the CFL over the last few years. This notwithstanding, the economics of the CFL have been on the downside since the golden days of the 1960s and 1970s. Average attendance, as shown in Table 11.1, is much lower than it used to be 25 or 30 years ago, despite fairly low ticket prices, and there has been no television bonanza in contrast to the NFL, since gate revenues still make for almost 75 percent of total revenues (O'Brien, 2004, p. 336). On the one hand, the CFL has managed to survive for a long period, despite a lack of consistent marketing efforts and an aborted expansion into the USA in the 1990s, whereas many other similar American minor football leagues—such as the USFL or the WLAF—have expanded and folded over these same years. On the other hand, CFL revenues and payrolls have dwarfed, relative to those of major league sports, as can be deduced from Table 11.2. This may be because of the current star system, whereby stars or star organizations catch all the attention, with televised NFL and all the new Canadian NHL or NBA franchises competing for the entertainment expenditures and the time of Canadian sports fans. There seems to be some improvement in the financial state of the league, however, as the payroll cap—which had dropped to as low as $2.1 million per team in 1996 (Barnes, 1996, p. 164)—later moved up to $2.5 million and then to $3.8 million in 2006. But the financial woes of the Ottawa Renegades, and their hypothetical survival, show that even though operating a CFL franchise costs only about $10 million per season, it can be a dicey venture.

Table 11.1   CFL Per-Game Attendance, per Period of Five Years

Average for Five-Season Period	Per-Game Attendance
1975–1979	29,600
1980–1984	29,240
1985–1989	25,625
1990–1994	24,070
1995–1999	Not available
2000–2004	25,330

Source: Author's computations from data compiled by http://www.kenn.com/sports/football/cfl.

Table 11.2   Average CFL Player Salary, in Canadian Dollars, as a Ratio of NFL Salary

Season	CFL Average Salary, C$	CFL/NFL Salary Ratio
1975	24,000	50%
1985	62,000	35%
1995	50,000	5.0%
2004	58,000	3.6%
2006	75,000	5.2%

Sources: Longley (2004, p. 211), O'Brien (2004, p. 458), and author's estimate based on 2006 new payroll cap (January 18, 2006).

have to help fans understand concepts like earnings before interest, taxes, depreciation, and amortization (EBITDA, or operating income); gross economic impact, and income multipliers when discussing team venues or major sporting events; as well as fast tax write-offs inducing new owners to purchase endangered franchises, like the Edmonton Oilers's. In the next few years, as Canadian cities like Hamilton, Winnipeg, or Quebec City will attempt to gain or regain an NHL franchise while others will make sure they preserve the ones they have, and as the construction boom induced by the Vancouver 2010 Olympics will come to the forefront, the discussion is most likely to stretch to include sporting facilities' building costs and who will get what revenues, as well as the contributions that sports venues are alleged to make to city-core redevelopment.

Although disillusioned Expos baseball fans could certainly argue otherwise, the biggest event in Canadian sports economics over the last few years has been the 2004–05 NHL lockout. It made headlines and was the source of an uninterrupted flow of news stories for 300 days! Nearly any Canadian, whatever his or her ethnic origin, had an opinion about who was to blame for the lockout, and many voiced their views about possible solutions. The present chapter intends to put the hockey lockout and the arguments of those involved in proper economic perspective. Once you have read this chapter, you should be able to explain the economic motives and constraints that rule NHL hockey, and you should be able to understand the main dynamics of any future labour conflict in team sports. While studying the implications of the NHL lockout, we will also examine the changing fortunes of the Canadian NHL teams, comparing the economics of NHL hockey with those of the other three major leagues in North America— namely, the National Basketball Association (NBA), the National Football League (NFL), and Major League Baseball (MLB). We will conclude by analyzing the impact of professional franchises and the possible involvement of the public sector.

BACKGROUND INFORMATION

The Root Cause of the 2004–05 NHL Lockout

The quotes that open the chapter seem to be distorted by some time warp. On first reading they would seem to apply quite well to the denouement of the 2004–05 lockout that team owners imposed on players of the NHL. After more than 300 days of lockout (a lockout is the mirror image of a strike, with the employer stopping its employees from working, to put pressure on the labour union), the negotiations ended in July 2005 with players taking an overall 24-percent pay cut, along with the imposition of the revenue-tied payroll ceiling that the NHL Players' Association (the NHLPA) had vowed never to accept (see Staudohar [2005] for a history of the lockout).

But in fact, as is obvious from the publishing dates of these quotes, all three authors purport to analyze the impact of the collective agreement signed following the *previous* NHL lockout, that of 1994–95. As the quotes show, and as Staudohar (2005, p. 24) reports, "the owners appeared to get much the better of the settlement, which was reported in the media as a solid victory on their part." Most experts initially thought that the 1995 agreement had put in place structures that would abate salary inflation in the NHL, by twisting bargaining power toward the owners and out of the hands of the players' agents. Indeed, still persuaded that the 1995 deal was a good one, the NHL owners decided to renew the agreement a few years later, when they could have asked for a new one. But by 2004, when it was clear to all that the NHL owners and players were up for a major clash and a long dispute, all hockey experts were claiming that the 1995 collective agreement had been a clear win for the players, bringing

NHL owners collectively on the brink of bankruptcy, and that something entirely new was needed. But this new financial arrangement could not just be imposed upon players, as it would be in a firm deprived of a labour union. It had to be negotiated through collective bargaining.

Collective Bargaining Agreements

In the North American major leagues, the relations between owners and players are regulated by a collective bargaining agreement (CBA), which is freely negotiated between representatives of the employer (the league commissioner) and the employees (the players' union). There is some irony about industrial relations in sports. In other industries, capitalists usually advocate free markets without restrictions and rigidities, arguing that unrestricted competition and flexible labour markets will bring about the best of possible worlds, while employees ask for protection against the consequences of free markets. In sports, where often owners are billionaires while their player employees are millionaires, players' unions ask that salaries be freely determined and that players be free to move from one team to another; team owners, by contrast, propose revenue sharing and argue that all sorts of impediments on labour movements and salary determination should be imposed, for the sake of the sport. This has given rise in the past to the *perpetual reserve clause*, whereby a player was forever forbidden to change teams without being traded by the owner, a clause that was successfully challenged in court, forcing team owners to negotiate CBAs with temporary reserve clauses (Barnes, 1996).

With current rules, only a subset of players are *bona fide unrestricted* free agents, able to move freely from one team to another. Most players are *restricted* free agents; that is, they can move to some other team but only at the end of their standard-length contract, and only if that other team pays some hefty penalty—up to five first-round draft choices. Other league rules designed to impede free labour markets include the draft of amateur players, whereby rookies can negotiate with only one team; caps on the individual salaries of rookies or those of star players; payroll ceilings, whereas salaries (adding or not benefits and bonuses) paid by teams cannot exceed a certain amount; and luxury taxes, whereby teams that spend more than a certain amount on salaries must pay back a tax to the league that is proportional to the excess amount. Revenue sharing, which as all other restrictions is officially designed to ensure that all league teams can compete fairly on the sporting scene, is another labour-market-impeding mechanism, since its effect is to discourage owners from competing with each other to acquire the best talent. In some cases, there are rules that provide countervailing power to the players, such as the possibility of going to salary arbitration in the case of restricted free agents, or the existence of exceptions in the case of salary or payroll caps. Different leagues have arrived at different mechanisms, for historical reasons.

While economics has a lot to say about income distribution between capitalists and workers under competitive conditions, economic theory is rather silent when a monopoly is facing a monopsony—which is the case in the labour market of major leagues, and particularly in the NHL. The monopoly is the players' union, the NHLPA: it is the sole supplier of hockey talent; the monopsony is the NHL: it is the sole source of demand for talented hockey players (European leagues put aside, as we saw during the lockout). What share of revenues hockey players get depends on the abilities and the bargaining power—whatever that means—of the two negotiating sides.

Salary Inflation

In the case of the NHL, as early as 1999 league commissioner Gary Bettman argued that the restrictions put in place in previous CBAs were no longer appropriate and that entirely new rules had to be put in place. Bettman pointed out that in the past NHL clubs had sought to

Table 11.3   Average Player Salaries in Four Major Sports (US dollars)

Season	MLB (Baseball)	NBA (Basketball)	NFL (Football)	NHL (Hockey)
1970, 1970–71	29,000	40,000	34,500	25,000
1980, 1980–81	143,000	190,000	69,000	110,000
1990, 1990–91	600,000	824,000	365,000	247,500
1993, 1993–94	1,076,000	1,250,000	683,000	543,000
2000, 2000–01	1,895,000	3,241,000	1,169,000	1,484,000
2004, 2003–04	2,372,000	3,783,000	1,250,000	1,830,000
2005, 2005–2006	2,632,000	4,037,000	1,250,000	1,460,000

Sources: Associated Press; Patricia's website; *Hockey News*; Lavoie (1997); http://www.plunkettresearch.com.

negotiate restrictions embedded in the CBA that would slow down the inflation of players' salaries. In 1995, this had been done by a three-pronged approach: (1) by maintaining restrictive free agency rules (the most restrictive of the four major league sports), (2) by introducing salary caps at the entry level; that is, on the salary of rookie players, and (3) by reducing arbitration rights, either by restricting its access or by allowing teams to avoid the rulings of arbitrators. Table 11.3 clearly shows that, from the point of view of the NHL owners, the 1995 CBA did not achieve its objectives. While the salaries of all major league sports did increase in the 1990s, those in hockey rose even more quickly.

The incredible increase in the purchasing power of NHL hockey players is highlighted in Table 11.4, where the average salary is put into Canadian dollars and compared to the average salary of Canadian employees. The ratio of these two averages reached its apex in 2001–02, in part due to the misfortunes of the Canadian dollar that dropped to its all-time low in January 2002 (see Figure 11.1 later in this chapter). The evolution of this ratio also might explain why most Canadians blamed players for a lockout that had been imposed by owners. Today, many Canadians are disenchanted with NHL hockey because players' salaries are out of touch with their own reality—86 percent of Canadian hockey fans believe hockey players are overpaid, whereas only 41 percent of the American fans believe the same (NHL, 2004b)—although this may be a misperception, as the most popular rock or pop stars earn much more than NHL stars. In addition, CEOs earn many times the average salary of their employees. In the United States, while CEOs earned only 42 times more in 1982, they earned 525 times more at the apex of the stock market in 2000, and this ratio was only down to 431 in 2004 (Desrosiers, 2005). Higher salaries in major leagues are just a reflection of the income distribution consequences of the current star system, where the winner takes it all.

Why did NHL salaries grow so much? Salaries were well under control before the creation in 1972 of the rival World Hockey Association (WHA) that broke the monopsony power of the NHL; they also rose slowly during the 1980s, when the NHL regained its monopsony position after the WHA folded in 1979. In December 1989, however, players decided to make their salaries public information—and this, with a new and more aggressive NHLPA led by Bob Goodenow in replacement of the owner-friendly Alan Eagleson, set off a new round of salary inflation. There were also key events that drove salaries upward, such as the 1988 trade that sent superstar Wayne Gretzky off to Los Angeles at double his previous salary, and an unprecedented $3-million deal obtained by a rookie, Eric Lindros, in 1992. After the 1995 agreement, many absurd contracts awarded to journeymen, restricted free agents, and rookies—granting huge bonuses to get around the newly imposed rookie salary cap—contributed to salary inflation.

Table 11.4 Average Salary of NHL Players and Average Salary of Canadian Employees, with Ratios (Canadian dollars)

Year	Average NHL Player's Salary, C$ (2)	Average Canadian Employee's Salary (3)	Ratio (2) / (3)
1970–71	26,000	6,050	4.3
1974–75	60,500	8,600	7.0
1979–80	118,000	13,700	8.6
1984–85	173,000	20,800	8.3
1989–90	233,000	24,950	9.3
1993–94	709,000	28,400	25.0
1999–2000	2,163,000	31,600	68.5
2001–02	2,720,000	33,500	81.2
2003–04	2,358,000	35,050	66.4
2005–06	1,683,000	37,180	45.0
2006–07	1,980,000	38,270	51.7

Sources: Lavoie, M. (1997); Table 1, Statistics Canada (Series V2415199 and V37426).

In addition, attempts to raid restricted free agents led to huge salary increases, such as that of Joe Sakic in 1997, when the Colorado Avalanche was forced to match the offer made by the New York Rangers. The NHLPA took full advantage of this by making a clever use of salary arbitration hearings. General managers also started to find ways to evade some of the restrictions that had been put in place to stop large-market teams from raiding more than once the rosters of small-market teams. This may be attributed to foolish management, but also to a change in the structure of ownership, whereas some newly rich American owners (e.g., Tom Hicks of the Dallas Stars, Ted Leonsis of the Washington Capitals, Bill Laurie of the St. Louis Blues) aimed at winning championships at great cost, even if this implied substantial financial losses. They did this to indulge in a fantasy or because winning generates profits in their other related operations—nine of the NHL owners are among the richest 400 Americans (Staudohar, 2005).

Revenues and Operating Losses

In contrast to the wisdom that attributes rising ticket prices to rising salaries, salary inflation was fuelled by the increased ability of teams to extort larger revenues through increases in ticket prices, new arenas, and corporate sponsorship. Teams get a few million dollars per year from "naming rights" with arenas taking the name of their corporate sponsors—Air Canada Centre, Rexall Place, Scotiabank Place (ex Corel Centre), General Motors Place, Bell Centre (ex Molson Centre). Licensed merchandise, for example team logos printed on jerseys, shirts, caps, cups, and other souvenirs, has generated revenues that have grown at a phenomenal pace, not to speak of food and drink sales or parking fees. Another factor in salary inflation was the additional funds—$570 million all together—that existing teams collected in the form of expansion fees in the 1990s from the nine new teams that were added to the league. But the latter were non-recurrent revenues, whereas the higher salaries granted were imbedded in the salary structure, and hence NHL expansion, retrospectively, had some features of Ponzi or pyramidal financing, where the profits of present firm owners are financed by selling shares to new owners, without the firm making any revenue of its own.

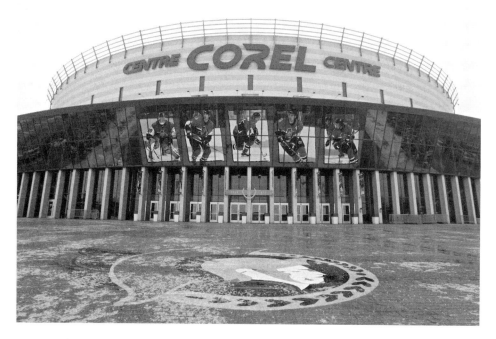

New sports facilities in Canada are built with money from both the private and public sectors.
JONATHAN HAYWARD/CP Images

But the most disappointing feature of NHL revenues was the inability of the NHL to contract a substantial national broadcasting deal in the United States. This had been the strategy upon which Gary Bettman and the Board of Governors had strived through—attempting to be part of all large television markets, including those of the southern states. But whereas the other major leagues have been getting huge revenues, shared equally by all teams, the NHL national television contracts are as small as ever, with only a few individual teams like the Toronto Maple Leafs pocketing large sums of money for local broadcasting rights, as shown in Table 11.5. Thus, one can say that the expansion toward the southern states has been a failure, since the league has been drawn into markets where hockey is an ephemeral fad rather than an ever-lasting cultural trait, without benefiting from any broadcasting bonanza. Perhaps related to this, attendance at NHL hockey games started to stagnate and even to drop during the two seasons preceding the lockout, as shown in Table 11.6.

The discrepancy between salary costs and recurrent revenues became ever more pronounced and worrying over the post–1995 agreement years. The NHL owners launched their campaign for a new CBA regime in February 2004, when its consultant, Arthur Levitt, a former chairman of the United States Securities and Exchange Commission, released his report on the financial woes of the NHL (Levitt, 2004). He claimed that only one-third of the teams had been profitable, with team owners overall having lost no less than $273 million over the 2002–03 season, a claim that was further reinforced when the NHL later found out that its team owners had lost an additional $225 million during the 2003–04 season. Levitt himself commented that "the league is on a treadmill to obscurity," adding that "I would neither underwrite as a banker any of these ventures, nor would I invest a dollar of my personal money in a business which to me appears to be heading south" (Spector, 2004). This led the media to offer support to the owners contra the NHLPA.

Table 11.5 Broadcasting National and Local Contracts for Each Major League, Amounts per Year per Team (US dollars)

	National Broadcasting Revenues	Local Broadcasting Revenues
MLB (Baseball)	ESPN, FOX, until 2006; $18.6 million per team/year	Huge revenues for some teams, often underestimated for tax purposes
NBA (Basketball)	ABC, ESPN, AOL until 2007; $31.7 million per team/year	Spread unequally
NFL (Football)	CBS, ABC, FOX, ESPN until 2005; $68.7 million per team/year CBS, NBC, ESPN 2006–2011; $115 million per team/year	None
NHL (Hockey)	Comcast (OLN) until 2008; $2.2 million per team/year. CBC, TSN until 2010; $2.7 million per team/year	Local revenues are about $12 million per team on average overall. Each Canadian teams gets between C$10 million (small-market) and C$40 million (the Leafs) per year

Sources: Merrigan & Trudel (2004: 193, 200); http://www.rodneyfort.com/SportsData/BizFrame.htm; inferences from other data.

Table 11.6 NHL Average Attendance per Game, 1975–2006

Season	Attendance per Game
1975–76	12,640
1985–86	13,835
1995–96	15,985
2000–01	16,550
2003–04	16,530
2005–06	16,955

Sources: www.Hockeyzone.com; data calculated from http://sports.espn.go.com/nhl/attendance.

Are NHL Owners Really Losing Money?

How reliable are the Levitt figures? This is a difficult question to answer. As we learned from the scandals that rocked the world of finance and auditing with companies as large as WorldCom and Enron, there is always some room for creative accounting. From the very start the NHLPA challenged the accuracy of the NHL figures, claiming that an audit of four individual teams had left them convinced that net revenues were underestimated by an average of $13 million per team. Notwithstanding the huge tax breaks provided by the ownership of a sports team (Fort, 2003), club owners pull various tricks to reduce their apparent profits. Firstly, they charge themselves hefty fees for running the team. This was reportedly done for several years by Barry Shenkarow, owner of the Winnipeg Jets, allowing him to earn substantial annual management fees while at the same time whining about the huge financial losses of the Jets, until the team departed to Phoenix (Silver, 1996).

Secondly, for team owners who also happen to be the owners of the cable company that broad-casts the team games, another strategy is to set low fees for television rights, thus lowering the rev-enues and profits of the team and increasing those of the cable company. Thirdly, a variant of this is available when club owners own their team arena, which is the case for 22 of the NHL clubs. The company owning the venue may set high rents and keep most of the revenues from events, thus lowering the profits of the team while raising those of the venue. In this manner, team owners can argue that the franchise is losing money, and ask for public funding under the threat of depar-ture to another city. This is precisely what owner Rod Bryden did. When Bryden attempted to sell the Ottawa Senators to a limited partnership in January 2002, he argued that the club's operating losses could easily be transformed into a break-even situation by amending the revenue-sharing agreement between the Senators and the Corel Centre, both of which he owned. While his fig-ures showed that the Senators were losing $6 million to $8 million (Canadian) a year, they also disclosed that the Corel Centre was making a $15-million annual gross profit, despite hosting a relatively small number of events besides hockey (Norfolk Capital and Triax, 2001). This is fairly common practice, according to a previous president of the NHL, Gil Stein (1997).

Following the Levitt report, all kinds of silly figures started to turn out in the media. For instance, based on obviously unreliable financial accounts, a reporter ran three successive sto-ries claiming that the Montreal Canadiens had lost $40 million in 2003 and $140 million over the 1998–2003 period (Blanchard, 2004). On the other hand, *Forbes* magazine ran its yearly revenue and value assessment of NHL franchises. The numbers for the 1993–94 and 2002–03 seasons are compared in Table 11.7. They show that the NHL and the Levitt report had exag-gerated operating losses to the tune of $5 million. However, the *Forbes* assessment also con-firmed that the financial situation of NHL teams had clearly deteriorated over the decade, and that teams overall were making operating losses; that is, they were losing money even before interest payments on the purchasing cost of the team were taken into account. In addition, while the NHL claimed that players got 75 percent of team revenues, *Forbes* data showed that the players' share was only 67 percent, although this was much higher than the 41 percent obtained before the 1995 CBA. There may be discrepancies in the figures provided by different sources, but they all pointed in the same direction: in the red!

The crippling financial state of the NHL was even more obvious when the NHL bottom line—operating profits or losses—was compared to that of the other major leagues, as shown in Table 11.8. It then became obvious that the financial state of the NHL had gone down over time not only in absolute terms but also relative to that of the other three major leagues. Obviously,

Table 11.7   NHL Revenues, Payroll Costs, and Profits per Team, Comparison of Independent and NHL Data

Season	1993–94		2002–03	
Source	**Financial World**	**NHL**	**Forbes**	**NHL**
Revenues (millions)	$31.4	$28.2	$70.0	$64.2
Player costs (millions)	$13.0	$15.9	$47.3	$48.6
Player costs share	41.3%	56.5%	67.5%	75.5%
Operating profit (millions)	$3.8	($1.5)	($4.1)	($9.1)
Profit share	12.1%	(5.3%)	(5.9%)	(14.2)%

Note: Negative numbers (losses) are in parentheses.

Sources: Data obtained from issues of *Financial World* (May 9, 1995) and *Forbes* (Forbes.com); NHL data released by the NHL in 2004 (http://www.nhlcbanews.com/historical_results.html).

Table 11.8 Evolution of Various Financial Measures, 1990–2004 (US dollars)

League Season	NFL (Football)			MLB (Baseball)			NBA (Basketball)			NHL (Hockey)		
	1990	1998	2003	1990	1998	2004	1989–90	1999–00	2003–04	1989–90	1999–00	2003–04
Revenues (millions $)	46.9	115.6	166.5	51.7	88.8	142.3	22.5	79.9	101.1	20.9	60.6	74.6
Gates (millions $)			39.3			50.0			35.2	12.2	24.2	34.1
Profits (millions $)	8.9	19.7	26.6	7.0	2.0	4.4	4.8	5.6	9.6	3.0	1.9	–3.2
Wage bill (millions $)	19.3	59.0	91.6	17.3	41.1	83.8	9.1	49.1	59.6	6.0	34.6	49.2
Salaries as % of revenues	41.2	51.0	55.0	33.5	46.3	58.8	40.5	61.5	59.0	28.7	57.0	66.0
Profit share %	18.9	17.0	16.0	13.5	2.2	3.0	21.3	7.0	9.5	14.3	3.1	–4.3

Sources: Various issues of the magazines *Financial World* (now defunct) and *Forbes*.

whereas the profit share in NHL revenues was in the same range as that of other leagues in 1989–90, it has long ceased to be the case. Other leagues, most notably the NFL, have managed to remain profitable. There were other indications that the financial situation of the NHL was bad at the time of the 2004–05 lockout. Several teams had gone through a bankruptcy procedure (Pittsburgh, Ottawa, Buffalo) before being salvaged, and several other teams—five in 2004—were being put under surveillance by their banks and asked to provide additional collateral.

NHL PROBLEMS AND THEIR SOLUTIONS

The strategy being pursued by the NHL was similar to that adopted by Major League Baseball in 2000, with the release, before starting negotiations with the players' union, of the report of the so-called Blue Ribbon panel on baseball economics, which "demonstrated" that the attempt by clubs to remain competitive led to salary and ticket price inflation, and to persistent operating losses to the tune of $10 million per team (Levin et al., 2000). The Blue Ribbon panel also claimed that free-market processes led to large and growing revenue disparities that were causing rising competitive imbalances. These, and the higher ticket prices, could potentially destroy fan interest in the game.

Gary Bettman and the NHL governors came up with very similar arguments (NHL, 2004). They argued that:

- Free-market mechanisms allow the foolish decisions of one or two clubs to have detrimental financial consequences on all clubs (this is called a *negative externality* in economics);
- The NHL needs "cost certainty," which turned out to mean a hard payroll cap, the value of which was linked to league-wide revenue;
- Revenue and payroll disparities have "widened to unprecedented levels," inducing competitive imbalance on the ice, thus requiring the creation of "an economic system where 30 clubs can ice a competitive team and be stable";
- A new economic system must also provide "entertainment to the fans at an affordable and competitive price," meaning lower ticket prices.

Financial and Competitive Balance

The last two points certainly appealed to fans. Fairness and competitive equity is an important issue among hockey fans (NHL, 2004b) and sports economists. But what has been the actual evolution of financial balance and competitive balance in ice hockey? Table 11.9 provides two dispersion measures each for revenue imbalance and payroll imbalance. The *coefficient of variation* is defined as the ratio of the standard deviation to the mean; the *range* is the differential between the maximum and the minimum values, divided by the mean. The range for 2005–06 is only 0.50 since the payroll ceiling is $39 million and the payroll floor is $21 million, while the average payroll was $36 million [0.50 = (39 − 21) / 36)]. The higher these measures, the larger are the imbalances.

My interpretation of the data is that the salary and revenue inflation that started in the 1990s did worsen payroll and revenue imbalances. However, while revenue imbalances in the new century are not as bad as they were toward the middle of the 1990s, payroll imbalances in the 2000s are clearly at their highest levels. Other statistical measures show that this must be mostly attributed to the behaviour of the high-payroll teams (Wakeford, 2003). There is thus

Table 11.9   Revenue and Payroll Imbalance, NHL, 1989–2004

Year	Revenue Imbalance		Payroll Imbalance	
------	Coefficient of Variation	Range	Coefficient of Variation	Range
1989–1990	0.23	0.84	0.17	0.75
1990–1991	0.23	0.84	0.24	0.81
1991–1992	0.31	1.29	0.23	0.82
1992–1993	0.34	1.08	0.21	0.80
1993–1994	0.35	1.24	0.28	1.02
1994–1995	0.37	1.54	0.27	0.94
1995–1996	0.33	1.24	0.24	1.04
1996–1997	0.28	1.07	0.27	1.02
1997–1998	0.28	1.08	0.28	1.00
1998–1999	0.28	1.14	0.25	1.16
1999–2000	0.27	0.94	0.32	1.36
2000–2001	0.26	1.01	0.31	1.13
2001–2002	0.29	1.06	0.37	1.34
2002–2003	0.27	0.96	0.32	1.39
2003–2004	0.27	0.90	0.35	1.24
Average	0.291	1.108	0.274	1.054

Sources: Wakeford (2003); author's calculations from data found on http://www.rodneyfort.com/SportsData/BizFrame.htm.

some validity to the concerns of the officials of the NHL: before the 2004–05 lockout, payroll imbalances were worse than ever, and could be linked to the irresponsible behaviour of some team owners and general managers. Indeed, the relationship between revenues and payroll is much tighter in the 2000s than it used to be, indicating that teams with large revenues managed to obtain and retain good players and did not hesitate to spend their cash. This could be interpreted as a move from profit maximizing to win-maximizing behaviour; or it could be due to owners being lured by the big payoff expected from successful playoff teams.

But does payroll imbalance lead to competitive imbalance? Payroll and winning percentages of a given team are indeed correlated. The average correlation coefficient between 1989 and 2002 was +0.43 (a positive ratio near unity would indicate that increases in payroll are nearly always associated with increases in performance; a correlation ratio of zero would show that there is no relationship whatsoever between payroll and performance; a negative correlation ratio would indicate that low payrolls are associated more often than not with high performance). However, competitive imbalance does not seem to have worsened. Table 11.10 shows a measure of winning percentage dispersion, given by the ratio of the standard deviation to the idealized standard deviation (to take into account the length of the season). In other words, the higher the dispersion, the higher the imbalance. Of course, other measures of competitive imbalance have been proposed, but we shall stick to this one. Winning dispersion in the 1990s is no worse than what it was in the "golden years" of ice hockey, and it is much reduced compared to the 1970s. In addition, the increase in payroll imbalance of the new century is associated with a *reduction* in performance imbalance.

It could be argued, however, as do officials of the NHL, that while competition in the NHL in a given year is now tighter than it used to be (reporters say that parity in the NHL has

Table 11.10   Dispersion Measure of Winning Percentage, NHL, 1920–2003

Time Period	Ratio
1920–1929	1.61
1930–1939	1.53
1940–1949	1.69
1950–1959	1.88
1960–1969	1.90
1970–1979	2.54
1980–1989	1.91
1990–1994	1.93
1995–1999	1.71
2000–2003	1.68

Note: The higher the ratio, the larger the performance imbalance within a season

Sources: Fort (2003, p. 155) for decade ratios, except the period after 1989, which comes from Wakeford (2003).

been achieved), the same clubs keep ending up at the top of the ladder. To account for this, some other approach is required, one that examines competitive imbalances *through time*. Studies by Richardson (2000) and Wakeford (2003) show that the correlation between present and future performance is much weaker than it used to be. In other words, it is harder for good teams to remain at the top, and poor teams improve more quickly. Hence, competitive balance through time has also improved. The major problems facing the NHL thus seem to be entirely financial, rather than related to a lack of competitive uncertainty on the ice.

The New 2005 Collective Agreement

It thus follows that the only valid reason for imposing a payroll cap was the need for team owners to get protection against themselves—the first two points made by Bettman (the issue of ticket prices will be discussed in the last section). While the players had vowed never to accept any payroll cap, the NHL lockout ended in July 2005 with the signing of a new collective agreement incorporating such a cap, valid from 2005 to 2011. Players were forced to surrender on all counts, ending up with less than they had been offered at some stage of the negotiations. Goodenow, the head of the NHLPA, had no choice but to resign a few weeks later. The quotes found at the beginning of the chapter would now seem to be fully appropriate. The main features of the new agreement can be summed up with six major points:

1. All existing salary contracts were automatically rolled back by 24 percent—a reduction that the players had already conceded to the owners in December 2004, in the hope of evading the payroll cap and saving the second half of the hockey season.
2. The owners imposed the much-sought-after payroll cap, which was set at $39 million, accompanied by a payroll floor of $22 million. Ironically, in February 2005 the players had turned down a cap offer at $42.5 million, but without the payroll floor.

3. To provide for true "cost certainty" in relation to revenues, the payroll cap is linked to league revenues: if revenues rise, so will the cap. In addition, players cannot earn more than 54 percent of league revenues; to insure this, an *escrow* tax has been put in place, similar but not identical to that of the NBA, with a certain percentage of players' salaries being withheld in case this ceiling has been exceeded (this percentage was set at 12 percent at the beginning of the 2005–06 season).
4. There is now a limit to the salary of an individual player: he can earn no more than 20 percent of his club total annual compensation.
5. Rookie salaries and their performance bonuses have been capped and more severely regulated, so that agents and team managers cannot evade the spirit of the collective agreement.
6. Qualifying offers and players' access to salary arbitration were further tightened, while owners were also given the right to bring overpaid players to salary arbitration.

The only good news items for the players are that the minimum salary has been pushed up to nearly half a million dollars and that the age required to access unrestricted free agency will be progressively lowered from 31 to 27 years old. But this seems like a vacuous gain now that a rigid payroll cap is in place, except that players will have better opportunities to move to teams and areas they prefer. Overall, as a rough estimate, $400 million has been transferred from the wallets of the players to those of the owners.

Payroll Caps and Revenue Sharing

All reporters to whom I talked during the lockout were quite in favour of payroll ceilings and could not understand why economists would only reluctantly support such a measure. More often than not these reporters pointed to the successful NFL, with its relatively hard payroll cap and its league parity on the field. What are the potential problems with a payroll cap?

The problem is that large-market teams, or owners operating successful clubs, can often increase their profits by spending more on players; that is, by acquiring talent either on the free-agent market or through unbalanced trades, thus going over the payroll cap. And under some conditions, it may also be the case that small-market teams can improve their profits by spending less than the payroll floor. There is thus some economic incentive for small-market teams to trade away some of their more established talented players to large-market teams, thus breaking the payroll minimum and maximum rules (Fort, 2003). Indeed, in the NBA, where competitive imbalance is highest among the four major leagues, the cap is completely ineffective, with nearly all teams going over the payroll cap thanks to various exceptions that have been put in place precisely to accommodate large-market teams and highly successful ones. A similar but less obvious pattern is observed in the NFL, with the cap also being violated through various omissions.

Thus, both in the NBA and the NFL the cap is a "soft" one, admitting circumvention. If the cap were to be truly "hard," then in all likelihood large-market teams or team owners intending to maximize winning would imagine all sorts of subterfuges to evade the enforcement of the cap. For instance, players might receive large financial compensation from another business run by an owner for some fictitious or menial work, or for some publicity stunt. If such hidden payments were to be found out, the owner could argue that this is not some kind of indirect salary that ought to be counted within the salary cap, but that instead it is part of the player's endorsement income.

This shirking problem is likely to be less serious if all teams have similar revenues, in which case the economic incentive to cheat is much smaller since the cap reflects fairly the capacity to spend of all teams, or if there exists a soft cap that allows rich teams to cheat legally. One reason that the NFL has a harder cap than the NBA is that a very large proportion of the NFL revenues arises from national broadcasting contracts and is shared (see Tables 11.5 and 11.8), so that revenue imbalance is smallest in the NFL. By contrast, revenue dispersion is high in the NHL, with little revenue being shared (Lavoie & Whitson, 2003). Although the 2005 CBA calls for a revenue-sharing arrangement that will redistribute money to clubs in the bottom half of league revenues that operate in metropolitan areas of 2.5 million or fewer TV households, neither the size nor the formula have yet (as of March 2006) been agreed upon. In all likelihood, rich NHL clubs like the Toronto Maple Leafs or the New York Rangers will have incentives to evade the payroll cap, just as they had incentives to circumvent the restrictions put in place in the 1995 CBA. Thus, while a hard cap undoubtedly should help to preserve or improve competitive balance, it might not be the panacea that everyone was looking for. In addition, Canadian fans who now rave about the payroll cap may become disenchanted when their home team, following a string of successful years, may have to dump players to remain under the cap before managing to win the coveted Stanley Cup, as already happened with the Ottawa Senators in 2006, when they had to let go Zdeno Chara, their star defenceman.

THE FUTURE OF CANADIAN NHL FRANCHISES

What is the future of NHL hockey? Some observers claim that it is bright since salaries, relative to revenues, are now under control. Others think that it is rather gloomy. The NHL owners themselves initially estimated that overall revenues in 2005–06 would decrease from $2,200 million to $2,000 million relative to the 2003–04 season, due to hockey falling into near oblivion in the sunbelt, as well as the negative response of frustrated fans located in the northern states or in Canada. But the latest reported figures show that this expected decrease in overall revenues did not occur, as overall NHL revenues in 2005–06 were just as high as those of the 2004–05 season. This is due in large part to the enforcement of rules on the ice, which has enhanced skill play and fast skating, as in Olympic play, to the detriment of hooking and fighting. These changes have made the game more exciting and seem to have seduced (Canadian) fans or ex-fans, making them more likely to watch games and fill arena seats.

A Reversal of Fortunes

The biggest change from our Canadian perspective is the new outlook for Canadian NHL franchises. Just a few years ago, many observers of the hockey scene were claiming that most Canadian franchises were bound to disappear. "During the past decade, no sports topic has received more attention in Canada than the notion that the National Hockey League was on thin ice in this country. . . . All of which gave credence to the idea that one day, the Toronto Maple Leafs might be the only Canadian entry in the 30-team league. Those who didn't see it this way were usually few and far between" (Naylor, 2004). Even the CEO of the Montreal Canadiens, as late as 2004, made the absurd claim that, without a salary cap, the existence of the Montreal team was "definitely threatened" (Labbé, 2004). In the previous edition of this book, we said instead that: "If the Canadian dollar could recover somewhat, if the Canadian economy could improve relative to that of the United States, and if Canadian teams outside Toronto can achieve better television revenues . . . it seems entirely possible that our current major league franchises could remain viable" (Lavoie & Whitson, 2003). Most of these conditions, as I write, are now fulfilled.

Figure 11.1   The Value of the American Dollar in Canadian Dollars, 1970–2005

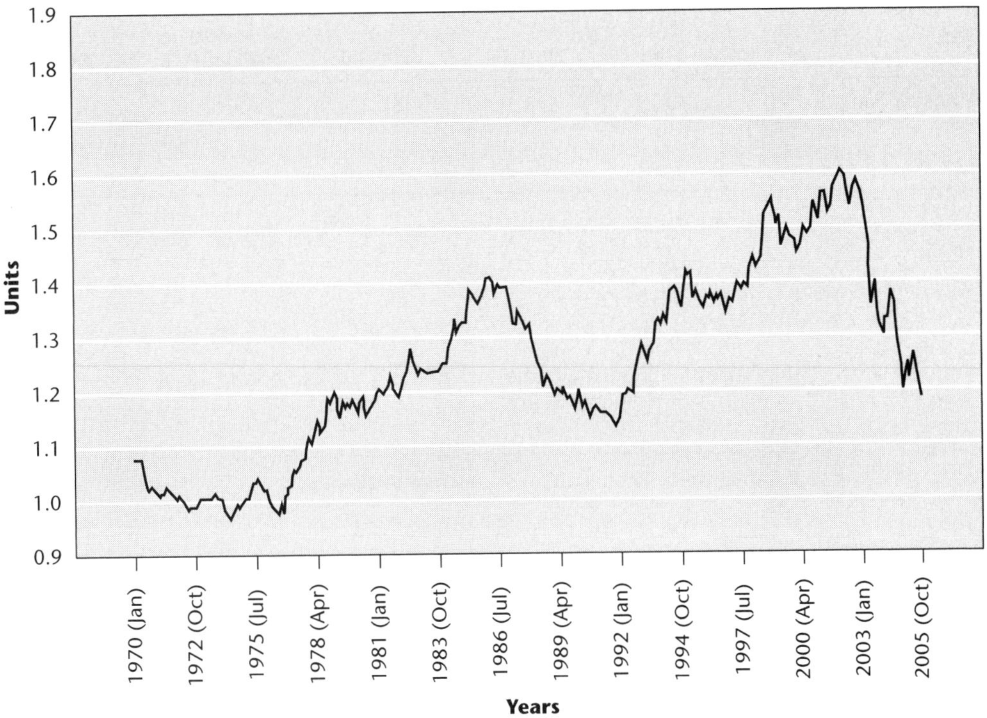

Note: When the Canadian dollar appreciates, this exchange rate falls.

Source: Based on data from the Statistics Canada CANSIM database <http://cansim2.statcan.ca>, Table 176-0064, Series V37426.

There is no doubt that the Canadian economy has improved relative to that of the United States. Figure 11.1 shows the evolution of the value of the American dollar, expressed in Canadian dollars, since 1970. The Canadian dollar has made a spectacular comeback, reaching levels that had last been seen around 1992, and in the early 1980s. When the Québec Nordiques and the Winnipeg Jets had to move south, one American dollar was worth about 1.40 Canadian dollar; the exchange rate is around 1.15 at the beginning of 2006, recovering from the all-time low of 1.60 in January 2002. As a result of the stronger dollar, Canadian teams all save $10 million or more on their payroll costs.

The dynamics of the league have changed considerably. This can be reflected under several areas. Consider first the evolution of ticket prices. Following the 2004–05 lockout, as shown in Table 11.11, NHL ticket prices have gone down, as fans had hoped they would when players' salaries were cut down by at least 24 percent. But ticket prices did not all go down equally. They went down by 8.4 percent on average in American cities, whereas they only decreased by 2.0 percent in Canadian cities (most of which was due to the reduction of Senators ticket prices). With the rising Canadian dollar, this means that Canadian clubs now nearly all rank among the top half in ticket prices, as shown in Table 11.12. In addition, all Canadian clubs now rank in the top half in average attendance per game, also as shown in

Table 11.11   Evolution of NHL Ticket Prices and Fan Cost Index, 1995–2006 (in US dollars)

	1995–96	2003–04	2005–06	Change 2005–06 Relative to 2003–04
Average ticket price	$34.70	$43.50	$41.20	–8.4% in U.S. cities
				–2.0% in six Canadian cities
Fan cost index	$203.30	$253.65	$247.30	

Note: Fan cost index includes the cost of four average tickets, hot dogs, soft drinks, beers, programs, caps, and parking.

Sources: www.teammarketing.com; author's calculations.

Table 11.12   Attendance Rank and Average Attendance per Game, and Ticket Price Rank, Canadian NHL Franchises, 2005–06

City	Attendance Rank	Average Attendance	Ticket Price Rank
Montreal	1st	21,273	7th
Ottawa	5th	19,473	17th
Toronto	6th	19,408	6th
Calgary	7th	19,289	15th
Vancouver	8th	18,630	3rd
Edmonton	15th	16,832	12th

Sources: http://sports.espn.go.com/nhl/attendance?year=2006; http://teammarketing.com.

Table 11.12. Indeed, five of the Canadian teams are ranked in the top eight clubs with respect to attendance per game, with Montreal being an easy number one.

The financial bottom line of Canadian franchises is also in much better shape than the average American franchise. This can be seen in Table 11.13, which describes the operating profits or losses of all major league Canadian franchises between 1989 and 2006. Canadian franchises did not do any worse than their American counterparts in the 1990s, and they did much better on average in the 2000s, before the 2004 lockout. After the lockout, while the profits of American teams averaged $2 million, those of Canadian teams excluding Toronto averaged $7 million, while the Toronto Maple Leafs made profits of $41 million. The fact that, in 2000–01, no Canadian or Québécois investors were willing to purchase the Molson Centre and the famed Montreal Canadiens franchise shows how much entrepreneurship and risk-taking is lacking among the more wealthy Canadians. The team ended up being picked up by an American *aventurier*, with the backing of a Quebec public bank! Fortunately, by contrast, Eugene Melnyk, one of the wealthiest persons in Canada, purchased the Ottawa Senators and the Corel Centre in 2003 at bargain prices.

Thus there has been a total reversal of fortunes, where small-market Canadian franchises are now in a much better financial situation than many American small-market franchises or franchises that do not benefit from fan loyalty. Besides the peculiar situation of the Pittsburgh Penguins, teams like Washington, the New York Islanders, and New Jersey are really doing poorly at the turnstiles, while sunbelt teams such as Atlanta, Carolina, Florida, Phoenix, and

Table 11.13 The Financial Bottom Line of Canadian Major League Franchises: Operating Income (Profits and Losses), 1990–2005

	1989–90	1990–91	1991–92	1992–93	1993–94	1994–95*	1995–96	1997–98	1998–99	1999–2000	2000–01	2001–02	2002–03	2003–04	2004–05	2005–06
Hockey																
Calgary	3.2	4.7	2.9	2.5	-0.3	2.7	7.8	0.6	0.7	1.9	2.1	-0.3	-4.1	-3.2	x	4.2
Edmonton	3.7	3.2	1.1	-2.3	-0.9	2.7	-0.1	2.3	2.7	3.6	2.5	-0.8	0	3.3	x	2.3
Montreal	4.9	6.9	5.5	4.9	6.6	-2.3	-0.4	8.3	5.8	12.7	12.2	6.4	-5.4	7.5	x	10.7
Ottawa					2.8	-2.6	0.1	1.2	1.4	-2.1	-4.5	2.0	-2.0	-5.0	x	17.5
Quebec	0	0.3	3.3	2.7	1.2	2.6	xx	xx	xx	xx	xx	xx	xx	xx	xx	4.2
Toronto	3.4	6.4	8.6	10.2	7.1	3.5	3.4	6.8	2.5	17.5	15.4	24.2	13.7	14.1	xx	xx
Vancouver	0.9	-0.8	0.4	0.8	1.4	0.9	-0.3	-10.4	-13.7	-11.3	-3.0	-0.8	0.7	1.3	x	41.5
Winnipeg	-0.4	-1.5	-2.5	-2.6	-3.6	-3.2	-11.7	xx	xx	xx	xx	xx	xx	xx	xx	1.1
Basketball																xx
Toronto							14.4	1.6	-8.0	1.2	5.1	4.5	10.6	9.5	7.4	
Vancouver							7.1	1.3	-12.4	-8.5	-13.3	xx	xx	xx	-1.3	xx
	1990	**1991**	**1992**	**1993**	**1994*****	**1995**	**1996**	**1997**	**1998**	**1999**	**2000**	**2001**	**2002**	**2003**	**2004**	**2005**
Baseball	7.0															12.0
Montreal	6.4	-4.2	11.8	12.4	-3.8	7.1	6.2	-3.7	5.6	1.9	-8.1	-2.4	-9.1	-8.3	-3.0	xx
Toronto	13.9	26.3	1.3	1.4	-1.6	14.5	-20.5	-9.5		-2.8	-5.9	-17.6	-23.9	0	7.8	29.7

Notes:

*NHL lockout in 1994–95 reduced season from 84 to 48 games; no play in 2004–05.

**NBA lockout in 1998–1999 reduced season from 82 to 50 games.

***MLB player strike in 1994 cut off-season by one month and a half, as well as the series.

Sources: Data from various issues of *Financial World* and *Forbes*. Positive numbers are profits; negative numbers are losses.

particularly Nashville and Anaheim seem vulnerable. Therefore the statement made nearly 20 years ago by Jones and Ferguson (1988, p. 456) to the effect that Canadian location "is simultaneously a proxy for Canadian sporting culture and a talisman for franchise survival," which seemed so misleading with the departure of the Jets and the Nordiques, may turn out to be true after all.

Indeed, if the Canadian dollar holds up, Winnipeg and Quebec City might regain their lost NHL franchises. They can be considered strong contenders to their rivals in American cities like Houston, Las Vegas, or Seattle. Winnipeg already has a state-of-the-art arena, the MTS Centre, although this city with its hard-core hockey fans has an arena that can accommodate only about 15,000 spectators. Quebec City could also support a team under the new economics of the NHL, but it would need to build a new arena, hopefully one similar to that of the Ottawa Senators. As Table 11.13 shows, the Nordiques team was relatively profitable until its departure. Finally, Hamilton is without a doubt a sizable hockey market, also with a viable arena, but it is a less likely candidate, having the drawback of being located within the Toronto Maple Leafs market area. But past experience shows that it would be preferable for any new owner to have very deep pockets.

The Role of the Public Sector

In the near future, readers will most likely witness groups lobbying to refurbish or construct NHL-viable arenas, in order to attract (or perhaps retain) NHL franchises in Canada. This brings us to the role of the public sector in the economic viability of Canadian professional sports teams. Most Canadians are now aware that the strategy favoured by owners, in trying to save a franchise afflicted by financial woes, is to ask for public financing. Whenever franchise owners threaten to leave a city, they ask some well-known accounting firm to produce an economic impact study, accompanied with enthusiastic statements about city pride, the business opportunities induced by the presence of a major league franchise, and the continent-wide tourist attraction brought about by the new venue. The study usually estimates the number of temporary jobs and amount of income benefits that would arise if some sporting venue were built or fully refurbished. The study also produces an estimate of the number of permanent jobs and amount of income benefits that would be forsaken were the team to leave the area. Similar studies are produced when a new franchise targets a city for public funding, as is most likely to happen if the NHL moves back North (and of course whenever there is an Olympic bid).

The consensus among academic sports economists, however, is that these commissioned studies are nearly useless. They routinely exaggerate the economic impact of professional sports, mainly because they use the gross impact of the franchise activity, rather than the much smaller net impact, typically 10 to 15 times smaller than the gross. For instance, these studies omit the fact that most of the money spent on season tickets would most likely be spent on some other activity within the local area if there were no team, and that team players spend only a small fraction of their revenues within the local community. The method is such that even if an NHL arena were constructed in the middle of Labrador, impact studies would still yield huge positive numbers.

Thus, the issue instead is whether local or provincial authorities believe that an NHL franchise provides enough psychological and social benefits to society that they are willing to build or help building a modern arena, with facilities that will also attract a few other entertaining events. The only real issue is whether the major league venue and its franchise bring about enough psychic income to the members of the home community, this psychic income being attributed to emotional excitement, social bonding, and enhanced collective self-esteem (Crompton, 2004).

In the United States, the construction of sports venues is heavily subsidized by the public sector, a rather paradoxical fact in the land of capitalism and free enterprise. Besides teams located in large markets, like the New York Rangers, financially successful teams play in recently built venues that are full of luxury boxes and opportunities for advertising revenues. These can be either owned by the team owners—but built largely at public expense—and carrying little or no property tax; or they can be state-of-the-art municipal venues—made available at below-market rents—with profitable management contracts that enable the team owners to accumulate lucrative revenues from advertising, catering, and other events. In these circumstances, Canadian team owners have been complaining, and with some justification, that they are not operating on a level playing field with their American-based competitors; they have lobbied every level of Canadian government (local, provincial, and federal) for financial assistance. Moreover, pressed by distressed fans and threatening owners, federal and provincial governments have considered intervening on the professional sports scene over the last few years. In 1999, Industry Minister John Manley announced that the federal government was prepared to offer temporary assistance to each of the six Canadian NHL teams. However, less than three days later, after an unprecedented public outcry, the Manley proposal was withdrawn (Whitson et al., 2000).

This example notwithstanding, public help has been provided by provincial authorities. In 1999, the Ontario government created a new property tax category that allowed municipalities to lower property taxes on sports venues; in turn, the city of Ottawa (but, notably, not Toronto) made use of this new category to diminish the Corel Centre property tax by nearly 90 percent, to a paltry $400,000. In 2001, just before the sale of the Montreal Canadiens, the city of Montreal cut in half the property tax assessment of the Bell Centre, although this tax is still around $7 million per year—the same amount paid for the Air Canada Centre. In Alberta, in 2002, the provincial government established a sports lottery and introduced an income tax on visiting players (which was rescinded at the end of 2005). Both measures have levied substantial amounts that were earmarked for the hockey teams of Calgary and Edmonton. Meanwhile, in both cities the teams play in arenas built (and recently refurbished) with public money, under terms that give many different kinds of revenue-generating opportunities to the teams. In other words, Albertan teams are just as much subsidized as American ones.

The new economics of the NHL make it less likely that future tax breaks or public subsidies will be forthcoming. With payroll caps and profitable teams, much of the justification for such help is gone. Still, in December 2005, the Quebec government was just about to reduce the tax assessment of the Bell Centre down to $1 million when the proposed bylaw was leaked to the media, leading to the quick and embarrassed withdrawal of the tax write-off.

CONCLUSIONS

The economics of the NHL have radically changed for Canadian franchises within the span of a few years. While the American economy was hit by a recession following the stock market crash of 2000, the Canadian economy barely slowed down and thus has caught up somewhat with its southern neighbour. Most importantly, the Canadian exchange rate has been boosted by good economic performance and a weakened American dollar, thus leading to a sharp reduction in the payroll cost of Canadian teams—as computed in Canadian dollars—as well as an increase in their revenues arising from merchandising, thus leading to a complete reversal in the relative financial situation of Canadian and American franchises. Whereas just a few years ago the survival of several small-market clubs such as Ottawa or Edmonton seemed in jeopardy (while other major league franchises such as the Vancouver Grizzlies and the

Montreal Expos did indeed depart in 2001 and 2005), there is now some genuine hope that cities like Winnipeg or Quebec City will recover an NHL team. Whether this is due to the adoption of the payroll cap in the 2005 collective bargaining agreement or due to the fact that the NHL is no longer a true major league in the United States, with television rankings below that of dart throwing or poker tournaments, is a moot point. It demonstrates that "expert opinion" can be off the mark, for few pundits would have forecast such a reversal. It also demonstrates that in economics, even though we may make decisions on the basis of historical data, the past is no indication of the future.

CRITICAL THINKING QUESTIONS

1. Imagine that you are an adviser to the provincial prime minister. Draw out the pros and cons of subsidizing or granting tax breaks to NHL teams in your province.
2. Imagine that you are an adviser to the mayor of a large Canadian city. Draw out the pros and cons of subsidizing the construction of a new venue to regain an NHL team.
3. It was suggested by the Mills Committee in 1999 that major league athletes playing in Canada ought to receive a tax credit to harmonize their income tax rates with the rates they would have paid in the United States. What do you think of the merits and the ethics of this proposal?
4. It was also proposed by the Mills Committee to grant a tax credit to cover the costs encountered by the parents of kids involved in amateur sport. Conservative leader Stephen Harper also made such a proposal during the 2006 election campaign. What do you think of such a proposal in light of the fact that recreational sport brings large health benefits, and in light of the fact that parents of kids taking art or music lessons also can encounter large costs? Should people with kids pay less income tax (or more) than people without kids?
5. Corporations or self-employed workers that purchase opera or hockey game tickets can use 50 percent of the cost of these tickets to reduce their taxable income. In the case of NHL hockey, it is estimated that this federal tax expenditure amounts to more than $20 million per year. Should such tax deductions be sustained?
6. To improve their financial situation, what should NHL team owners be looking for when bargaining during the next collective agreement? Should they be concerned with improving the competitive balance in the NHL?
7. Imagine that you are advising a business intending to bring back an NHL team to Winnipeg. What possible financial risks would you highlight?
8. Major league hockey players earned, on average, $1.7 million (Canadian) in 2005–06, while Canadian high school teachers earned on average slightly more than $50,000 per year. Discuss whether you believe this to be fair. Discuss the advantages and the drawbacks of an economic system that leads to such discrepancies.
9. What benefits, and drawbacks, do you see in the 2010 Winter Olympic Games in Vancouver–Whistler?

SUGGESTED READINGS

Andreff, W., & Szymanski, S. (Eds.). (2006). *Handbook on the economics of sport*. Cheltenham: Edward Elgar.

Cagan, J., & de Mause, N. (1998). *Field of schemes: How the great stadium swindle turns public money into private profit*. Monroe, ME: Common Courage Press.

Edge, M. (2004). *Red line. Blue line. Bottom line*. Vancouver: New Stars.

Fizel, J. (Ed.). (2005). *Handbook of sports economics*. Armonk, NJ: M.E. Sharpe.

Fort, R. (2006). *Sports economics*, 2nd ed. Upper Saddle River, NJ: Pearson Education.

Fort, R., & Fizel, J. (Eds.). (2004). *International sports economics*. Westport, CT: Praeger.

Leeds, M., & von Allmen, P. (2002). *The economics of sports*. Boston: Addison-Wesley.

Rosentraub, M. S. (1997). *Major league losers: The real cost of sport and who is paying for it*. New York: Basic Books.

WEB LINKS

The Economics of Sports

http://wps.aw.com/aw_leedsvonal_econsports_1/

A site set up by the authors of the first undergraduate textbook on the economics of sport, with quizzes and several other links to sports economics websites.

Rodney Fort's Web Pages

http://www.rodneyfort.com/

Fort is also the author of a textbook on the economics of sport. This is probably the most complete website on the business of sports, with extensive data sets and plenty of information.

HockeyZonePlus

http://www.HockeyZonePlus.com

This bilingual site operated by François Coulombe is devoted to hockey. It contains a large business section on hockey, including a large historical data bank on the salaries of all NHL players, but part of the site has not been updated.

The National Hockey League Players' Association

http://www.nhlpa.com

This site provides the latest salaries of all NHL players, as well as their year-by-year statistics.

Patricia's Basketball Website

http://www.dfw.net/~patricia/

This site contains the most complete data banks on basketball.

CHAPTER 12

SPORT, POLITICS, AND POLICY

Jean Harvey

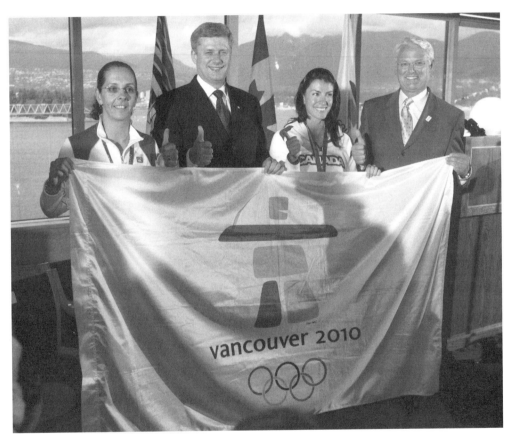

Politicians do not miss any opportunity to increase their political capital by associating themselves with high-performance sport.

CHUCK STOODY/CP Images

The issue of government intervention is not whether or not governments should be involved in sport, but the extent and nature of that involvement.

Canada, 1992, p. 187

To a great extent, the idea that "sport doesn't mix with politics" has now vanished. The most visible aspect of the link between sport and politics is the increasing government intervention in the funding and regulation of sport. Today, national sport organizations (NSOs), provincial sport organizations (PSOs), and local sport clubs call on their respective levels of government to help them develop, fund, and administer competitive regional, provincial, national, and international teams. Government funding is also expected for grassroots sports, as well as for venues for hosting global megasport events such as soccer's World Cup and the Summer and Winter Olympic Games. Regulations developed by international sport organizations such as the World Anti-Doping Agency (WADA) and the International Olympic Committee (IOC) not only command the attention of governments but also, to a certain degree, provoke specific modifications to provincial/territorial national sport policies. Given such interrelationships, the issue is not whether the state should intervene in sport, but rather what state intervention and public policies are needed for contemporary sport.

But fundamentally, the relationship between sport and politics is much more complex, as it is deeply rooted in the social nature of sport. As stated in Chapter 1, sport is a contested terrain.

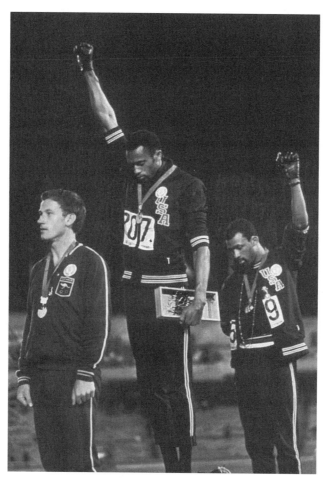

Sport can be a site of political resistance.

AP/CP Images

The relationship of politics to sport prompts numerous questions: What is the definition of sport? Which social values should orient sport? Who should have access to participation in sport? How should sport be structured? for what ends? Should sport be the responsibility of the state? All these questions speak to the relationship between sport and politics. As sport is closely entrenched in societal power relations, it has the potential to be a tool both for the reproduction of dominant power relations and for political resistance and change. For example, when governments invest heavily in high-performance sport, they hope the victories of the athletes will bolster dominant views about national identity. Conversely, at the Mexico 1968 Olympics, when U.S. athletes Tommie Smith and John Carlos raised their gloved fists as they stood on the podium, their Black Power salute was meant as an act of resistance to existing racial power relations in their country (see Zirin, 2005; see also the photo on page 222).

The history of the modern Olympics also provides various examples of encounters between sport and politics, through boycotts, protests, and the banning of countries. Indeed, since their beginnings in Ancient Greece and their resurrection by Pierre de Coubertin in 1894, the Olympic Games have been and are deliberately used by national states for international policy purposes. For example, under the leadership of Adolf Hitler, the 1936 Berlin Games were meant to showcase to the world the cause of National Socialism, Nazi ideology and the superiority of the Aryan race. Several countries threatened to boycott the games, as Hitler did not want Jews and Black people to participate. In Canada, for example, the Workers' Sports Association, as well as religious, university, and veterans' group leaders, were in favour of boycotting the Nazi Olympics (Kidd, 1996b). Eventually, Hitler was forced to concede to international pressure and lifted some restrictions. Ironically, his orchestrated display of white superiority was ruined by the outstanding performance of African American Jesse Owens, who won four gold medals in track and field. In a tragic turn of history, when the Olympics returned to Germany in 1972 Israeli athletes and trainers were taken hostage by Palestinian extremists, a disastrous series of events that received renewed attention in 1999 with the Academy Award–winning documentary *One Day in September*.

Intense public protest by various anti-racist movements, most notably the 1964 banning of South Africa from the IOC in protest against apartheid, is a strong example of the ways in which sport is used as a means of putting diplomatic pressure on countries. The isolation of South Africa from international competition became almost all-encompassing after the General Assembly of United Nations (UN) passed a resolution in 1971 inviting countries not to participate or compete with those upholding discrimination or apartheid laws and policies. This provision led to a request to ban New Zealand from the 1976 Montreal Games in protest against a series of rugby matches played between New Zealand and South Africa. New Zealand was not banned, and as a result most African countries boycotted the Montreal Olympics. The next Olympic Games, held in Moscow in 1980, were also marked by a boycott, this time by the United States and several Western countries in protest of the invasion of Afghanistan by the Soviet Union. Countries from the former Eastern Bloc, with the exception of Romania, exacted their revenge four years later by boycotting the 1984 Los Angeles Olympic Games, alleging that the United States was not safe for their athletes.

Government involvement in sport in Canada is far from new. In the second half of the nineteenth century, local governments in big cities like Montreal and Toronto created municipal parks; for several decades, these parks played a major role in preventing the working class from participating in sport through regulations that restricted the types of sports allowed on their grounds (Gruneau, 1983). While municipal parks were mainly conceived as peaceful and quiet retreats from the busy streets for the benefit of the urban elite, working-class sports were often banned from these places. The enactment of the Lord's Day Act by the federal government in 1906 banning the practise of sport on Sundays was another state intervention that limited opportunities for the working class to play sports (Kidd, 1996b). At the beginning of the twentieth century municipalities started to play a different role, initially as a result of pressures from different elite groups, like the National Council of Women of Canada, lobbying for vacation schools and supervised playgrounds as ways to prevent youth delinquency. As a result, over the last century municipalities got increasingly involved in recreational sport through the subsidization of playground associations and local clubs, as well as through the development and maintenance of increasingly large numbers of sport fields and venues. First, lobbied by the bourgeoisie to control urban masses after World War II, municipalities became increasingly involved in providing sport participation opportunities for their citizens, a role they still play today. Indeed, parks and recreation represent a significant item in current municipal budgets.

The Great Depression of the 1930s prompted federal and provincial involvement in sport and recreation as the growing numbers of unemployed youth and adults, in their unrest, represented fertile material for leftist movements, reformist groups, and various forms of political resistance. Again, these interventions were exclusively meant as social control measures. In December 1936, the National Employment Commission of Canada prompted the Minister of Labour to establish young men's physical training centres, the goal of which was to help unemployed young men develop good levels of mental and physical fitness in order to maintain their employability. The Minister soon agreed to this recommendation and provisions were made to create training centres under the Unemployment and Agriculture Act, 1937, as well as under the 1939 Youth Training Act. The programs involved agreements with participating provinces in order to fund a wide variety of youth training opportunities often involving gymnastics and sports (Harvey, 1988). For constitutional reasons, however, not all provinces agreed to participate in these programs, a point we shall return to later on. During World War II, the federal government turned its attention to fitness for war. To that end, the National Physical Fitness Act was passed in 1943, to be repealed in 1954.

The reconstruction effort at the end of the war created a context for the transformation of the Canadian state into a welfare state. A welfare state is one in which organized power is deliberately used to play a more active role in society, providing, for example, a minimum income for all, as well as some state-financed social services like education and health insurance. This renewed role of the Canadian state set the stage for a more active intervention into sport. But, according to Macintosh, Bedecki, and Frank (1987), the adoption in 1961 of Bill C-131, an Act to Encourage Fitness and Amateur Sport, was predominantly the result of an increased preoccupation of the government toward high-performance sport and the promotion of Canadian nationalism through sport. Since the adoption of Bill C-131, the federal government has been increasingly active in the sport field. Moreover, several events attracted the attention of the House of Commons, such as the 1972 Canada–USSR hockey series and the 1988 Ben Johnson doping scandal. The Canada–USSR hockey series in 1972 was a highly volatile moment for Canadian sport and for Parliament Hill in Ottawa—not just a symbolic confrontation between East and West, but also an event expected to restore Canadian nationalism via victory in its national winter sport. The Ben Johnson doping scandal at the 1988 Seoul Olympics also commanded great attention and intense debate in the House of Commons, leading to the striking of a Royal Commission, commonly referred to as the Dubin Inquiry, with a mandate for investigating the Johnson affair and the broader use of performance-enhancing drugs in Canadian sport (Dubin, 1990). The report recommended that the Canadian government adopt a strict anti-doping policy and prompted the creation of an arm's-length organization to control and police the use of performance-enhancing drugs in sport.

In summary, the relationships between sport and politics are complex and multifaceted. In this chapter, I will focus specifically on an overview of current sport policies and programs in Canada, although, as we shall see, it is difficult in our globalized world to understand national policy without considering the larger international context. I will try to answer the following questions: What motivates nation-states, such as Canada, to get involved in sport? What constitutional and political contexts at the domestic and international levels influence the development of sport policies in Canada? What are the key current sport policies in Canada? Before answering these questions, a brief review of some key concepts is in order.

DEFINING SOME MAIN CONCEPTS

State, power, government, politics, policy, and programs—it is easy to become swamped and overwhelmed by political science and political sociology terminology. Giddens defines politics as: "The means by which power is used to influence the nature and content of governmental activities" (1989, p. 729). This definition, by itself, speaks to the broad social reality that is covered by the word *politics*. The definition also refers to another concept: the state. For Giddens, a state, is "a political apparatus (governmental institutions, such as court, parliament, civil service, officials) ruling over a given territory, whose authority is backed by the legal system and by the capacity to use force to implement its policies" (p. 732). Main characteristics of a modern nation-state are its sovereignty over a given territory; its monopoly of the use of force; its legitimacy, mainly provided by its democratic electoral system; and the fact that its constituents are defined as citizens having both formal rights and duties and who generally recognize themselves as part of a given nation. A key question to ask, then, is What is the role of the state in contemporary society? Before attempting to answer this question, it is important to emphasize that any social institution is the product of history; that is, a result of power relations among social classes, gender, race, and so on. This is an important point to remember when examining theoretical traditions in political science and their differing visions of the role of the state.

For the purpose of this chapter, I wish to limit the discussion to the two main and opposing theoretical positions. For pluralists, the state is a neutral referee of competing social interests. For them, in theory, no specific organized interest has more persuasive power than others on the orientation or direction of state policies. For Marxists, the state is the instrument of the ruling capitalist class in its domination of society (refer back to Chapter 2 for more on this). Although many nuances have added to that bold statement, the Marxist approach is a better reflection of the unequal influence different social classes have on the state. More specifically, the advanced capitalist state has three overall functions. The first is to adopt measures that allow the accumulation of capital, for example through investments in transportation infrastructure, the adoption of labour laws that will keep salaries at the lowest possible levels for Canadian companies to remain competitive, and taxation that will attract private investment. The second function is to preserve social cohesion. This is achieved through measures that ease tensions between the interests of the dominant class and the dominated classes. At the minimum the state has to give the impression that it is not the sole servant of the dominant class if it wants to keep its legitimacy. Finally, the third function of the state is one of coercion, as the state has a monopoly over the use of force in order to preserve social order (Harvey & Proulx, 1988).

Modern nation-states have sovereignty over a given territory but interact with other nation-states as part of their international relations. In addition, a panoply of supra-national organizations, such as the United Nations, the G8, the World Trade Organization, and treaties such as the North American Free Trade Agreement (NAFTA) create a context influencing the actions of nation-states. In the current context of globalization, many authors argue that nation-states are losing even more sovereignty (e.g., see Harvey & Houle, 1994), as national policies have to be at least partially in line with the international context. For example, the

Canadian sport doping policy has to follow WADA regulations in order for Canada to be able to compete in the Olympics and most amateur international sport events.

Building on our basic understanding of the concepts of politics and the state, let's explore the concepts of government, policy, and programs. Returning to Giddens (1989), who states that "government refers to the regular enactment of policies and decisions on the part of officials within a political apparatus . . . we can speak of government as a process, or of *the* government, referring to the apparatus responsible for the administrative process" (p. 301). While politics concerns the means by which power is used, policy or public policy refers to "a course of action or inaction chosen by public authorities to address a given problem or interrelated set of problems" (Pal, 2006, p. 2). It is important to emphasize here in Pal's definition of politics the point that a decision by a government not to act on a specific issue is often, by itself, a policy. Finally, there is a fine line between programs and policies. Policies are mostly "guides to a range of related actions in a given field" (Pal, 2006, p. 2), while programs are the specific courses of action taken in view of fulfilling the goals of a policy. Governments do possess a wide variety of action tools or policy instruments for the implementation of policies and programs. Although there are a wide variety of policy instruments typologies, let us adapt Pal's (2006) classification system for the purposes of this chapter (see Figure 12.1). The first broad category refers to tools of *indirect action:* information is the first tool in this category. Information can be the preferred course of action in the case of health promotion, for example. Such was the case with ParticipAction, a program whose focus was to encourage Canadians to become more physically active. The second type of tool in the indirect actions category is expenditures, which can take several forms as listed in Figure 12.1. Government funding for national, provincial, and local associations fall into this category. The third type of tool in this category relates to regulations that are made to promote or discourage certain types of behaviour. For example, anti-doping policies prohibit the use of banned performance-enhancing substances.

The second main category in Pal's classification system (see Figure 12.1) refers to tools of *direct action*. State agencies are created to implement policies where the state is the delivery provider, such as the case of provincial departments of education and of health and social

Figure 12.1 Classification of Policy Instruments

Indirect Action	Direct Action
Information	*State agency*
	Department
	Social agency
Expenditures	
Cash transfer	
Grants	*State corporation*
Subsidies, loan	
Tax expenditures	*Third-party partnership/contract*
Voucher	Nongovernmental organization
Tax	Nonprofit corporation
User fees	Company
Fines	
Regulations	
Permissions	
Licences	
Criminal and non-criminal prohibitions	

Source: From *Beyond Policy Analysis*, Third Edition, by PAL, 2006. Reprinted with permission of Nelson, a division of Thomson Learning: www.thomsonrights.com. Fax 800-730-2215.

services. State or Crown corporations, such as Canada Post and CBC–Radio Canada, are arm's-length agencies that offer direct public services in lieu of the state and are responsible to the House of Commons for their actions. Finally, in our neo-liberal times, where state-provided public services are increasingly criticized by right-wing forces, third-party arrangements like public–private partnerships are believed within right-wing circles to be the best tool for efficient intervention. In short, tools for state intervention are numerous, but as I will outline later in the chapter, the choice of possible tools varies widely from one policy field to another as a function of the perceived overall role of the state in each of these fields. Now that we have a minimal basis for understanding politics and policy in our society, I wish to turn to the specific domain of sport and politics—which, like any other domain, has its own specificities, issues, and problems that influence and are influenced by state intervention.

REASONS FOR STATE INTERVENTION IN SPORT

At the beginning of this chapter, I provided several examples of state intervention in sport. I wish to return to that point here in order to discuss issues and problems specific to state intervention in sport. One good way of getting an organized perspective of this issue is to identify what generally motivates the state to intervene in sport. Over the course of history, these motivations obviously change as new problems and issues arise but they also change as social forces influence what constitutes the legitimate role of the state in society. For example, compared to the nineteenth century, the Canadian state is now much more interventionist in its actions. In the first known book on sport and politics, Jean Meynaud (1966) identified three major motives for public authorities to intervene in sport: to safeguard public order; to improve the physical fitness of the citizens; and to affirm national prestige. According to Meynaud, the safeguarding of public order is an issue for the state since hosting major sport events involves security issues and because sport is sometimes the cause of violence, on or off the field. For Meynaud, doping in sport also constitutes an issue of public order since it sometimes involves the use of banned substances. Four decades after Meynaud's work, sport has become an ever more important social phenomenon and reasons for state intervention in sport have diversified.

I have regrouped these contemporary motives for state intervention in sport into four main categories. First, governments see sport as an instrument of social cohesion. For example, high-performance sport is considered an important tool for the promotion of national unity. Governments perceive that medals and trophies earned by Canadian athletes around the globe contribute to fostering national pride as well as Canadian identity. Sport is also perceived as a tool of social cohesion for at-risk populations, particularly at-risk youth, since it allegedly contributes to the prevention of delinquency. In that instance, sport also serves as a function of social control. Second, governments increasingly recognize sport as an instrument of economic development (or, according to our theory section, capital accumulation). For example, hosting mega-sporting events allegedly contributes to the tourism industry by attracting athletes and fans to the host cities. Moreover, hosting major events or having professional sport franchises are widely believed by governments to have a high economic and symbolic impact, helping cities to showcase themselves as world-class tourist destinations and ideal locations for all kinds of businesses and industries (see Chapter 13, Globalization). Third, sport policy is a tool of foreign policy. To this end, states use sport to push specific agendas, as we have seen earlier with the international struggle against apartheid. Conversely, states see sport as an instrument to foster international cooperation, such as is the case with the Commonwealth Games and the Jeux de la Francophonie, whose functions are to increase political and economic relationships among "communities" of countries. The final motivation for state intervention in sport is related to social development and the promotion of social inclusion. Sport is popularly believed to contribute to the education and health of individuals and to their participation in society as active citizens. To that end, inclusive policies are put in place to reduce social and economic barriers, to promote equity for women and men and for visible and cultural minorities. The above description provides a wide overview of the motives of modern advanced capitalist states to deliberately intervene in sport, but not all interventions are planned or premeditated. At times, governments are forced to react and act quickly as a result of a sudden crisis, as was the case with the Ben Johnson scandal in 1988.

THE SPORT–POLICY CONTEXT

In order to better understand the shape and direction of current federal sport policies and programs, I wish to return briefly to general considerations about the constitutional as well as the specific political contexts that forge sport policy in this country. First, it is of utmost importance to remember that by its constitution, Canada is a federal state with two major orders of government: the federal and the provincial/territorial. As such, municipalities are the creation of provinces/territories. The constitution defines, although not always clearly, the jurisdiction of the federal government and of the provinces/territories, *but* there is nothing in the constitution on sport. However, sport is generally associated with social policies, particularly education and health policy, both of which are under provincial/territorial jurisdiction. International sport is linked to Canada's foreign policy, which is clearly under federal jurisdiction. The High Performance Athlete Development in Canada Agreement of 1985 and the National Recreation Statement of 1987 were passed to delineate more precisely the mutual roles of the federal and provincial/territorial governments. The 1985 agreement recognized the jurisdiction of the federal government on the national and international levels, while provinces and territories maintained their control over and responsibility for the provincial/territorial and municipal levels of the sport system. The 1987 legislation recognized the primary role of the provinces and territories in the area of recreation, including sport, but opened the field to the federal government for support to national organizations, international representation, and providing directly to citizens promotional documents and documentation encouraging participation in sport. Presented in this manner, the situation appears very clear and straightforward.

Unfortunately, this was and is not the case. For example, hosting major international sport events primarily involves the cities orchestrating the bid process, but international sport falls under the jurisdiction of the federal government. Cities cannot bid for the event without the permission of the provinces/territories and without the financial help of the higher levels of government. Any federal government intervention in municipalities needs provincial approval. While several provinces have a history of flexibility on these arrangements when the federal government has money to spend within their borders, other provinces are very strict in the preservation of their jurisdiction. As far as foreign policy is concerned, some provinces do request a presence on the international scene—such is the case with the Jeux de la Francophonie, where Quebec, New Brunswick, and Ontario play an important role.

The other set of considerations I wish to underline here touches on what we call a policy field. Each policy has a specific culture, a set of norms and values about the general role of the state in that field at a given time in history. For each field, there is generally a state agency under the responsibility of a cabinet minister and, moreover, a specific set of social forces or interest groups that are active. Having different agendas, these social forces constantly lobby government for their view to be considered. Arguably, sport constitutes in itself a specific policy field, although it is related to education, health, and foreign policy. In this country, according to the current dominant neo-liberal vision, the state should not intervene too directly in sport. Indeed, major interest groups like the Canadian Olympic Committee (COC) and national sport organizations (NSOs) are constantly lobbying for more funding by the federal government and, at the same time, less government control. However, other groups such as the Canadian Association for the Advancement of Women and Sport and Physical Activity (CAAWS) are in favour of strong government regulations to force sport organizations to implement stronger gender-equity programs. With regard to professional sport as a private enterprise, it normally does not want state intervention in its business affairs. That is not always the case, however, as we will see with the events that led to the most recent piece of Canadian sport legislation. Given the characteristics of the field, it would probably appear inappropriate for the Canadian state to take control of the Canadian sport system through the creation of, for example, a Crown corporation. Most state interventions in the form of Crown corporations have to preserve some arm's-length relationship between the federal government and the sport milieu, which is difficult given that the government plays an increasingly prominent role in the governance of Canadian sport, namely through the imposition of strict conditions and criteria as part of the financial support it provides to NSOs and national multi-sport and service organizations (MSOs).

This leads to the last set of considerations regarding the context of sport policy. It is very rare that the state does not put in place a formal administrative unit in charge of the delivery of policies and programs. Sport is no exception. With the adoption of Bill C-131 in the early 1960s, a Fitness and Amateur Sport Program emerged under the Ministry of Health and Welfare. In 1971, two separate units were created under the Fitness and Amateur Sport Directorate: Sport Canada and Recreation Canada. With Sport Canada, the federal government created for itself an administrative unit to intervene in the world of high-performance sport, until then the exclusive territory of NSOs and MSOs. Currently, two separate units in two different departments are in charge of sport and physical activity. Sport Canada is a branch of Heritage Canada and remains almost exclusively in charge of high-performance sport. The Physical Activity Unit is a division of the Public Health Agency of Canada and is in charge of promoting physical activity, in its broadest sense, for Canadians. Indeed, because the federal government, starting with Pierre Elliott Trudeau's in 1968, is increasingly viewing high-performance sport as a vehicle for the promotion of national unity and international prestige on the world sporting stage, high-performance sport becomes the priority over mass participation. In summary, a complex range of constitutional, political, and administrative structures and forces, as well as pressure from organized interest groups, make up state intervention in any policy field in Canadian society.

FROM THE MILLS COMMITTEE TO BILL C-12

Before presenting an overview of the federal government's sport policies and programs, I wish to focus in this section on the economic and political context that led to the adoption of the 2002 Canadian Sport Policy and the enactment of Bill C-12, the law that governs sport policy in Canada. Their story started in 1997, with meetings between NHL Commissioner Gary Bettman and the mayors of Canadian cities with an NHL franchise. Bettman's message, in short, was that Canadian teams were facing financial difficulties and governments should be prepared to help if they wanted to keep their franchises. He argued that many U.S.–based teams play in publicly funded facilities virtually rent-free, enjoy generous tax exemptions, and their players pay less tax on their large incomes. Moreover, Canadian franchises paid their players in U.S. dollars at a period in time when exchange rates between the United States and the Canadian dollar were at a disadvantage for Canadian teams. In other words, his message was that the owners of Canadian franchises were looking for subsidies and tax exemptions in order to make sufficient profits and government should do something to financially assist these teams in order to avoid a mass exodus to the U.S., such as was the case with the Québec Nordiques and the Winnipeg Jets.

As a first response to the NHL-instigated "crisis," the government formed a sub-committee, dubbed the Mills committee under the leadership of Liberal MP Dennis Mills, to study sport in Canada. The focus of the committee was to demonstrate that sport, as an industry, had an important economic impact and therefore qualified for governmental financial aid as did other industrial sectors, like the tourism industry. As expected, the report tabled in November 1998 recognized that "high-level commercial sport is an important contributor to the country's economy as well as to its cultural identity" (Sub-Committee, 1998, p. 101) and included a "Sport Pact"—a "Canadian professional sport stabilization program" that involved providing tax assistance (a type of expenditure) to Canadian NHL franchises. The report was immediately criticized from both within and outside the Commons and was eventually rejected by the government in April 1999. Indeed, all opposition parties, which had representatives on the sub-committee, issued dissenting reports that mainly argued against the Sport Pact. Nonetheless, under the pressure of team owners like Rob Bryden of the Ottawa Senators, in the summer of 1999 discussions resumed between the federal government and the Canadian hockey teams leading to what is commonly referred to as the Manley proposals (named after then–Minister of Industry John Manley). The Manley proposals consisted of an assistance package to professional hockey teams with contributions from the provinces and municipalities. On January 18, 2000, three days after the announcement of the proposal, the plan was withdrawn in the face of wide public protest. Canadians of all walks of life—through mail, letters to newspaper editors, protests in the streets, e-mail messages, and so on—made it clear to the government that professional hockey in North America is a rich private industry and therefore doesn't deserve public subsidies. (For a more detailed account of the Manley affair, see Whitson, Harvey, & Lavoie, 2000.) The NHL's dramatic stunt for government subsidies and tax exemptions is a good example of how the Canadian bourgeoisie can easily press the federal government to put one of its demands on the political agenda.

Despite its main focus on the professional/commercial sport industry and its obvious bias in favour of subsidizing professional sport (see Rail, 2000), the Mills committee also had the mandate to overview the scope of the federal involvement in sport in Canada and to see how sport's contribution to Canadian national unity could be enhanced. The committee did receive numerous briefs from NSOs, MSOs, and PSOs, as well as from academics, and as a result held extensive discussions pertaining to mass and high-performance sport. The committee report included a section on the social and cultural aspects of sport, dealing mostly with ethics in sport, sport participation, and youth at risk. It also included numerous recommendations for high-performance sport, focusing on NSOs, coaching, sponsorship, the hosting of major sport events, issues of sport and physical activity accessibility, and the need for stronger intergovernmental cooperation to solidify the sport system. Basically, the report asked for stronger financial involvement from the federal government to increase access to mass sport and to provide more services and support to high-performance athletes and to NSOs. The government positively received the recommendations, but did not support the idea of more funding. Nevertheless, the winds of reform were blowing. Canadian athletes were not performing well in international sport events such as the Olympics; NSOs and MSOs were requesting more funds for athletes and coaches. In addition, national organizations were complaining about the lack of federal funding for the promotion of participation in physical activity in the face of a perceived epidemic of obesity.

In 2000, the newly appointed Secretary of State (Amateur Sport), Denis Coderre, launched a vast series of consultations with provincial governments, NSOs, MSOs, and athletes that culminated in a National Summit in Ottawa in April 2001. The summit ended with a proposed new sport policy for Canada that was agreed upon by the provinces and territories in May 2002. The main feature of the policy was its four pillars, or goals, of enhanced participation, excellence, capacity, and interaction.

The *enhanced participation* pillar sought to promote the personal and social benefits of sport participation, support sport organizations to increase participation, increase children's exposure to sport in schools, encourage communities to increase sport participation, and increase access and equity in sport for underrepresented groups. Since the 1970s Sport Canada has primarily been preoccupied with high-performance sport, and the enhanced participation pillar opens a new field of intervention for Sport Canada geared at Canadians from all segments of society involved in sport activities at all levels and forms.

In the *enhanced excellence* pillar, governments would establish targets for major games, increase the number of qualified, fully employed female and male coaches, increase accessibility for high-performance athletes to key services like financial support, and confirm the role of the Canada Games as a platform for future high-performance athletes. The purpose of this pillar was to assist athletes to achieve world-class results at the highest levels of international competition through fair and ethical means.

The third pillar, *enhanced capacity,* meant that governments would ensure the essential components of the sport system are in place to fulfill the goals of the two first pillars, promote safety and ethical behaviour, develop a long-term strategic approach to hosting major sport events, and support the development of volunteers.

The goal of the final pillar, enhanced interaction, was to increase collaboration, communication, and cooperation among levels of governments, as well as with the partners in the sport community. It was expected that provinces and territories would endorse the Canadian Sport Policy and sign individual agreements with the federal government to implement that policy throughout Canada. Since then, provinces and territories have signed such agreements. The four pillars of the Canadian Sport Policy represented a mix of consensus reached throughout the extensive consultation phase leading to the 2002 Summit and of the will of the federal government to take an even more active role in Canadian sport, while remaining at arm's length with regard to the delivery of policies and programs. Moreover, throughout the process the government underlined that increased funding would come with a higher accountability to MSOs and NSOs to follow Sport Canada funding criteria, for example regarding doping, dispute resolution, women, and bilingualism.

With the enactment of Bill C-12 in 2003, the Canadian Sport Policy became entrenched in the law. The current Canadian Sport Policy and Bill C-12 are the result of a convergence of specific lobby efforts, first by corporate professional sport, followed by a wide range of MSOs and NSOs. Political parties also had their input in the process. For example, throughout the meetings of the Mills committee the Bloc Québécois was very active in resisting the will of the majority party to subsidize professional sport and in the end was successful in convincing the other opposition parties to adopt the same position. The three dissenting reports indeed had their impact on the outcome of this issue. All opposition parties also underlined the importance to provide more funds for Canadian athletes and to support mass participation in sport and physical activity. While Bill C-12 constitutes a significant legislative change in replacing Bill C-131, notably through the specific objectives of the four pillars, it nevertheless didn't provide a solution to all issues. The most important one relates to grassroots sport and the promotion of physical activity. As noted above, the dismantling of the Fitness and Amateur Sport Directorate that left Fitness Canada with Health Canada and sent Sport Canada to the new

Heritage Ministry created a situation in which relationships and joint initiatives between the two former units of the same directorate became impossible. In the decade following the separation of the two units a considerable rift built up between them. On the one side, as noted earlier, Sport Canada focused on high-performance sport as an element of promoting national unity. On the other side of the agenda, the Physical Activity Unit of the Public Health Agency of Canada (former Fitness Canada) is now entrenched within the Canadian Strategy for Healthy Living. This strategy includes the promotion of sport education and all forms of physical activities, but sport is understood as only one element of physical activity and healthy living. Behind the increased participation pillar was in fact an attempt to regroup the two units into a new Sport Ministry. But that failed, notably as a result of disagreements between Health Minister Alan Rock, who would not let go of his health promotion portfolio, and Heritage Minister Sheila Copps, who loved the opportunities to gain political capital provided by high-performance sport. As a result, Bill C-12 includes two sets of objectives, one for sport and one for physical activity, and is the responsibility of two cabinet ministers.

CURRENT POLICIES AND PROGRAMS

In this section I will discuss the specific policies and programs administered by Sport Canada. Since the enactment of Bill C-12, several programs and policies have been redesigned or are still under review. New policies also came to life. For example, a new Sport Participation Development Program (SPDP) has been put in place marking the renewed interest of the federal government for participation in sport. In 2003, the federal budget allocated $45 million over five years to Sport Canada to increase sport participation. The funds are made available to those NSOs and MSOs developing new strategies to increase participation in their sport through the SPDP. The new money also funds the federal/provincial/territorial bilateral agreements. The other important element is the adoption in May 2005 of Sport Canada's policy on Aboriginal people's participation in sport. As for the SPDP, the latter policies reflect the pillars of the Canadian Sport Policy and its main goals to promote inclusion and equitable access and reduce barriers to participation in sport for Aboriginal peoples at all levels of the sport system.

Sport Canada programs and policies form an intricate network of intervention mechanisms that fall into the category of expenditures. As we shall see, even if expenditures are instruments of indirect action, the funding criteria adopted by Sport Canada over the last two decades result in an increasing indirect control over MSOs and NSOs. Indeed, more funding from the federal government meant increased dependency for these organizations, which have to align their policies and programs to obtain their funding. Given the length of this chapter, it is not possible to describe and analyze in depth each aspect of these policies and programs (see Figure 12.2). Therefore, I will provide only an overview of some of the most salient. The greatest proportion of Sport Canada budget goes to three funding programs: (1) the NSOs and MSOs, (2) the athletes, and (3) hosting sport events (see Table 12.1). A large proportion of the budget of these organizations depends on federal funding.

Sport Funding and Accountability Framework

The first and most important regulation is the Sport Funding and Accountability Framework (SFAF), which is the process by which the federal government identifies which NSOs and MSOs are eligible for Sport Canada contribution programs. It also determines in what areas, at what levels, and under what conditions these organizations qualify for funding. Introduced

Figure 12.2 Federal Sport Policies, Programs, and Regulations

Policies and Programs

- The Canadian Sport Policy (2002)
- Policy on Aboriginal Peoples' Participation in Sport (2005)
- Athlete Assistance Program: Policies, Procedures and Guidelines (2005)
- Canadian Policy Against Doping in Sport (June 2004)
- The Canadian Strategy for Ethical Conduct in Sport (2002)
- Federal Policy for Hosting International Sport Events (Hosting Policy 2000)
- Women in Sport Policy (1986)
- Federal Government Policy on Tobacco Sponsorship of National Sport Organizations (1985)
- Treasury Board Policy on Official Languages
- Sport Policy Research Initiative

Funding programs

- Athlete Assistance Programs
- Sport Funding Accountability Framework
  - Contribution Guidelines for NSOs
  - Contribution Guidelines for MSOs
  - Project Stream Component
- Hosting Program

Source: Sport Canada (2002). *The Canadian sport policy.* The Department of Canadian Heritage. Reproduced with the permission of the Minister of Public Works and Government Services Canada, 2006.

Table 12.1   Overview of Sport Canada Expenditures ($000)

	1998–99	1999–00	2000–01	2001–02	2002–03	2003–04	2004–05	2005–06
Total operating	3,947	8,471	6,215	9,821	7,824	7,666	8,266	9,470
Sport support program	34,889	35,468	42,356	43,864	48,312	55,594	81,948	91,428
International relations— games/hosting	14,494	8,285	24,849	31,646	15,745	25,270	21,481	17,672
Athletes assistance program	8,038	9,010	14,749	15,117	15,108	15,199	19,845	24,800
Special authorities	65	127	108	325	55	22	0	0
Total grants and contributions	57,487	52,890	82,064	90,953	79,222	96,086	123,275	133,901
Total expenditures	61,435	61,361	88,279	100,775	87,047	103,752	131,541	143,372

Source: The Department of Canadian Heritage. Reproduced with the permission of the Minister of Public Works and Government Services Canada, 2006.

in 1995, the first SFAF was a means to determine which sport organization should receive federal funding in the face of severe budget cuts applied to sport. SFAFIII, the current framework, is the third of its kind and will run until 2010. Through this mechanism and its accompanying contribution guidelines, Sport Canada has a tool that has a great influence on the policies and programs of each organization it provides funding to. There are 17 general eligibility criteria that NSOs must meet to receive federal funding. Some of them relate to the nature and the structure of the NSO itself. For example, it must be the single national governing body for that sport, have a democratically elected volunteer leadership, be athlete-centred, and have an appeal mechanism. But most of the criteria relate to commitments the NSO must have for several Sport Canada policies and programs. For example, the NSO must have adopted the Canadian Policy on Doping in Sport, it must be committed to ethical officiating and coaching education and conduct, and it must have formal policy on bilingualism, access and equity, women, persons with a disability, and Aboriginal people, as well as a policy against harassment and abuse.

Through these criteria, Sport Canada tries to make sure all its policies, programs, and regulations are implemented throughout the sport system. As a result, through its eligibility and contribution guidelines Sport Canada makes sure that all its policies and priorities are followed by the organizations that receive funding. If Sport Canada doesn't intervene directly in the daily life of the MSOs and NSOs, it nevertheless enforces a series of strict rules of conduct.

The Athlete Assistance Program

The second federal major funding program is the Athlete Assistance Program (AAP). Through a carding system, the program identifies and financially supports athletes in the top 16 in the world in their sport or those athletes who have been identified as having the potential to reach that level of performance. The program consists of a monthly living and training allowance and post-secondary tuition support if applicable. The program also helps athletes in post-sport career transition. Roughly speaking, the carding system includes two major categories: the senior cards provide an allowance of $1,500 per month, and the development cards provide an allowance of $900 per month. In 2004–05, 468 athletes had development cards, 736 had senior national cards, and 362 had senior international cards, for a total of 1,566 cards in 75 different sport disciplines. However, the current carding system doesn't match the needs of all high-performance athletes. Athletes CAN, a lobby organization for athletes funded by Sport Canada, argues that more funding is needed and that athletes are still living under the poverty line. This is the case especially of those who haven't yet made it to the international level and those who are unable to access scarce private sponsorship funding.

In the early 1970s, direct financial help to athletes was considered against the dominant vision of amateur sport, but reality made this view increasingly impossible to support. The AAP originated from a previous program put in place in 1973 by the Canadian Olympic Association, now known as the Canadian Olympic Committee (COC), in preparation for the 1976 Montreal Olympic Games and as a result of extensive pressure and demands by Canadian Olympic athletes. After the Montreal Olympics, the initiative was taken over by the government and became the current program (Macintosh et al., 1987). Increased pressure was put on the federal government to put more money into the program, because the cost of living, training, and travelling to international competitions kept growing. Moreover, the low level of support to Canadian athletes contrasted sharply in the 1970s and the 1980s with the state system followed by the Eastern Bloc countries, where athletes trained virtually full time. To compete with the athletes of the Eastern Bloc, most developed countries put in place comprehensive athlete support systems. While the pressures increased for Canadian athletes to perform on the world stage, the AAP funding was virtually frozen at the level of $4–5 million between 1984 and 1994. Most of the 1990s were also considered dark years for athlete financial support, as funding to NSOs and MSOs was cut because the government deficit was increasing. After the Mills report, however, and in preparation for the Vancouver Winter Olympics in 2010, financial support to athletes has recently virtually doubled through the *Own the Podium* initiative (see Table 12.1), although that money is concentrated in selected disciplines.

The needs of Canadian athletes are not limited to the issues of financial support, however. In the early 1980s, an increasing number of abuses of power by coaches and NSOs were documented. A report on athlete rights in Canada argued that basic human rights, like the right to defend oneself in the case of an alleged arbitrary decision, are often not respected. Mechanisms were proposed to correct this situation, but the situation didn't improve enough for athletes (Kidd & Eberts, 1982). Bill C-12 created the Sport Dispute Resolution Centre of Canada (SDRC) in order to provide a non-judicial dispute resolution system to Canadian athletes and sport organizations. As we saw earlier, the SFAFIII required that each NSO and MSO adhere to the dispute resolution centre's structure to get federal funding for athletes to have access to the AAP. It can be said that the SDRC constitutes an improvement for athletes as it provides them with a tool that offers some protection from arbitrary decisions or abuse by their NSO, MSO, or coaches. Also, it has the advantage of being a much quicker decision process than the judicial system. On the other side, the mechanism has the advantage of relieving the federal authorities from the necessity to step up and take a position on most of the controversial files.

The Hosting Program

The third federal major funding program is the Hosting Program, which Sport Canada considers a key instrument in the government's approach to enhancing sport capacity and development. Its purpose is to assist sport organizations or organizing committees in hosting national sport events, such as the Canada Games, or international sport events. It is widely believed in the sport community and government circles that these events produce significant sport, economic, social, and cultural benefits. The program is also seen as a contributor to other government goals, such as promoting Canadian identity, and fostering the international image of Canada and of Canadian cities. The current Hosting International Sport Events Policy of 2000 also places an emphasis on legacies. Indeed, sport organizations and organizing committees must include provisions for the legacies (bursary funds, installations, etc.) in their candidacy submissions in order to qualify for funding. Table 12.1 shows relatively modest budgets dedicated to hosting, considering that both international events and the Olympic Games are included in the amounts. However, it is important to note that hosting major events also often implies significant public investment, notably in infrastructure. For example, the cost of the Sea to Sky Highway between Vancouver and Whistler is, by itself, a huge infrastructure investment that should be included in the expenses section of the Games budget. A growing amount of literature on the outcomes of hosting world-class events demonstrates that benefits are largely overestimated, costs are underestimated, and social benefits are often modest if not negative, as shown in the report evaluation of the 2001 International Amateur Athletics Federation World Championship in Edmonton (Heritage Canada, 2002; see also Chapter 13, Globalization).

Other Policies, Programs, and Regulations

I will now briefly present the other policies, programs, and regulations listed in Figure 12.2. Policy on women in sport dates from 1986 and takes a liberal feminist approach to the issue of women in sport. The policy is mainly a series of objective statements encouraging gender equity in sport, and these objectives are operationalized in the structure of funding programs. For example, as shown earlier one of the SFAFIII criteria requires that NSOs and MSOs have policies demonstrating commitment to equity and access for women. According to the policy, Sport Canada is dedicated to increasing the number of women in power positions within the Canadian sport system, to the provision of equal access to competition and services (e.g., coaching, travel) for women, and to the development of more opportunities for women to participate in sport. Sport Canada is in dialogue with organizations such as the Canadian Association for the Advancement of Women and Sport and Physical Activity (CAAWS), launched in 1981, which gets most of its funding from Sport Canada.

The Canadian Strategy for Ethical Conduct in Sport and the Canadian Policy Against Doping in Sport both originated from the recommendations of the Dubin commission. Indeed, the report documented that the measures put in place by the government of Canada with the Sport Medicine Council of Canada were not sufficient and that the existing anti-doping policy had to be revised. Justice Dubin was not in favour of direct state intervention in the daily administration of sport organizations, and thus he suggested that a state-funded independent organization be put in place to implement a new and improved anti-doping policy. Currently, the organization in charge of implementing the policy, including anti-drug testing, is the Canadian Centre for Ethics in Sport (CCES)—born from the merger between the Canadian Centre for Drug-free Sport and Fair Play Canada.

The CCES is responsible for a range of issues including fair play, drug-free sport, equity, safety, and non-violence in Canadian sport. Again, ethical conduct and anti-doping are among the general criteria of SFAFIII. Canada is not the only country dealing with doping problems—the issue is a global one. In 1999, after doping scandals in cycling, the IOC decided to convene a conference in Lausanne, Switzerland. An outcome of the conference was to recommend the creation of WADA as an independent international organization dedicated to anti-doping and equally funded by the IOC and nation-states. Housed in Lausanne, WADA moved its headquarters to Montreal in 2002 after the Canadian government lobbied to house the organization. This was seen as an opportunity for Canada to make its presence known in international sport and to foster its views on international anti-doping policies. In 2004, WADA adopted the World Anti-Doping Code.

In addition to gender equity and doping initiatives, another important hurdle facing the Canadian sport system rests in the area of language, specifically the lack of bilingualism. Although French and English have been recognized as Canada's two official languages for decades, sport organizations continue to blame their inability to provide adequate bilingual services to their members as a function of limited financial resources for translation and to their status as independent, not-for profit organizations that should not be subjected to federal government legislation. Counterarguments to these claims point out that these national organizations have to adhere to the constitution of the country if they wish to be recognized as *the* national organization in their sport. Besides, these organizations receive an increasingly important amount of public funding provided by taxpayers from both linguistic communities. Over the years, numerous complaints have been filed, mostly by French-speaking athletes, about the lack of bilingual services—for example, unilingual coaching services, the forced relocation of national-team athletes to where bilingual schooling is not available, and perceived linguistic discrimination. In 2000, the office of the Commissioner of Official Languages published a document called *The Official Languages in the Canadian Sports System,* describing these incidents and outlining the intense debates that arose over language politics in Canadian sport. Given the lack of action from the government, a follow-up report was issued by the Commissioner in 2003. Now, as has been discussed, a bilingual strategy for NSOs and MSOs is a criterion of the SFAFIII.

CONCLUSIONS

Sport, especially at the international level, has a highly metaphoric power of identification for countries and therefore can serve very important political goals. High-performance sport, as well as grassroots sport, involves the distribution of collective resources and thus implicates the state. In this chapter, I have tried to demonstrate that sport and politics are not mutually exclusive and that sport policy is a complex and important area of contemporary sport. Through an overview of some current policies and programs, I have intended to show the complexity of the federal government's intervention in sport. I have underlined how private organizations like NSOs and MSOs interact with the state in the governance of Canada's sport system. At this point I wish to underline that even if federal government funding to sport organizations is increasingly contingent, NSOs and MSOs are nevertheless organizations that still have a great deal of autonomy and often resist Sport Canada policies. My overview has also demonstrated how, since Bill C-131, the federal government has concentrated its action into high-performance sport mainly for the promotion of Canada's national unity and social cohesion. Discrimination and inequalities are still thriving in Canada's sport system in terms of class, gender, race, ethnicity, and language. Only through action by citizens and by organized pressure groups will the politics of sport improve in Canada. What issues will governments face in the future? Increasing amounts of public funding will continue to be requested by sport system participants as long as the quest for Olympic medals and World Cup titles remains at the centre of state preoccupations. On the other hand, the so-called obesity crisis, the aging population, and inequalities of access to sport participation opportunities call for more state intervention in order to tackle these issues. Indeed, the problem is not whether the state should intervene in sport, but rather what public policies should be adopted for the benefit of all Canadians.

CRITICAL THINKING QUESTIONS

1. What are the main reasons why governments increasingly intervene in sport? Should that course be continued or reversed? If so, how?
2. Should the federal government continue to put the emphasis on high performance or switch to improve sport participation for all?
3. What has to be done to improve current sport policies in Canada?
4. Can national sport organizations survive without state funding?
5. Should Canada play an active role on the international sport scene? If so, what should that role be?
6. Since an increasing number of athletes and sport organization are now sponsored by private corporations, should the government reduce its funding?

SUGGESTED READINGS

Macintosh, D., & Whitson, D. (1990). *The game planners*. Montreal: McGill–Queen's University Press.

Macintosh, D., Bedecki, T., & Franks, C. E. S. (1987). *Sport and politics in Canada*. Montreal: McGill–Queen's University Press.

Zirin, D. (2005). *What's my name, fool? Sports and resistance in the United States*. Chicago: Haymarket Books.

WEB LINKS

Sport Canada
http://www.pch.gc.ca/sportcanada/
Information on Canada's sport policies and programs.

International Olympic Committee
http://www.olympic.org/
Detailed and constantly updated information on the Olympics.

Physical Activity Unit
http://www.phac-aspc.gc.ca/pau-uap/fitness/about.html
Detailed information on the Canadian Public Health Agency's policies and programs.

CHAPTER 13

GLOBALIZATION

David Whitson

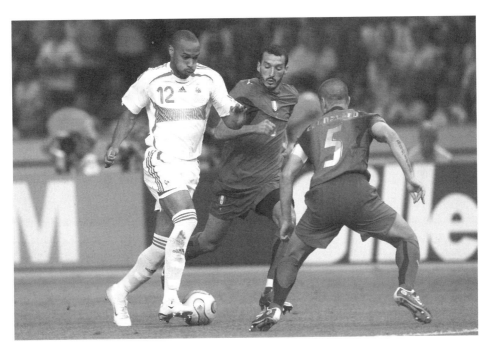

The 2006 World Cup of Soccer was a truly global event, with 32 nations qualifying.

© Stephane Reix/For Picture/Corbis

Yes, OK, soccer is the most "popular" game in the world. And rice is the most "popular" food in the world. So what? Maybe other countries can't afford football, basketball, and baseball leagues: maybe if they could afford these other sports, they'd enjoy them even more.
Alan Barra, *Wall Street Journal* (cited in F. Foer, *How Soccer Explains the World*, p. 243)

It felt like another day in the era of globalization. The economy keeps expanding heartily and people's lives keep getting harder.
Rick Salutin, *The Globe and Mail*, April 21, 2006

In 2004, Franklin Foer, a political journalist for the American magazine *The New Republic*, published a book called *How Soccer Explains the World: An {Unlikely} Theory of Globalization*. In a series of provocative and entertaining essays, Foer explores topics as diverse as soccer clubs' historical connections with political and regional rivalries in Spain and the former Yugoslavia; the wealth and commercial ambition that are creating new rivalries today and diminishing the meaning of traditional ones; the flood of players from Latin America and Africa to European clubs while domestic leagues in their own countries struggle to survive; and the antipathy toward the game held by some influential American sports journalists, notably ESPN radio host Jim Rome. Foer cites *New York Times* columnist Thomas Friedman (1999), who has written widely of globalization as a force both inevitable and beneficent, enabling unprecedented standards of living for both nations and individuals. But Foer goes on to question some of this breathless enthusiasm for the "new world order." He argues that, in soccer at least, even though there is more money at the top, the promised prosperity has never materialized for a great many players and clubs. On the contrary, in fact, the gap between the rich and the poor has widened into a chasm in soccer just as it has in the world itself for many individuals and nations.

I introduce my own discussion of globalization with this brief overview of Foer's book because I believe that soccer offers some extraordinarily good illustrations of globalization in sport, and in the sports business.[1] As I was writing this chapter, in the spring of 2006, I had the pleasure of viewing several big matches from the 2006 European Champions League competition on satellite TV. The Edmonton sports bar that screened the matches was packed with expatriates from England, Italy, and Latin America, but also with Canadians like myself who had not grown up with the game. I couldn't help but be struck by how satellite television has expanded the sporting horizons and interests of Canadians, and indeed the Canadian media. Canadian sportscasts and sports pages now regularly report major European soccer results, whereas 30 years ago it was rare to find even the NBA covered in the Canadian media.

Having noted this small example of globalization, though, I want to add immediately that the excitement of a small core of soccer fans in Edmonton was nothing in comparison with the passion that gripped the city as the Oilers progressed through the 2006 Stanley Cup playoffs, upsetting Detroit, San Jose, and Anaheim before losing the final to Carolina in seven games. Indeed, for a brief few days in late April, when it seemed as if Edmonton and Calgary might renew the "Battle of Alberta" and Ottawa and Montreal might also meet in the second round, one couldn't help being reminded that hockey arouses Canada's sporting passions like no other sport, and that there is no other country where hockey takes over public attention like it does in Canada. There are limits to globalization, in other words, and even though there are many Canadians who welcome opportunities to follow other sports, there are others (almost certainly more) for whom it is our traditional sport, hockey, and our own regional rivalries that still matter most.

GLOBALIZATION: A CONCEPTUAL OVERVIEW

The literature on globalization has grown substantially in recent years, even within the sociology of sport (see, for example, Harvey et al., 1996, and Rowe et al., 1994). In fact, there has been an active debate in sport sociology about whether some of the developments often associated with the term "globalization" are better understood as modernization, or as the Americanization of sport in other countries (Donnelly, 1996). Other, more specific discussions about global phenomena—about, for example, the growth of the Olympics as a television spectacle, the global appeal of Michael Jordan (Andrews, 2001), or the global manufacturing activities of Nike (Sage, 2004)—not surprisingly reflect the theoretical assumptions and research interests of their authors (see Chapter 2 for an overview of some of the most influential theoretical perspectives in sport sociology). For our purposes here, though, we will define globalization simply as a process or combination of processes through which the world is becoming a more integrated place (Robertson, 1992). As investments and goods, ideas and news, and even people (with some important qualifications) flow across international boundaries in unprecedented ways, the world is becoming one in which more people are aware of events in distant places (including sports events) and more people are affected by decisions taken in distant places—by transnational corporations or by international bodies like the World Trade Organization (WTO)—than was true for earlier generations.[2]

If our starting point, then, involves thinking about globalization as a combination of processes, it is also helpful to think of economic processes, political processes, and cultural processes—as well as the relationships among them (Short & Kim, 1999). It is beyond the scope of this chapter to explore these in detail; however, some illustrations will hopefully encourage readers to think of examples in their own lives. In the economic realm, the most basic idea to grasp is that money (especially investment capital) and products (whether raw materials, manufactured goods, or services) now move around the world more quickly and easily than ever before. In the case of money, we now have global financial markets and a host of new financial products (like mutual funds) that facilitate investment in other parts of the world. In addition, the concerted effort over the last quarter-century to promote "freer" global trade has meant that companies can try to promote their products in other countries (whether hard goods like cars or shoes, or "soft goods" like films, sports television, or advertising), without the tariffs or other barriers that once protected domestic products. This has led to opportunities for ambitious companies to establish themselves as global brand names, while other (typically locally based) companies have failed because of new competition. It has also led to corporate mergers and takeovers, and the phenomenon of transnational corporations (like Nike, News Corp., and Toyota) doing business in many countries at once. None of this is unprecedented. International trade and corporate empires both date way back to the days of

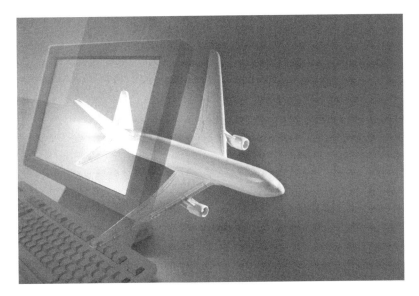

Communications technologies make the world a smaller place.
© Comstock/SuperStock

colonies and The Hudson's Bay Company. However, computer technology has facilitated both the rapid movement of money and the management of far-flung empires, and the post-1980 period represents a new phase in the economic pressures that encourage globalization (e.g., competition, and the drive for growth).

Shifting our attention to the political processes that are part of globalization, the most obvious might be the growth in importance of transnational bodies like the WTO and the International Monetary Fund (IMF), as well as regional institutions like the European Union (EU) and NAFTA (North American Free Trade Agreement). However, we should also recognize that much of the economic integration discussed in the previous paragraph was facilitated by the withdrawal of governments from economic functions that used to be considered essential to national autonomy. Many governments, for example, have privatized what were once publicly owned national airlines (like Air Canada) and other public utilities (electricity, and sometimes water). In addition, although it may be hard for those born since 1980 to appreciate this, Canada (and other governments) once strictly regulated foreign investment in key sectors of the economy, instead of welcoming it. Canada also routinely employed industrial policies including tariffs, tax incentives and grants for Canadian companies, and "buy local" government procurement policies, all intended to encourage the growth of home-based industries. In the trade agreements of the 1980s and 1990s, though, national governments signed away much of their power to "manage" their economies in return for freer access for their companies to foreign capital and foreign markets.

This was consistent with the neo-liberal ideology shared by many governments in those years, which believes in the efficiency of markets and believes that the private sector can provide services more efficiently than can governments. Critics of neo-liberalism contend that privatization and de-regulation amount to abandoning the idea of a national economy, in the hope that Canadians will be "winners" in the global economy. What is widely agreed is that these new limits on what governments can do have altered relationships between governments and investors so that governments at all levels (city and regional governments, as well as national ones) now find themselves chasing after highly mobile investment capital. We have seen this phenomenon in sports in the efforts of cities to attract or keep professional sports franchises.

In the cultural sphere, most of us—at least in the Western world—are experiencing new kinds of transnational connectedness (Hannerz, 1996). Satellite television makes possible the global broadcasting of news and sports events, while the Internet and cheaper travel enable us to connect with like-minded persons in most parts of the world, for purposes that vary from music to politics to sex. In these circumstances, national cultures (or cultural practices once associated with particular countries, like cuisine, or sports) can no longer be associated quite so closely with their places of origin. Rather, they are carried to many places as people move around the world, taking their cultural interests and skills with them. For example, C. L. R. James (1963) and Eduardo Galeano (1998) have described how European colonizers took the games of cricket and soccer to the West Indies and Latin America, respectively, and how these sports developed new styles of play, and sometimes new social meanings, in these "New World" societies.[3] Conversely, some recent migrants to Canada from societies where sport is not a part of childhood or where sport is not encouraged among women have feared the "Westernizing" influences of Canadian sports, and worried that sports were taking their children away from the values and role models preferred in their own cultures (see Chapter 5).

At another level, as some cultural practices have been turned into entertainment products—professional sports, music, and film are the clearest instances—they have become big businesses, marketed around the globe (Butsch, 1990). American popular culture offers the most familiar examples of the marketing of cultural products, and often provokes criticism of

American cultural "hegemony" (see Chapter 2). Yet it is simplistic to assume that American culture is spreading inexorably around the globe (Lull, 2000). Consider, for example, the global popularity of Italian and Chinese food, and the newer fashions for world music and ethnic clothing, much of each originating in French-speaking Africa or Latin America. Consider, also, the ways in which cities like London or Paris are no longer English or French so much as "world cities," encompassing large communities from parts of Asia, Africa, and other parts of Europe. Consider, finally, the global passion for "association football" (or soccer) everywhere outside North America, despite American indifference to the game and despite attempts to promote American football. Hannerz thus invites us to see cultural globalization as a multi-polar process in which some regions and countries participate more actively than others, and in different ways.

Each of these processes through which traditional links between culture and place are loosened—the transportation of cultures that follows from migration, and the promotion of new cultural "products" in the electronic media—are leading to unprecedented cultural heterogeneity in some places, and beyond this, to cultural hybridity, which Hannerz defines as the production of *new culture*, when peoples and cultures blend together to produce new and original syntheses. Again, it's important to recognize that the effects of cultural globalization are not equally felt everywhere. It is the affluent countries of the global "North"—particularly Western Europe and North America—that are being transformed most visibly by immigration, and these same affluent countries where more homes have personal computers and satellite television. Even within Canada, though, evidence of cultural heterogeneity is all around us in cities like Toronto and Vancouver, but less present in small towns and rural regions that are getting older, poorer, and whiter. Thus, one visitor to Canada has remarked that while Vancouver and Toronto are among the most multicultural cities in the world, "villages only forty-five minutes away [seemed] undisturbed in their white-bread, Protestant, nineteenth century pasts" (Iyer, 2000, p. 124). Others, meanwhile, express concern that an urban/rural divide is developing in Canada that has racial and cultural overtones. In parts of the prairie provinces, in northern B.C. and in northwestern Ontario, and in northern Quebec and parts of Atlantic Canada, rural populations that include fast-growing Aboriginal communities as well as aging settler communities (farm communities, logging communities, fishing communities)—neither of which can offer a promising future to their young—are becoming culturally and politically detached from the multicultural cities that will be the engines of economic growth (see Epp & Whitson, 2001).

What's important to emphasize here is that the processes of globalization, whether cultural or economic, are characterized by "uneven development." At one level, this refers simply to the uneven spatial distribution of the effects of globalization. Some countries and, especially, cities (London, for example, and Los Angeles) become financial and cultural centres through which money and ideas flow: centres where capital is concentrated and cultural products are produced, and where value is added to everything (not least property) as a result of lucrative "new economy" activities (Short & Kim, 1999). Other countries, meanwhile, and even whole regions (much of sub-Saharan Africa, Hannerz suggests) remain largely untouched, except insofar as they are impoverished by a steady outflow of natural resources and people. In addition, the stark contrasts associated with uneven development also invite us to see globalization as a set of processes that produces winners and losers, and increases socioeconomic polarization not only between societies, but also within them. Most evidence would suggest that the affluent countries of the "North" have been net beneficiaries of globalization, as are many societies in Asia where urban standards of living are increasing rapidly. Nonetheless, both Asia and North America have significant areas of rural poverty alongside their booming cities, while North Americans even in urban areas are all too familiar with the phenomenon of the "jobless recovery," in which more wealth is produced without producing more jobs.

Such increases in both wealth *and* poverty invite critics to ask who benefits (and who benefits most) from globalization, and whether more cannot be done to mitigate some of its harmful effects. Economic globalization has produced huge profits for corporations that operate successfully on a global scale (whether in mining, or televised entertainment), and this translates into well-paying jobs for most of their employees. It has also increased the market for "producer services" (accounting and other financial services, management consultants, and various kinds of technical/scientific and advertising/marketing expertise), all providing employment for a growing cadre of educated, "knowledge economy" workers, with good salaries and high standards of living (Short & Kim, 1999). Yet political integration has proceeded much more haltingly than economic integration, in the NAFTA countries as well as the European Union, and while companies can move production across borders very easily, barriers to the movement of workers and their families still remain. The debate in the United States Congress in 2006 about policing along the Mexican border illustrates clearly that migrants from poor countries who try to reach countries where there are better employment prospects (whether in America or in Europe) still face legal and political obstacles, and often grave physical dangers as well.

I cannot do justice here to what are large and ongoing debates, and I refer readers to some of the questions concerning social conflict, power, and ideology that are raised in Chapters 2 and 4. However, I want to leave readers with two ideas to consider during our subsequent discussions of globalization in sport. The first is simply that it's important to understand both the upsides and downsides of globalization, to think about who are the winners and losers and why there are people who fiercely oppose it as well as enthusiastic advocates. The second, directly related, idea is that some of the processes of globalization (like "free trade," for example) result from political decisions, and therefore their consequences are legitimately matters for political debate. Some of globalization's advocates present it as an inevitable process, a historical trend that is inexorable and therefore beyond political control (see Friedman, 1999). However, although there are new technologies that raise standards of living and that most people in most societies will want to incorporate into their lives (the Internet, television, and safe drinking water), governments can still make decisions about how we access these services and how much the public can be expected to pay. They can also monitor the results, and hold corporate service providers accountable. These are legitimate matters of public policy, therefore, and we should not treat as inevitable any "trend" that has controversial social consequences.

GLOBALIZATION AND SPORT

Conceptualizing globalization as a complex and contested process, with economic, cultural, and political dimensions, lays a foundation for exploring some of the changes we have seen in sport over the last quarter century. Some of the more significant of these changes might include the expansion of the NBA into Canada and the NHL into the southern United States; the staging of soccer's World Cup in America in 1994 and in Asia in 2002; the growth of the Olympics into a global event and a massive commercial spectacle; and the migration of professional athletes from poorer countries to those where the highest salaries are paid, a phenomenon we can see just as clearly in the NHL as we can in European soccer. This list does not pretend to be exhaustive; however, what is common to all of these examples, I suggest, is a search for new audiences, new markets, new jobs—in short, for opportunities to make more money from sport. This is the economic dimension, very clearly. What should become clearer, though, as we proceed, is that cultural changes follow directly from these economic ambitions.

In the first two examples offered above, the pattern is clearly that the organizations and financial interests that manage each sport as a business[4] were seeking to expand the markets for their products by promoting these sports in places where they were not historically part of the local popular culture. The NHL, the NBA, and FIFA (the Fédération Internationale de Football Association) each saw opportunities to dramatically "grow" their respective games, developing potentially lucrative new markets for merchandise and television packages, in addition to live audiences. For this potential to be realized, though, required that NHL hockey, for example, be actively promoted in the southern United States. The same was true for NBA basketball in Canada, and for soccer in both the United States and Asia. Readers can debate how well these economic ambitions have been fulfilled (all three, arguably, remain works in progress). My point here, though, is simply that for new sports to become popular on an enduring basis requires cultural changes in the places where sports entrepreneurs hope to promote new leisure choices. People have to get interested in these new activities, and if they do, this means less time and less money for the games they enjoyed before. The new cultural choices associated with globalization compete directly, in other words, for people's time and attention—and money—with entertainment forms and spending habits that are traditional to those places.

The last two examples highlight slightly different dynamics. In the Olympic example, we have an organization—the International Olympic Committee (IOC)—that is not commercial in quite the same sense as the NBA or FIFA. Neither do the Olympics, as a quadrennial event, effect lasting changes in the sporting cultures of nations. However, anyone with any interest in the subject will know that the Olympic Games have become a global television extravaganza, that corporations are willing to pay higher and higher sums to be associated with the Olympics as advertisers and sponsors, and that the IOC, under the leadership of Juan Antonio Samaranch and Richard Pound, put a strategic priority on promoting the value of the Olympic "brand" (Barney et al., 2002). Among the reasons for the global appeal of the Olympics are that they provide a stage for many small countries that cannot support the "major leagues," and for athletes (especially women) who don't otherwise get the media exposure enjoyed by the major professional sports. The Olympic movement promotes values—internationalism, inclusiveness, excellence—that many people admire and want to be part of. The Olympic Games are a unique institution, in other words, and have a history of promoting sport around the world.

The final phenomenon flagged above, the increasingly global movement of professional athletes, will be the subject of a more extended discussion in a moment. For now, though, a striking example will suffice. Foer estimates that there are now more than 5,000 Brazilian soccer players plying their trade in other countries. Of the 22 players who represented Brazil in the 2002 World Cup, only seven still played their club soccer in Brazil.[5] This exodus of Brazilian soccer players is, he suggests, "one of the great migrations of talent in recent history, the sports equivalent of the post-Soviet brain drain" (2004, p. 131). Most would agree that these Brazilian migrants have improved the standard of play—and the entertainment value—of the foreign leagues they now play in, and the economic advantage for the individual players is obvious: higher salaries than they could hope for at home, in a country whose largely poor population cannot support the richer economy of professional sport that exists in Europe, in Japan, and in America. However, an exodus of talent on this scale has had predictable effects on the domestic game. Brazilian fans seldom get to see their top players, and the quality of Brazilian league play has suffered. For Uruguayan writer Eduardo Galeano, this exodus of good players from Brazil, Argentina, and Uruguay has led to "mediocre professional leagues (at home), and ever fewer, ever less fervent fans. People desert the stadiums to watch foreign matches on television" (1998, p. 206). It is thus not unusual now, Foer notes, for a Brazilian league match in Rio de Janeiro's famous Maracanã stadium (capacity more than 100,000) to have only a few thousand spectators.

There are many interesting examples and comparisons one could pursue—far too many to proceed in this fashion. In an effort to distill the arguments, the discussion that follows will focus on three aspects of globalization in sport, involving phenomena that can be observed in a number of sports and in many different countries. First, we will proceed with our discussion of player migration, and the globalization of the labour market in professional sports. From there, the argument will move to an examination of globalization in the sports business, including the growth of transnational ownership and investment, the search for global television audiences, and the experience of several sports with global marketing strategies. The final subsection will focus on fans, and examine the effects of the first two changes on the ways that fans relate to teams, to players, and to sports themselves. The chapter will conclude with some observations on the extent to which sports interests have been successful in constructing the "global consumer," and enquire into the cultural implications of changes in the sports business. Returning to questions raised in our conceptual overview of globalization, we will also enquire into who wins and loses as a consequence of the increasing global integration that we find in many sports.

Professionalization and Globalization in the Sports Labour Market

We've noted above the diaspora of Brazilian footballers now playing in better-paying leagues in Europe, and this is also true for Argentina and, to a lesser extent, other Latin American nations (e.g., Mexico, Paraguay, Peru). The rich leagues of Western Europe—Spain, England, Italy, and to a lesser extent, Germany, France, Portugal, and the Netherlands—now include substantial numbers of Latin American players, as well as players from Africa and from former East Bloc countries, where player salaries also remain low. Indeed, the labour market for soccer players has now become so transnational that in the 2006 Champions League final, the English representative, Arsenal, fielded only two English players. Their starting lineup included players from France, Spain, Sweden, Germany, Belarus, and Ivory Coast. Their opponents, FC Barcelona, fielded a lineup that featured a majority of Spaniards; however, it also included star players from Brazil, Cameroon, and Mexico.

In the North American major league sports, similar trends can be observed over the last quarter century. Canadian readers will be aware that NHL teams began to employ European players in the 1970s, initially as a response to the World Hockey Association (WHA) and the competition for elite players that the new league introduced. Before 1990, though, the numbers were still fairly small, and most came from Sweden and Finland—players like Börje Salming, Mats Näslund, Jari Kurri, and Esa Tikkanen. Refugees from the state-supported hockey systems of Eastern Europe like Fetisov (from Russia) and the Stastny brothers (from Czechoslovakia) were exceptions to this pattern. With the collapse of the Soviet Union, though, and turmoil in Czechoslovakia, many players from Russia and the Czech and Slovak Republics sought their fortunes in North America, and now many NHL lineups include players from a variety of European nations, as well as increasing numbers of Americans. The NBA is less international than the NHL, remaining overwhelmingly American. However, there are now small numbers of NBA players from Croatia and Serbia, from Lithuania, from Spain and Argentina, and from China (as well as Canada and Australia). Major League Baseball has had increasing numbers of players from a small core of Latin American countries, as well as Japan, for a number of years.[6]

If a global labour market is the new "normal" in the major team sports, though, why should this be an issue? To understand how globalization departs from established practices, and alters some of the meanings traditionally associated with intercommunity competition, requires looking back almost a hundred years to the early days of "representative" sports. Alan Ingham has noted in an influential essay that sporting contests have provided dramatic representations of "us" and "them," and that the historical popularity of team sports derives from their capacity to dramatize communal identities and rivalries (Ingham et al., 1988, p. 437). In the early days of spectator sports, indeed, cheering for the home team meant cheering for teams comprised of local talent, and this gave credibility to popular beliefs that sporting success reflected favourably on the community that had produced them.[7] However, as hiring a few "travelling players" to bolster the local side, and then hiring whole squads of professional players became standard practice, the relationships between teams and the communities they represented began to take on a different character, which Ingham et al. depict as more akin to a merchant–customer relationship. Fan support is solicited for the best representation that local owners can provide. Now, though, team success no longer reflects the quality of local players, let alone the characteristics of local people. Instead, it reflects the wealth of the owners and—crucially, today—the wealth of a city's economy and its capacity to yield the revenues that support competitive salaries (Whitson, 2001).

For the greater part of the twentieth century, then, professionalism was the norm in North American major league sports. However, although this meant that those playing for a city have very seldom been raised in that city (in 2006, Fernando Pisani was the only one of the Edmonton Oilers to have been raised in Edmonton), several factors continued to encourage fans to identify with players and to see them as representatives of their communities. To begin with, until recent decades, restrictive player contracts bound professional athletes to the teams they began their careers with, unless those teams chose to trade them or cut them. Team rosters, in these circumstances, were more stable than they are today, and fans learned to identify with players who represented the city for many years and often had made their homes there. However, baseball's "reserve clause" was overturned by the United States courts in 1976, and ever since then player unions in all the major leagues have negotiated steadily lower barriers to free agency (see Weiler, 2000). Predictably, this has led to steadily increased player mobility.

The history of globalization in the soccer labour market, not surprisingly, is different. The most obvious difference, perhaps, is that instead of one major league in each sport, as has been the case in North America (except in those brief periods when "rival" leagues have attempted to compete), there has been serious financial competition among teams based in Spain, England, and Italy to sign elite players from each other and from anywhere else in the world. The other obvious difference is that, with soccer played on a much more global basis than any of the North American games, the talent pool is more genuinely global, with many good players now coming from Africa and, especially, Latin America. However, a third important difference is that even though player associations have pushed over the years to ease restrictions on player mobility, they have been historically weaker than their North American counterparts, with the result that major change did not come until 1995 (much later than in North America), following a ruling by the European Court of Justice (ECJ). The Court ruled in favour of a minor-league Belgian player named Jean-Marc Bosman, saying that rules which the major European soccer leagues had enforced that had limited teams to three foreign-born players contravened the rights of players who were EU citizens to pursue their trade in any EU country (Ammirante, 2006). This opened the door for ambitious English teams, for example, to scout and sign players from France and Portugal, leading to the overwhelmingly foreign Arsenal and Chelsea sides that represented London in the 2006 Champions League competition. It has also encouraged players from French- and English-speaking Africa, and from Brazil and Argentina (many of whom have Spanish or Italian ancestry), to seek resident status in these European Union countries.

Increased player mobility has thus led to important changes in professional sports, in both North America and Europe. On the positive side, it has led to markedly higher player salaries (though some might argue that the stars, at least, now make too much money), and it has radically altered the relationships between players and teams, undermining the absolute control that managers used to have over a player's career. It has enabled fans, at least in those countries where the top leagues play, to regularly see the world's best players, and to enjoy the skills of Brazilian soccer players or Czech hockey players on a regular basis. It also speaks to ideas of human rights that wonderful players from small countries, players like Jaromir Jagr and Samuel Eto'o (the Cameroon-born star who now plays for Spanish soccer champions FC Barcelona), are able to earn salaries commensurate with their abilities.[8]

On the negative side, however, we've noted that this same phenomenon has reduced the Brazilian and Argentine soccer leagues to the status of minor leagues, staffed mostly by hopefuls and has-beens, with a corresponding decline in fan interest. The same observation could fairly be made of Czech and Russian hockey in the last decade or so (Cantelon, 2006). In the top leagues, increased player mobility has produced a situation in which good players often switch teams at the end of each contract, and players rarely stay with the same team for their entire career. This new pattern has meant a re-shaping of relationships among players, teams, and the communities they are supposed to "represent." It may also be changing the meanings of fan allegiances and loyalties, in ways we shall explore shortly.

Before leaving the phenomenon of increased player mobility behind, though, we need to reflect on the fact that globalization in the sports labour market is so far mostly a one-way street, with players from poorer countries, or at least countries where the structure of professional sport does not support "major league" salaries, migrating to those countries where the salaries are highest. There is, as yet, very little traffic in the other direction. There have always, to be sure, been small numbers of North American university hockey players and basketball players (many of them "too small" by NHL and NBA standards) who have gone on to play in Europe. However, the European leagues in these sports do not generate either the arena revenues or the television revenues (see below) that would enable them to pay North American–style salaries, even in those Western European countries that support major league salaries in soccer. A further barrier to the movement of Canadian and American athletes to Europe, moreover, has been the unwillingness of many unilingual North Americans to make the sorts of cultural adjustments (including mastery of another language) that we routinely expect of European or Hispanic players coming here. Both of these issues were highlighted in the recent NHL lockout, when some NHL athletes started to play in Europe but came home early, complaining of poor conditions or simply the "foreign-ness" of the living environment (Cantelon, 2006).

Finally, here, I want to challenge one of the arguments sometimes made by advocates of globalization, namely that the increased presence of players from other lands in our midst and the increased visibility of heroes of "other" races will lead inexorably to increased tolerance, and ultimately the disappearance of racism. Even though there are bits of evidence that appear to support this thesis—the increasing number of Black players in professional sports in both Europe and North America, and France's celebration of its victorious team in the 1998 World Cup (a team made up predominantly of Black players from France's former colonies)—the larger picture is discouraging. Riots in French cities in early 2006 revealed how short-lived this goodwill was, and how deeply ingrained in French society are anti-Black and anti-Arab attitudes. In addition, soccer matches in Spain, Italy, England, and the Ukraine have been marred by ugly episodes of racist chanting by fans (see Foer, 2004, pp. 38, 154). In North America, the presence of Black stars in professional sports is of longer standing and hence more familiar. However, the NHL (and the major junior Ontario Hockey League) has had racist incidents in very recent years (Pitter, 2006). There is also a constituency in Canadian hockey that has regularly given European players (Swedes and Russians, in particular) a rough reception, sometimes on the grounds that "foreigners" are taking Canadian jobs. My point here is simply that although racism and xenophobia cannot be blamed on globalization (they clearly predate globalization by many centuries), increased player migration has led to some ugly reactions. Globalization, therefore, has not led to the tolerance that some predicted, and "global culture" is not—or not yet, at any rate—a culture in which people of all colours are readily accepted for their accomplishments.

Corporate Strategies: The Promotion of Sports "Product"

Turning from player mobility to owners, and the increasingly global horizons of professional sports entrepreneurs, we can see even greater changes in the business of sport over a period of about 40 years. The first change to note is in the kinds of people who are owners. The traditional team owner was typically a rich local businessman, for whom sports ownership was part of being a prominent local citizen, or simply a prestigious hobby. From about the 1980s on, though, it became more common to find sports teams owned by corporations, or by major investors from outside the community.[9] The underlying factor here is that sports came to be viewed as an investment that could potentially pay off in a big way. Instead of a business in which the revenues came primarily from gate receipts—and indeed from cheap seats (or, in many European soccer stadiums before the 1980s, from standing room admissions)—leagues in all sports began to follow a business model pioneered in the NFL and the NBA, in which new "revenue streams" were actively developed. Luxury boxes, more expensive food, and new forms of electronic advertising all increased the revenues available within the stadium (or arena) itself. Of even greater potential value, though, were the revenues to be gained outside the venue: from the promotion of licensed merchandise, from the sale of television products among the much larger audiences who don't often attend live games, and from the capital gains that could be realized from increases in the values of franchises or shares (Horne, 2006; Whitson, 2001).

In the case of merchandise, of course, sports clubs have sold jerseys and other clothing bearing team insignia and colours for many years. However, most such sales were to faithful fans, and sales were mostly limited to the city or region where the team was based. The market, in other words, was local. There were a few exceptional teams that developed national followings: the New York Yankees and the Montreal Canadiens, for example. However, even for these, merchandise sales were a relatively small factor in team incomes. In the 1980s, though, the NBA and the NFL demonstrated that merchandise could be promoted in a much more systematic manner, and with the celebrity drawing power of Michael Jordan, Chicago Bulls gear was sold around the world, much of it to people who had never seen Jordan play. In Europe, major soccer clubs like Manchester United and Real Madrid have moved even more aggressively into the marketing of merchandise, promoting sales not only in their home countries but in the Americas and Asia, too. Real Madrid is alleged to have signed English midfielder David Beckham as much to promote merchandise sales in the Asian market as for his abilities on the field, while both Madrid and Manchester United (Beckham's former club) now regularly report higher earnings from merchandising and sponsorship than they do from gate receipts (Ammirante, 2006). In both Europe and America, teams that once attracted national followings due to their histories of success (the Dallas Cowboys and the Los Angeles Lakers would be additional examples) now seek to establish themselves as globally recognized "brands" (Horne, 2006).

It is television, of course, that has made such commercial ambitions feasible. Satellite television has created the prospect of worldwide audiences for the most prestigious leagues (the English Premier League and Italy's Serie A in soccer, and NBA basketball), as well as for events like the Masters in golf and Wimbledon in tennis. It is satellite television, likewise, that has made possible worldwide audiences for the Olympics and the FIFA World Cup, audiences that attract rights fees now valued at more than a billion dollars. Television took these events into homes around the world, creating a version of "global culture" in which people around the world now follow the same global entertainment events, and talk and care about the fates of the same global celebrities. Television also multiplied the value of any advertising that is visible to its cameras (on team jerseys, as well as around the playing surface), thus greatly expanding the potential income from advertising and sponsorships (Bellamy, 1998; see also Chapter 10).

However, if satellite-fed broadcast television had dramatically expanded the revenues available to sports in the 1960s, both in North America and Europe, the real bonanza would not come until the late 1980s, with the arrival of pay television as a commercial reality. The introduction of successive forms of pay television—cable and satellite subscriptions, and later pay-per-view—together with the channel capacity that these technologies provide, opened up a succession of new possibilities in the sale of televised sports entertainment. These include the now familiar sports networks (TSN, ESPN, SkySports in Europe), as well as more specialized channels devoted to particular sports (golf, fishing) and even particular teams (Real Madrid, for example, and the Toronto Maple Leafs). This growth of *narrow-casting,* or special-interest channels aimed at niche markets—other examples would be channels devoted to religious programming, or to mysteries—created demand for more sports programming than the broadcast networks had ever shown and opportunities for new kinds of sports "product," notably pay-per-view channels (Bellamy, 1998). In Europe and Australia, moreover, where cable and satellite did not become established until the 1990s, having exclusive rights to televise the most popular sports (soccer in Europe, and rugby league in Australia) also proved an effective vehicle for selling millions of satellite subscriptions and dishes (Williams, 1994). This all led to increases in the rights fees available to the most popular sports, and it illustrates the extent to which sport has become incorporated into "circuits of promotion," in a culture where the value of any event to advertisers can be calibrated according to its capacity to promote the major products and personalities associated with it (Whitson, 1998).

It has also led the major sports, and the television interests now intimately connected with them, to actively seek global audiences. In both Europe and America, the home audiences for the major sports leagues—the English and Italian soccer leagues, the NBA, the NFL—had reached saturation points, or something very close to this. Thus, if further growth was to take place, the greatest potential clearly lay abroad, through the sale of television packages in markets that had not previously followed the English Premier League (EPL) or the NBA, for example, in any numbers. This is why EPL matches are now available on Canadian (and Japanese) television throughout the season. Another innovation has seen the creation of new competitions (the Champions League soccer competition, for example, or the World Cup of Rugby) that are aimed specifically at international television audiences, as well as the traditional territories for these sports. Indeed, televised sport has demonstrated that, with rare exceptions, the appeal of sport crosses international boundaries more reliably than do other forms of popular entertainment—like drama or comedy—that rely more heavily on language skills and culturally specific knowledge. The Internet is also a source of up-to-the-minute sports information.

At the same time, the optimism of some expansion-minded enthusiasts that, with the right marketing, any sport could be sold anywhere has to be viewed with some skepticism. Despite the very real successes of soccer's biggest clubs in promoting themselves in Asia, the world's most popular game has made only small inroads in the United States. Likewise, despite three decades of NHL efforts to expand hockey's footprint in American popular culture, the results remain disappointing (Mason, 2006). Americans remain resistant to sports that didn't originate there; or perhaps they remain resolutely loyal to their own sporting traditions? At the same time, despite efforts by the other U.S.-based major leagues to establish markets for their products in Europe and other continents, these have achieved fairly limited success. It can be hypothesized, then, that global marketing runs up against entrenched cultural tastes and loyalties everywhere.

Fans: Constructing the Global Consumer?

For many fans, though, and especially younger fans, the dynamics described above have arguably led to a "de-localization" of sporting interests and loyalties—an idea that suggests that people are becoming less and less attached to the sporting practices and institutions historically associated with the places they live in (Wilson, 2006). At one level, this is illustrated in the growth of transnational television audiences for the major leagues (English and Italian soccer, as well as the North American professional sports), and a corresponding decline in fan support for smaller clubs in provincial cities. It is also registered in the growth of global interest in famous teams (Manchester United, Real Madrid, the Dallas Cowboys, the Los Angeles Raiders), and a rise in "elective affinities" among young fans: supporting teams other than their local representatives on the basis of team success, "attitude," or—increasingly—celebrity players like David Beckham. Since Real Madrid signed Beckham in 2003, income from sponsorship, advertising, and merchandising has multiplied, and the club has launched its own 24-hour satellite television channel and a website in English, Japanese, and Spanish (Ammirante, 2006). What's going on here is that fan allegiances rooted in place (the practice of rooting for the home team) and in *social* choices (class or ethnic identities, for example, or regional loyalties) are being undermined by the language of consumer choice, in which fans everywhere are encouraged to identify with "world class" teams and players (Whitson, 1998, pp. 65–6).

At a deeper level, though, de-localization also means that traditional national (or regional) sports must now compete with sports imported from other countries, if they are to retain their audiences and their cultural significance, especially among young people. Thus, as the major professional sports expand and go global, *as businesses,* the kinds of national and regional rivalries that once defined the meanings of sports in popular culture are supplanted by the attitudes and practices of consumer choice, and of global youth culture and fashion. What is emerging may be a global sporting culture in which the media industry plays a significant part, and audiences around the world (or the affluent world, at least) are invited to take an interest in the same sports events and celebrities. Canadians, for example, now have access to a wider range of sports entertainment than we had in the past, including not only NBA basketball and Champions League soccer but also sports like cycling and rugby that were once very difficult to find on Canadian television. Canadian sports audiences, like audiences in other countries, are being addressed as free-floating consumers, who might switch teams and even develop new sporting interests if we are given access to world-class sporting entertainment.

The claim of promoters of cultural globalization, indeed, is that "as people gain access to global information, so they develop global needs and demand global commodities, thereby becoming global citizens."[10] For critics of globalization, however, this road leads inexorably to the loss of cultural diversity, as the expensively produced cultural events that the mainstream media publicize—the major professional sports and the Olympics, Hollywood films and U.S. television dramas, musicians on the major labels—make less well-funded cultural productions look unprofessional, even homespun, by comparison. It should be recognized here that the purpose of marketing is precisely to create demand for new products, and that global marketing sets out to reshape patterns of cultural consumption and to "grow" the markets for the products of transnational corporations (Fawcett, 1992). However, we need to examine the rhetoric through which this is accomplished, in particular the now familiar notion of "world class" products.

I want to propose here that the label of "world class" seeks to connect global brand names with ideas of excellence, specifically the idea of being the best of its kind in the world. What global brands purport to offer—whether an event like the Olympic Games or the World Cup, or the products of the global corporations that associate themselves with such events—are famous names, state of the art production, and products that are supposed to be the best of their kind in the world. We need to distinguish, though, between excellence and fame, especially where the latter is a product of expensive publicity machines (consider *The Da Vinci Code*). Think also about how difficult it is to determine "the best" when considering cultural products (like films or books, or sports) that may be difficult to compare. The term "world class" was once meaningfully applied to athletics or swimming performances that were measurably the best in the world in a given year. However, it is now used as a claim to superiority in so many other contexts, ranging from orchestras to universities to cities—contexts where qualitative comparisons are difficult, and criteria of excellence open to debate—that it has come to be devoid of concrete meaning. It can be suggested, indeed, that the label "world class" now denotes nothing so clearly as self-promotion, and indeed the status of an aspirant as opposed to an established claimant.

CONCLUSIONS

I have presented globalization as a complex of processes that combine to make the world a more integrated place, and I have tried to distinguish, for the sake of clarity, between economic or business processes (e.g., freer trade, or transnational corporate integration) and cultural processes (e.g., the spread of heterogeneity and loosening of historical ties between cultures and places). It remains crucial, though, in thinking about globalization, to remember the linkages between economic and cultural processes. For example, it is the drive on the part of sports businesses to construct global markets that has taken us some ways toward the creation of a global sporting culture. "The global expansion of the leisure and entertainment industries undoubtedly brings new opportunities to many of us—opportunities to watch or even practice sports that were once not available to us in our home countries—and this development is heralded by those who want to celebrate the benefits of increased consumer choice" (Ammirante, 2006, p. 240). However, for critics of globalization, among whom Ammirante would certainly number himself, this is a dubious benefit. He points to "the metropolitan derivation of most of the cultural products (and the lifestyles) that attain worldwide promotion and distribution" and to the fact that global soccer is increasingly dominated by a handful of super-rich clubs. It is important, therefore, to understand that in the entertainment industry, just as in other industries, globalization is an agenda promoted by the biggest of businesses, and indeed that the entertainment industry is one of globalization's most effective boosters (Fawcett, 1992).

Here we have, in capsule form, the essence of economic globalization, as well as the standard objection to it: the takeover of our most popular sports by super-rich individuals and media corporations, and their management of these popular institutions with more thought given to the bottom line than to the traditions of the team or the sport. Examples include the marketing of leagues like the English Premier League and the National Basketball Association, teams like Real Madrid and Manchester United, and celebrities like Michael Jordan and David Beckham. It's important, nonetheless, to see the continuities as well as the changes. Professional sport was a business from its inception, in both Europe and North America. However, the sports business in America began in the 1960s to adopt business models and practices being used with success elsewhere in American business (franchising, expansion, and national marketing are the best examples of this). In Europe and Australia, in contrast, teams and national governing bodies continued to operate along more traditional lines for another quarter century, and traditional ways of doing things often trumped commercial logic. Since the early 1990s, however, and the advent of pay TV, sports entrepreneurs in Europe, as well as Australia and parts of Asia, have quickly moved to adopt similar money-making strategies, and the outcome is the global spread of a more frankly commercial approach to sport (Horne, 2006, pp. 29–30). Nonetheless, globalization in the sports business has not meant the spread of American sports around the world, as some feared, so much as it has seen the spread of American business and marketing practices, practices that originated in the United States but are no longer uniquely American.

Turning to cultural globalization, it can be suggested that, as above, the threat is less the inexorable spread of U.S. popular culture than it is the steady detachment of culture from place, as a result of a combination of migration, media, and market forces. To the extent that this continues, one might predict that some once-local cultural traditions will be commercialized, and will be marketed around the world (West African and Cuban music might be examples of this in music, as is rugby in sport). Others, meanwhile, will die out, and the world's cultural diversity will be diminished. Both of these trends—that is, the commercialization of "folk" culture and the loss of cultural diversity—will be seen by some as troubling developments, and this includes not just anti-globalization activists but also some traditional "conservatives" who care about the survival of local traditions. Indeed, Foer proposes that "the innovation of the anti-globalization left is its embrace of traditionalism: its worry that global tastes and brands will steamroll indigenous cultures," and that global marketing by Real Madrid and Nike will succeed in "prying fans away from their old allegiances" (2004, pp. 4–5).

Such fears must be credited with having some grounds, for most of us will be able to see in our own experience some evidence of cultural homogenization. However, Foer goes on to observe that in his own research into the globalization of soccer, cultural homogenization turned out to be less than he had anticipated. On the contrary, many of soccer's quirky local cultures—and blood feuds—appear to be flourishing despite globalization. And in Canada, too, we can find lots of evidence of local traditions and enthusiasms, as well as regional allegiances and rivalries that seem alive and well. We've already noted the passion with which Canadians followed the fortunes of the Oilers during the 2006 Stanley Cup playoffs (like the progress of the Calgary Flames to the 2004 Stanley Cup finals), and we should register the passionate enthusiasm for hockey that persists in the many smaller cities across Canada where the junior game is thriving: places like Kamloops and Cranbrook, Red Deer and Brandon, Peterborough and London, and Rimouski and Moncton. We might also recognize the continued place of curling in the culture of rural Canada and some prairie cities (see Mott & Allardyce, 1989), as well as the revival of enthusiasm for the Canadian Football League.[11]

Foer also warns us, finally, against the temptation to see the past through highly selective glasses. He clearly enjoys many of the cultural traditions associated with soccer, and regrets that in trying to move the game "up-market" soccer's new investors have destroyed some of the game's working-class atmosphere. Yet he also remarks that the nostalgia he encountered in some quarters for the game's good old days uncritically celebrated traditions of bigotry, drunkenness, and violence against "others" that were better left behind. It also appeared to gloss over the fact that the old-fashioned terraces where working-class male fans gathered to shout their partisan allegiances and hatreds were places where fans were often treated like cattle and where, in too many tragic instances, significant numbers of fans were injured and even killed. The cultural effects of change aren't all bad, in other words, and we should be careful about glorifying "tradition" in an uncritical way (2004, pp. 96–98).

With these caveats—reminders that the effects of globalization may have good and bad elements and, in any event, may often be exaggerated—I want to close by returning to a point made in the introduction to this chapter, namely that both economic and cultural globalization raise issues of public policy. In our first free trade agreement with America in the 1980s as well as the subsequent NAFTA, Canada did everything it could to keep culture off the table, because the economics of cultural reproduction and distribution give enormous advantages to the American film, music, television, and publishing industries (Grant & Wood, 2004). Canada thus fought successfully for a "cultural exemption" that allows us to continue to support our cultural industries: our music industry, our publishers, our film industry. Such policies are continually challenged by the American cultural industries, which tend to see the Canadian market almost as an extension of their own domestic market (predominantly English-speaking, already familiar with American entertainment products and personalities). However, we need to remember that culture represents a different kind of product from wheat or auto parts. Our culture is part of our identity, and our authors and athletes and musicians and filmmakers constitute a big part of what keeps us different—from our neighbours to the south, and from everyone else. This is what makes the protection of Canada's ability to produce our own culture, and of cultural diversity within Canada, matters of more than academic interest and matters of more than entertainment, too.

ENDNOTES

1. I use "soccer" throughout, for a Canadian audience. However, readers should be aware that everywhere outside the United States and Canada, this game is known as football (or *futbol,* in Spanish-speaking nations).
2. Following Hannerz (1996), I use "international" to refer to relations or bodies that involve nation states, and "transnational" to describe other kinds of connections (e.g., corporate, or interpersonal).
3. Brazilian soccer, like West Indian cricket, is known for its offence-oriented, almost flamboyant style of play. Both James and Galeano also relate how cricket in the West Indies and soccer in many Latin American countries (notably Brazil and Argentina) have become tied up with national identity in ways very similar to the role that hockey plays in Canada.
4. We need to understand here that sports don't have interests of their own, distinct from the interests of those who own teams, televise games, and so on. Thus, whenever we hear people talking about the "interests of the sport" (in expansion, for example, or in appearing drug-free) we should recognize that this really means the interests of those who are in the business of selling that particular sport as entertainment.
5. By 2006, all of Brazil's 11 starters were European-based.
6. See Alan Klein (1991, 1997) for accounts of baseball in the Dominican Republic and Mexico, respectively, and the effects of major league baseball on baseball in these countries.
7. As an example, during the Edmonton Oilers' successes in the 2006 Stanley Cup playoffs, Mayor Stephen Mandel suggested that the team reflected the city itself: industrious, feisty, and with a never say die determination.
8. A qualifying note is important here. Some readers will have noticed that this discussion, which is focused on the most popular professional team sports, has said nothing about global opportunities for women athletes. This is because there are no women's professional leagues, as yet, that attract the media coverage and television audiences that would support the salary levels of the West European soccer leagues or the North American major league sports. Neither is there the competition for players described above. The Canadian and American women's soccer teams now draw substantial stadium audiences for international matches, and a very few leading athletes in some of the individual Olympic sports (notably skiing and track) can make significant prize money in international circuit competition. However, tennis and golf are still the only women's sports to have generated sufficient media audiences to support year-round circuit competition and the sorts of earnings commensurate with this.
9. English soccer in the last three years has seen two of its biggest clubs taken over by foreign tycoons: Chelsea by Russian billionaire Roman Abramovich, and Manchester United by American Malcolm Glazer, the owner of the NFL's Tampa Bay Buccaneers. On a smaller scale, the NHL's Ottawa Senators were "rescued" (i.e., taken over and kept in Ottawa) by Toronto pharmaceutical magnate Eugene Melnyk.
10. Theodore Levitt (1983). *The Marketing Imagination.* London: Collier Macmillan, cited in K. Robins (1991). Tradition and translation: National cultures in a global context. In *Enterprise and Heritage: Crosscurrents of National Culture.* J. Corner & S. Harvey (eds.). London: Routledge, pp. 26–27.

11. Curling in Canada underwent some commercialization in the 1990s, with the advent of cash bonspiels that made possible professional careers for a handful of the country's leading players. It's also a sport that is now part of the Winter Olympics program and has annual World Championships (for both men and women), events at which Canada is usually a favourite but doesn't always win. The processes of commercialization and globalization are not nearly as advanced, though, as they are in the other sports that have been the focus of this chapter.

CRITICAL THINKING QUESTIONS

1. Consider the popular idea that hockey is "Canada's game" in the light of how many countries the game is now played very well in. Compare hockey and soccer as global games.
2. Is globalization leading to a greater diversity of sporting choices or to the dominance of a small handful of men's professional sports?
3. What are the differences between sports fans of 40 years ago and those of today? Is the expansion of consumer choice an important advance? What are the limitations of consumer sovereignty?
4. What are the meanings of "world class"? in relation to sports? cities? universities?
5. What does it mean to be a global citizen? How might this go beyond being a global consumer?

SUGGESTED READINGS

Foer, F. (2004). *How soccer explains the world: An (unlikely) theory of globalization*. New York: Harper Perennial.
Horne, J. (2006). *Sport in consumer culture*. London: Palgrave Macmillan.
King, A. (2003). *The European ritual: Football in the new Europe*. Burlington, VT: Ashgate.
Tomlinson, J. (1999). *Globalization and culture*. Chicago: University of Chicago Press.
Whitson, D. (2001). *Hockey and Canadian identities: From frozen rivers to revenue streams*. In D. Taras and B. Rasporich (Eds.), *A passion for identity: Canadian studies for the 21st century*. Toronto: Nelson.
Whitson, D., & Gruneau, R. (Eds.), (2006). *Artificial ice: Hockey, culture, and commerce*. Peterborough, ON: Broadview Press.

WEB LINKS

The International Forum on Globalization
http://www.ifg.org
A forum to stimulate new thinking and public education in response to economic globalization.

The Canadian Centre for Policy Alternatives
http://www.policyalternatives.ca
Independent, non-partisan research concerned with issues of social and economic justice.

New Internationalist
http://www.newint.org
Independent, provocative information about the fight for global justice.

The Guardian Unlimited
http://sport.guardian.co.uk
Sports articles from a British daily newspaper.

Goal.com
http://www.goal.com
Coverage of European soccer leagues and competitions.

Northeastern University, Sport in Society
http://www.northeastern.edu/csss/rgrc.html
Analysis of hiring practices of women and people of colour in American sports leagues.

National Consortium for Academics & Sports
http://www.ncasports.org/articles.htm
Discussion focusing on educational attainment and the use of sport to positively effect social change.

The Globalist
http://www.theglobalist.com/DBWeb/Community.aspx?FeatureId=42
Information dedicated to promoting the understanding of global issues.

Play the Game
http://www.playthegame.org/
Advocates integrity and the countering of corruption in the world of sport.

CHAPTER 14

SPORT AND RELIGION

Christopher L. Stevenson

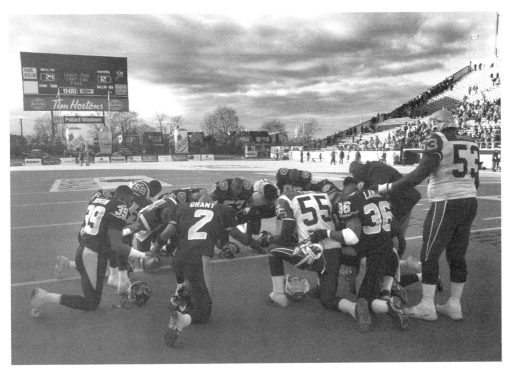

This prayer huddle after a football touchdown illustrates the connection between religion and sport.

CP PHOTO/Frank Gunn

The Lord delighteth in a pair of sturdy legs.

Leslie Stephen (Maitland, 1906, p. 138)

This chapter is titled "Sport and Religion," but more properly this should really read "Sport and *Christianity*," because it is Christianity and its relationship with sport that will be our specific focus. The reason for concentrating on Christianity rather than on Islam, Judaism, or Buddhism is because it has been Christian beliefs and values that have had such a powerful influence on the development of societies in Europe and in North America. And, more particularly, these Christian beliefs and values have had an enormous influence on the development of sport in these societies. The values that are enshrined in modern European and North American legal systems, political systems, and social structures—the foundations upon which these societies have developed—were specifically derived from Christianity. And so the kind of society that Canadians developed from the seventeenth century onward was built on Christian ideals and ideas.

No one can doubt that other faith traditions were also present during the development of modern societies and modern sport, but these faith traditions—whether Native spirituality in North America or rabbinical Judaism in Europe—were rather marginal factors in the development of modern societies and of modern sport. The ideas and ideals of rabbinical Judaism, for example, had little impact on the ways in which European societies developed through the seventeenth, eighteenth, and nineteenth centuries. Similarly, the values and beliefs of the Aboriginal peoples of North America had little influence on the ways in which North American societies developed. The reason is simple—these faith traditions were both very much marginalized groups within these societies and had very limited access to any form of social power. Christians, on the other hand, predominated in these societies and held firmly onto the levers of power, and so their values, ideals, and ideas became the foundations of these modern societies.

Now it is certainly the case that societies change, and indeed we see such changes in the religious affiliation of Canadians, as represented in their responses to census inquiries (see the Statistics Canada 2001 Census "Religions in Canada" analytic series, available online at http://www12.statcan.ca/english/census01/Products/Analytic/companion/rel/canada.cfm). These data indicate that the percentage of Canadians who are willing to self-identify with a Christian religion has dropped from 82.8 percent in the 1991 census to 76.6 percent in the 2001 census. On the other hand, the percentage of those Canadians who self-identify with any number of non-Christian religions (Hindu, Sikh, Islam, Judaism, etc.) has increased from 3.8 percent in 1991 to 6.0 percent in 2001, while the percentage of those who claim to have "no religion" has also increased, from 12.3 percent in 1991 to 16.2 percent in 2001. Nevertheless, despite such changes in religious affiliation in Canadian society, there have been limited consequences for the fundamental philosophical, value-based underpinnings of organized sport. As we will see in this chapter, the values that were embedded in organized sport from its beginnings were derived from nineteenth-century Christianity, and although each generation of athletes and participants has to some extent struggled with them, these values have yet to change substantially.

The organization of this chapter is as follows. First, we will look at the evidence that sport and religion have had a long history of interrelationships. Second, we will focus very specifically on the defining influence that one particular strand of Protestant Christianity—"muscular Christianity"—has had on the development of "modern sport." Finally, we will examine some of the contemporary issues surrounding the relationship between Christianity and elite, competitive sport.

SPORT IS RELIGION

One of the first issues we must deal with is the claim made by some authors that sport *is* religion. Sport, says Charles Prebish (1984)—particularly sport in its modern, commercialized, spectacular form—acts *as* a religion, is viewed by its fans *like* a religion, and so really *is* a

Box 14.1   A Sociological Approach to the Study of Religion

Malcolm B. Hamilton (1995) has described the purpose of a sociological approach to the study of religion, which is what this chapter is all about:

> [T]he sociology of religion poses the questions of the role and significance of religion in general, in human society . . . . [and] to further the understanding of the role of religion in society, to analyze its significance in and impact upon human history, and to understand its diversity and the social forces and influences that shape it. (pp. 1–2)

religion. Other scholars have argued similarly, that since sport has all of the characteristics of a religion, then it needs to be recognized *as* a religion. Frank Deford, writing in *Sports Illustrated* (1980), coined the phrase "Sportianity" to capture these ideas.

So what are these characteristics of a religion that sport shares? Michael Novak (1976, pp. 29–31) has offered the following suggestions: (1) that a religion (a) is organized and structured, (b) begins with ceremonies, at which a few surrogates perform for all, (c) consecrates certain hours as sacred time, (d) has heroic forms for its followers to emulate, and (e) is built upon ascecis and the development of character through self-denial, repetition, and experiment; and (2) that in official ceremonies, (a) sacred vestments are used, rituals are prescribed, customs are developed, with actions that are highly formalized, (b) right ways and wrong ways of acting are plainly marked out, and professional watchdogs supervise formal correctness, and (c) moments of silence are observed, and concentration and intensity are indispensable. The proponents of sport-as-religion claim that sport does, indeed, demonstrate these characteristics; that sport does have notions of "sacred time" and "sacred space" (that is, space and time set aside specially and reverently for the game), that it has a number of "sacred rituals," that its participants (its "priests") undergo long and difficult periods of preparation, while its fans (its "congregation") often organize their leisure time around its festivals, many of whom experience strong emotional feelings, even states of ecstasy, and often make sizeable donations to support it (either as spectator fees, or as actual contributions to sponsor teams or individual participants). All of these characteristics, the proponents say, are those of a religion.

Of course, there are many other scholars and theologians who disagree! These writers argue that sport is most definitely *not* a religion, even if it does occasionally under some circumstances demonstrate some superficial similarity to a religion. These scholars would rather focus on the root purpose of religions as social institutions: that of dealing with questions of ultimate meaning, for which they attempt to provide answers (for example, Chandler, 1992). Sport cannot deal with such questions; sport "cannot tell us where we came from, where we are going, nor how we are to behave while here; sport exists to entertain us, not to disturb us with questions about our destiny" (Chandler, 1992, p. 59). And when one looks at some of Michael Novak's (1976, p. 30) other characteristics of religion, that a religion "places us in the presence of powers greater than ourselves, and seeks to reconcile us to them," and "makes explicit the almost nameless dreads of daily human life; aging, dying, failure under pressure, cowardice, betrayal, and guilt," it seems that sport has little to do with these fundamental issues either.

Furthermore, Chandler (1992) argues that people are not simply spectators during religious rituals, whether they are Christian or Navajo; rather, either "Grace is conferred on Christians, [or] Navajos are brought in to harmony with the universe" (p. 58). In either case, an external power is invoked to produce this transformation, whereas in sport no such change is required or expected. Sport rituals, in fact, Chandler argues, "are designed simply to assert superiority," and such "rituals of dominance simply underscore the sporting participants' objective: to win" (p. 58).

SPORT AND RELIGION IN EARLY SOCIETIES AND CULTURES

But if sport is not a religion, it is still important to appreciate that sport and games have nevertheless long been associated with religion. Indeed, in many societies, sport, games, and religion have been closely intertwined and interdependent. Allen Guttmann (1978) has emphasized this point. He suggests that there is "plentiful evidence" that most early or historical societies "incorporated running, jumping, throwing, wrestling, and even ball playing in their religious rituals and ceremonies" (p. 16). He points back to Ancient Greece, and explains that the various sporting festivals or games, such as the Olympic, Pythian, Isthmian, and Nemean games, were indeed "sacred festivals, [and] integral aspects of the religious life" (p. 21) of the Greek culture of the time. Guttmann quotes Ludwig Deubner as saying: "The Olympic games were sacred games, staged in a sacred space and at a sacred festival; they were a religious act in honour of the deity. Those who took part did so in order to serve the god and the prizes which they won came from the god . . . The Olympic games had their roots in religion" (p. 21).

And if we consider the various indigenous cultures in the Americas as another example, here, too, we find considerable evidence of the use of games *in* and *as* religious rituals and ceremonies. Stewart Culin, an early American anthropologist, wrote about the games of the Plain Indian culture, which were played "usually at fixed seasons as the accompaniment of certain festivals or religious rites" (Guttmann, 1978, p. 17). Culin suggested that, "in general, games appear to be played ceremonially, as pleasing to the gods, with the object of securing fertility, causing rain, giving and prolonging life, expelling demons, or curing sickness." Similarly, Guttmann pointed to the relay races of the Jicarilla Apaches of the United States Southwest, the "log races" of the Timbira Indians of Brazil, and the ball games of the Maya and Aztecs—all of which, as far as we can discern, were intimately related to their religious practices and ceremonies.

Sport, Games, and the Early Christian Church

But what of the early Christian societies—what was their attitude toward such games and contests? It seems quite clear that the general attitude of the early Christian church toward games, physical contests, and recreational pastimes was largely negative. By late in the fourth century CE, when the Roman Empire had become officially Christian, the church was so strongly opposed to such mass spectacles as the Roman Games that they were officially abolished in 393 CE (Barney, 1996). The Games were viewed not only as decadent but also as cruel and barbaric, with their emphasis on such spectacles as fights between wild beasts as well as gladiatorial fights to the death.

This was partly the double legacy of the teachings of St. Paul and St. Augustine. St. Paul's attitude toward the body, or the "flesh," in his language, was that the flesh corrupts—thus, while one's "spirit" might be true to God's teachings and wants to put these into practice, it is the "flesh" that corrupts these pure desires and causes us to turn away from God and toward perversions and evil (*Galatians*, 5: 16–26). St. Augustine also had a strongly negative attitude toward "the body" and anything associated with it—sexuality, gluttony, drunkenness, and so on. This attitude derived, so he tells us, from his own experiences as a young man, when he enjoyed all sorts of bodily pleasures. Augustine eventually turned away from such things, repented of them, and then condemned them vigorously in his writings and his teachings

(*Confessions*). The influence of both of these "saints" was powerful in the early church (even, indeed, into the modern era) and resulted in a fundamental Christian attitude of suspicion toward anything to do with the body.

And so from the early church, and for nearly 1900 years thereafter, the Christian attitude toward games and sport has been one of distrust. It has been the soul that has had the highest value, the highest priority, with the body and its physical passions and desires very much treated as a hindrance to true spirituality. Some strands of Christianity have even promoted the mortification of the flesh—deliberate mutilations, or deliberately ignoring disease or injury—as a means of overcoming bodily passions and becoming more in tune with the mind of God. It has been only when "use" or "need" could be argued that the church has given its approval to games and physical contests and recreations. Let us look at a particular example of this in the case of the Puritans.

The Puritans

The Puritans were a group of Christians who have come to have a rather unpleasant reputation. The popular notion of Puritans is that they were against anything and everything that gave pleasure! In a word, "Killjoys"! Lord Macaulay had a famous saying, that "The Puritan hated bear-baiting, not because it gave pain to the bear, but because it gave pleasure to the spectators" (Firth, 1968, p. 142). This is rather unfortunate, because, as most stereotypes, it is largely inaccurate. Certainly, the Puritans of the 1570s to the 1640s were a people who strove to live pure, "holy," Christian lives, and tried hard to focus on "purifying" themselves spiritually—hence their name, Puritan. And they certainly established rules for living in order to better achieve their spiritual goals, but these rules were primarily for themselves and not necessarily for everyone else. The objective was for each person *individually* to achieve holiness.

The popular ideas about Puritans as killjoys come from the behaviour of some branches of Puritanism in the late 1500s and early 1600s. When the Puritans established their communities in the New World, in Massachusetts and Connecticut, and so on, they established laws for these communities in accordance with their values and beliefs. They were concerned for the sanctity of the Sabbath Day, and were appalled that others would spend the day "full heathenishly, in taverning, tippling, gaming, playing and beholding of bear-baitings and stage-plays" (Guttmann, 1988, p. 26). And so when they had the power to do so, they instituted laws to govern community behaviour on Sundays. Guttmann (1988) tells us, for example, of the Act of 1644, which established "That no person or persons shall hereafter upon the Lords-Day, use, exercise, keep, maintain, or be present at any wraslings, shooting, Bowling, ringing of Bells for Pleasure or Pastime, Masque, Wake, otherwise called Feasts, Church-Ale, Dancing, Games, Sport or Pastime whatsoever" (p. 27). In Massachusetts Bay in 1630, John Baker was "whipped for shooteing att fowle on the Sabbath day" (p. 27), and "Vermonters who ran, rode, jumped, or danced on Sunday were subject to ten lashes and a 40 shilling fine" (p. 28). It is on such evidence that some historians have come to the conclusion that "the Puritans saw their mission to erase all sport and play from men's lives" (Brailsford, 1969, p. 141).

However, a closer look at the writings of the Puritans suggests that their attitudes to physical activity were not entirely negative. They certainly recognized that people needed recreation from their labours—but it had to be a purposeful and godly recreation. The key here, therefore, is that if recreational activities can be claimed to be "useful," such as rest or recreation—then they are acceptable. Guttmann (1988) provides us with evidence of this approach by Puritan thinkers from the seventeenth century; thus, Perkins, in 1614, believed that "rest from labour with the refreshing of bodie and mind, is necessary," and listed a number of activities as "verie commendable, and not to be disliked" (p. 30). Elton, in 1625, agreed: "There are such movings of the body as bee honest and delightfull exercise of the minde, and serve to the refreshing of the body and minde, as Shooting, Tennis-playing, Stoolball-playing, Wrestling, Running, and such like" (p. 30). And in 1726, Cotton Mather declared:

> We would not be misunderstood . . . that a due Pursuit of Religion is inconsistent with all manner of Diversion: No, we suppose there are Diversions undoubtedly innocent, yea profitable and of use, *to fit us for Service*, by enlivening and fortifying our frail Nature, Invigorating the Animal Spirits, and Brightening the Mind, when tired with close Application to Business. (Wagner, 1976, p. 144; my emphasis added)

What was implied in these pronouncements was that the purpose for participating in such activities *must be* a useful one. The judgment must be, according to Richard Baxter, that "the *end* to which you really intend in using it, must be to fit you for your *service to God*" (Guttmann, 1988, p. 31). Usefulness, then, was a legitimate rationale for justifying the playing of games and sport—even for the Puritans! But usefulness within limits: there was to be no playing on the Sabbath, complete avoidance of any association with cruelty, and no gambling, no drinking, and no idleness or wastefulness.

RELIGION AND THE DEVELOPMENT OF MODERN SPORT

But surely these cultures of the past and their fusion of religion and games have little relevance to today's modern sport. Not so! In fact, modern sports might not exist—at least in their present form and in their present dominance—if it had not been for the influence of a particular set of ideas contained in Protestant Christianity: "muscular Christianity." And "usefulness" was certainly a large part of the justifications for which supported the development of modern sports.

What I am suggesting is that there was a historical moment, a window of opportunity, when the possibility of the development of "modern sport" occurred. I do not mean the very day or the very hour when this happened; rather, there was a period of time—not very long, but long enough in terms of a decade or so—when significant influences came into alignment creating the possibility that the "modern" forms of sport could evolve. This historical moment was obviously somewhat different for different sports, but by and large many of the beginnings of modern sport occurred sometime between the 1830s and the 1880s.

A number of scholars have argued that in order for traditional folk games to be changed into the beginnings of modern sport, society needed to see itself and the natural world around it differently; that is, it had to take on "modern" attitudes and values, based on a secular, rational, and scientific world view (see Guttmann, 1978, pp. 80–9). But there also needed to be a change in the reasons *why* people played these games and sports, and this reason (in the new scientific, rational, world order) had to be that of *usefulness*. Sports could be permitted, even accepted, *if* they were seen as *useful*.

In order to appreciate the enormity of what happened in the development of modern sport, it is important to understand the huge transformation between the early 1800s and the 1880s in the ways in which sports and games were played. Traditional folk games and sporting recreations were wild and unruly affairs, minimally organized and played irregularly—often once or twice a year and mostly associated with local festivals and country fairs, and characterized by much drunkenness, gambling, and violent behaviour. For example, the result of a sixteenth-century "football" game was that "much harme was done, some in the great thronge falling into a trance, some having their bodies bruised and crushed; some their arms, heades or legges broken, and some otherwise maimed or in peril of their lives" (Dunning & Sheard, 1979, pp. 23–4).

Box 14.2   The Development of Hockey: The Struggle between the "Montreal Rules" and the "Halifax Rules"

While there were as many different ways of playing "hockey" as there were places with ice-covered rivers and ponds in North America, the two main contenders for rules-supremacy seem to have been the "Montreal rules," established in order to play the now-famous first game in the Victoria Rink in Montreal in 1875, and the "Halifax rules," which developed in the Halifax–Dartmouth area throughout the early 1800s. (There were a number of differences between these two sets of rules—but perhaps the key differences were the degree of physicality permitted and whether or not a forward pass was allowed.) We now know that the Montreal rules won the day, perhaps because their proponents were better organized or because they were the first set of hockey rules to be printed and therefore available to everyone. But the situation was still fluid in 1889, when the Dartmouth Chebuctos hockey team travelled up from Nova Scotia to Quebec City to play against the Montreal and Quebec City teams. This entailed a 1,900-kilometre journey by the Intercolonial Railway, and then negotiation over whose rules they would use in the games—the Halifax rules or the Montreal rules? Eventually, pragmatism reigned and a game was played by each set of rules—Montreal and Quebec City teams winning the games that were played according to the Montreal rules and Dartmouth winning the games played according to the Halifax rules (Vaughan, 1996, p. 56).

Each community had its own version of these games, with rules and customs peculiar to itself, to which there was much local loyalty. There could be any number of participants playing at one time, there was nothing consistent about the size of playing surface or the types of balls or sticks or goals that could be used, there were different ways in which players could score, and "goals" could be situated in different places on and around the playing area. There were many different types of early forms of stick and ball games played on ice in Europe, in Canada, and in North America generally through the 1700s and into the early 1800s—games called shinney, ricket, and hurling—well before any one game called "hockey" emerged to be the dominant form of the sport (see Gruneau & Whitson, 1993). All of this rich diversity meant that inter-community competition was a rarity, partly because of the daunting logistics of travel to another community, either by foot or by horseback, and because it meant playing by someone else's rules and customs.

Yet out of this chaotic mix of many different ways of playing football, hockey, baseball, and all sorts of other games, the modern form of sport emerged; that is, a way of playing these games evolved that was qualitatively and quantitatively different from the old, traditional ways of playing. Guttmann (1978) has argued that modern sports have a particular set of characteristics; thus (1) participation in these sports is not limited to only certain social groups or classes, (2) sports skills, techniques, and training methods become highly specialized and "scientific" in nature, (3) the playing and training systems which are used in these sports are highly efficient and focused, (4) sports' organizational structures are bureaucratic in nature, (5) the highly sophisticated and complex measurement of performance is a central feature of the competition, and (6) records are kept. So, out of the irregular, crude, idiosyncratic, traditional sports, a new efficient, standardized, rationalized, "modern" type of sport evolved.

Guttmann (1978, 1988) argues that this development of "modern" sport was but one part of the changes that were taking place in Western societies from the seventeenth century onward. There was a growing acceptance of a secular and scientific world view that was associated with new forms of rationality and the concomitant development of industrial economies and bureaucracies, above all with an emphasis on "achievement." These ideas influenced all aspects of social life, including the types of activities with which one filled one's recreational, non-working time. And so the evolution of modern sport out of its roots in traditional folk games was the result of the slow development of this "modern," rational, and scientific world view.

But the final piece of the puzzle had to be the justification that the new "modern" sports were *useful*. It is here that Christianity, in the guise of a particular logic called "muscular Christianity," played a critical role. There had always been considerable resistance from the socially elite groups in society to the traditional games played by the lower classes—seeing them as depraved and depraving, a waste of time, and associated with gambling, drinking, riotous behaviour, and physical violence. They simply deplored them; there was no place for such activities in a modern society. So, somehow, these negative attitudes toward sport had to change in order for modern sport to become socially accepted and, indeed, encouraged. What was essential was to frame these emerging sports in such a way that the old negative connotations were dispensed with and new, positive, "modern" rationales adopted—and the watchword was "usefulness."

Muscular Christianity provided that rationale at a particularly crucial moment in the development of modern sport. During the 1850s in England, two writers, Thomas Hughes and Charles Kingsley, both active Christians, wrote a number of novels and essays in which they promoted the ideas and the values that came to be known as muscular Christianity. This was a Christianity that was robust and active, in which honesty, openness, strength of character, and a dedication to one's country were celebrated as the highest of virtues. The muscular Christian, it was said, "has hold of the old chivalrous and Christian belief, that a man's body is given to him to be trained and brought into subjection, and then used for the protection of the weak, the advancement of all righteous causes, and the subduing of the earth which God has given to the children of men" (Hughes, 1861, p. 83). And—surprise!—this was a Christianity whose virtues could be demonstrated par excellence in sports. In books like *Tom Brown's School-days*, Thomas Hughes promoted the idea that strength of character, piety, and manliness were learned on the sports field. For, according to Charles Kingsley: "Games conduce not merely to physical, but to moral health; that in the playing-fields boys acquire virtues which no books can give them; not merely daring and endurance, but, better still, temper, self-restraint, fairness, honour, unenvious approbation of another's success and all that 'give and take' of life which stand a man in such good stead when he goes forth into the world" (Haley, 1978, p. 119).

Muscular Christianity, then, provided an argument that said sports are useful because they contribute to building up of the participant's morality, character, manliness, piety, and patriotism. Through the playing of the new forms of "modern" sport, character is built—and not just any "character," but the most desirable of Christian characters. As one of Tom Brown's teachers says about the game of cricket, "the discipline and reliance on one another which it teaches is so valuable . . . It merges the individual into the eleven; he doesn't play so that he may win, but that his side may" (Hughes, 1994, p. 349).

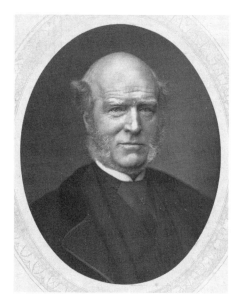

Thomas Hughes—Christian, novelist, and social reformer.

© Hulton-Deutsch Collection/CORBIS

It was this collection of ideas that provided the last piece of the puzzle in setting the stage for the development of modern sports. Muscular Christianity provided the most positive function possible for the playing of sport—and it quickly caught on. Sport became an accepted feature of school life, played by the students, guided by the teachers, and praised for its character-transforming qualities by the headmasters. Schools throughout England, and then throughout the British Empire and into Canada and North America, used the arguments of muscular Christianity to justify the introduction of sports into schools. It became commonplace for teachers to be hired according to their abilities in sport, rather than their command of their academic subject matter. By the 1880s the "games ethic" was supreme throughout the English-speaking world, and schools in North America—and particularly those private boarding schools designed to educate the sons of the elites—had introduced sports into the recreational times of their students. Schools such as Upper Canada College in Ontario (established in 1829) and Rothesay Collegiate School in New Brunswick (established in 1891) are striking examples of schools in which sports were (and still are!) promoted as building the desirable character in the sons (and, more recently, the daughters—see Box 14.3) of the leading families in the Dominion.

This belief that games and sports could positively influence a participant's character, converting him into a person of morality, self-discipline, and with an obedient nature, was also seized upon as a solution to the increasingly difficult social problems of the growing towns and cities in Europe, Canada, and North America. These cities, growing in population because of huge migrations in from rural areas and increasing immigrations from all parts of Europe and beyond, were faced with serious social problems—overcrowded urban spaces, and the rapidly growing prevalence of drunkenness, gambling, and various riotous behaviours. Civic leaders tried various reform measures and municipal ordinances to deal with these problems, to little or no avail.

Box 14.3   Gender and Muscular Christianity

It must be understood that the ideas and values that made up the notion of muscular Christianity in the late nineteenth century and into the twentieth century was much influenced by both gender and social class. That is, the focus was exclusively upon boys and men from the upper and upper-middle classes—the boys who were attending the private, elite schools, who were taking part in the school sports, and who would be the future social elites in their societies. The education of women and girls (to the extent that it actually occurred in an organized manner) took place primarily in the home, with an emphasis upon training in those feminine and wifely arts thought necessary for a wife to possess so that she might provide the most comfortable home possible for her husband. The writers and the preachers who developed and codified the ideas of muscular Christianity were very much interested in the development of the attributes of "manliness" in boys and young men. Manliness was, they believed, the quintessential character of the muscular Christian—and as such was expressed through the characteristics of honesty, openness, fairness, self-restraint, strength of character, and patriotism. And it was also their belief that it was through the moral influences of both school and school sports that manliness could be developed in young men.

It was much, much later in the process of development of modern sports and modern school sports—in some societies, not until the late twentieth century—that the benefits of sport participation came to be seen as also appropriate to women and girls. But first, of course, the beliefs and ideas about manliness as the prime outcome of participation in sport had to have been de-emphasized and then generalized to non–gender specific attributes of character.

What these civic leaders needed was some way to divert the new urban working classes away from their dissolute and destructive activities and to turn them toward alternative, socially and morally improving activities. And muscular Christianity, as linked with sport, seemed to fit the bill—with its emphasis on morality and other Christian virtues. In many cities, civic leaders took the new "modern" forms of sport, and promoted them in the organizations that were working with the urban working-class populations. The YMCAs, for example, soon began to use sports in addition to their traditional activities of bible studies and meetings, as both a means of attracting young men into their buildings and as a means of moulding their characters. Whether or not sport was successful as a means of urban social control, society's enthusiasm for sport nevertheless grew by leaps and bounds.

Muscular Christianity, therefore, played a critical role in the development of modern sport—the role of providing the acceptable justifications for participating in sport. Without these justifications, it is conceivable that the modern forms of sport that were just beginning to emerge might not have been accepted by the schools of the time, nor by the influential civic

---

Box 14.4   The Domestication of Christmas

Sports were not the only site of struggle between older traditions and celebrations and the emerging values and concerns of the growing middle classes; the celebration of Christmas was the site of another such struggle.

Critics of our twentieth- and twenty-first-century Christmases decry the overwhelming emphasis on consumption associated with it, with producers using Christmas symbols to sell their products, and consumers spending billions of dollars annually. Such critics often lament the loss of an earlier and supposedly "purer" form of Christmas, a pious-yet-joyful, religious celebration of the birth of Jesus Christ. But there never were such Christmases! In fact, there have always been struggles over the meaning of Christmas and over the behaviours that are deemed appropriate to it.

For example, in the sixteenth and seventeenth centuries, some of the more "fundamentalist" Protestant groups (see the Puritans above) were able to ban Christmas entirely in certain places in Europe and North America—banning the singing of carols, Christmas trees, and other decorative greenery—while in other places Christmas survived as the opportunity for a wild, drunken, noisy, and violent community holiday.

Stephen Nissenbaum, in his book *The Battleground for Christmas* (1996), has illustrated the struggle that was occurring in eighteenth-century America between the expectations of the middle classes for their Christmas celebrations and those of the lower classes. Bowler (2005) has described the conflict between these different approaches to Christmas thus:

> Respectable folk were woken at night by bands of drunken roisters, banging on doors, breaking windows and treating the neighbourhood to . . . loud and offensive 'beating on tin pans, blowing horns, shouts, groans and catcalls,' [which were] meant to mock their betters and keep them from their sleep. Gangs swarmed out of the urban slums to disturb church services, invade wealthy districts and brawl with the watchmen hired to keep the peace. (p. D55)

Nissenbaum has described the ways in which such rambunctious Christmas traditions were eventually domesticated thorough the efforts of concerned civic leaders, who managed to reinvent its meanings and created new, safer (for the middle classes) traditions, such as re-inventing the traditional, edgy, and judgmental St. Nicolas as the harmless yet jolly "Santa Claus," and developing new notions of more family-centred and domestic celebrations.

leaders, opinion-makers, and reformers of the time. The probability is that our present social reality would be something quite different, and possibly sports—in the forms that we know them today and with the meanings we attribute to them today—would also be quite different.

What is also significant about muscular Christianity is that its central ideas and beliefs still remain with us *today*. The idea that "sports build character" comes directly from muscular Christianity; the idea that somehow those who play sports well also have moral characters that are beyond reproach comes from muscular Christianity; the idea that sports can be used to train qualities of leadership, obedience to authority, and self-discipline comes from muscular Christianity; the idea that sports provide an ideal training ground in masculinity—that sport, and particularly extreme contact sport, transforms young boys into men—comes from muscular Christianity; the idea of sacrificing oneself for the success of one's team, one's school, or one's country comes from muscular Christianity. All of these ideas have come from muscular Christianity and still have currency in justifying the presence of sport in a variety of today's social settings, including schools, colleges and universities, management training courses, juvenile delinquency programs, and inner-city projects.

Of course, it must be stressed that this development of the notion of muscular Christianity, the belief about the efficacy of sports in creating the qualities of the muscular Christian, and the historical and continuing influence of these ideas, has little to do with whether or not participation in sporting activities is *actually effective* in "building character" in young men and women. Indeed, some critics of intercollegiate athletics (especially as these are practised in the United States) have argued that the socialization outcomes of such sports are more likely to be *undesirable* personal characteristics than desirable ones. When we look at the research in the sociological literature, however, we find that it is quite ambivalent over whether participation in sport influences a person's "character"—his or her values, attributes, beliefs, and so on—but certainly there does not appear to be any overwhelmingly convincing positive evidence (see Stevenson, 1986). However, as Coakley and Donnelly (2004a) have cautioned, "[the] failure [of research] to find consistent, measurable effects of sport participation on specific character traits *does not mean* that sports and sport experiences have no impact on people's lives" (p. 95). After all, as the so-called "Thomas theorem" puts it: "If men define situations as real they are real in their consequences" (Thomas and Thomas, 1929, p. 572). That is, in this case, if we believe that sports build character, then we act as if they do and we treat sports participants as if their character has indeed been positively affected.

CONTEMPORARY TOPICS

Let us now turn to the present day and look at some of the contemporary issues surrounding sport and Christianity. We will look a number of topics, beginning with superstition and sport; next, we will look at some issues around the contemporary interaction between these two, apparently quite contradictory, value systems—elite, competitive sport and Christianity; and, finally, we will examine some of the critiques of Evangelical Christianity's use of sport as part of their marketing techniques for evangelistic crusades and events.

Superstition and Sport

Sport, in many ways, is a hotbed of superstition. Players, coaches, fans—all have their own particular "lucky" charms and "lucky" rituals, which they believe or at least hope contribute to a positive outcome for their team in the game. The Canadian hockey teams at the 2000 Salt Lake City Winter Olympic Games had a "lucky" loonie hidden at centre ice—and they won both men's and women's gold medals! But what do we know about these superstitions, and why do people have them and use them?

Most people have some experience with superstitions: a black cat crossing your path brings bad luck, but a four-leaf clover brings good luck. Newspaper reports often provide examples of the many (often bizarre) superstitions that are rampant in the world of sports, including athletes insistent on always eating the same meal before a game, always performing the same pregame routines, always wearing the same clothes that they wore when they last won a game, never stepping on the lines on the field, and so on. Some athletes carry around talismans—the "lucky" t-shirt, the "lucky" sneakers, the "lucky" stuffed bear, the "lucky" coin, and many others. Jack McCallum (1992) has described the superstitions of Bill Parcells, when he was head coach of the NFL's New York Giants. Parcells, McCallum says, "doesn't want any of his players or staff to precede him into the locker room, and he always wants to see the same players—Phil Simms, Brad Benson and Chris Godfrey—before he sees anyone else. He'll never pick up a penny that has tails facing up" (p. 204).

Womack (1992) has analyzed some of these rituals and talismans and has identified four different types. First of all, there are the *day-of-game* rituals. Womack quotes a professional hockey player as saying: "When you win you try not to change anything. Nothing. You do everything exactly the same as you did the whole day of your win . . . Get up on the same side of the bed. Eat the same meals, at the same places . . . If your salad was dry, order it dry again. . . . You leave at the same times, take the same routes, park in the same place, enter through the same door" (p. 196). For example, Stéphane Lebeau has described his rituals on the day of an NHL game:

> On the day of a game, I get up at 8.30am. I have my usual breakfast, orange juice, oatmeal, two slices of bread, and a glass of milk. Then I head off to team training. When I get back, I always eat a hamburger steak and watch a show on TV. I have a 90-minute nap in the afternoon. Four hours before the game, I eat a plate of spaghetti. I arrive at the locker room at around 5pm and I put on my underwear. In the two and a half hours before warm-up, I chew 20 to 25 sticks of gum and drink lots of water. I tape up my three or four sticks for the game and, before every game, I jump in the dressing room spa for three or four minutes. Then I put on the rest of my equipment. (Lebeau, 2006)

But when a ritual "fails"—that is, the team or the athlete loses a game—then the rituals are changed as the athlete searches for a new pattern of behaviour that will "ensure" a win.

Second, there are the *pregame* rituals: These are rituals associated with getting ready for the game—getting the equipment together, getting dressed, being prepared by the medical staff, and so on. For example, says Womack, "some hockey players dress the entire left side of their bodies first—socks, skates, kneepads, etc.—before dressing the right side" (p. 197). Indeed, Wayne Gretzky has been quoted as saying:

> I always put my equipment on the same way: left shin pad, left stocking, right shin pad, right stocking. Then pants, left skate, right skate, shoulder pads, elbow pads, first the left, then the right; and finally, the jersey, with the right side tucked into my pants.
> During the warm-up, I always shoot my first puck way off to the right of the goal. I go back to the dressing room and drink a Diet Coke, a glass of iced water, a Gatorade, and another Diet Coke. (Lebeau, 2006)

Another player, Jocelyn Thibault, has described his routine as: "Before a game, I always lay my equipment out on the floor in the same way and six and half minutes before the game, I pour water over my head" (Lebeau, 2006). McCallam (1992) reports that Wade Boggs, when he played for the Boston Red Sox, had an extremely precise set of rituals in preparing for a game, including "[ending] the grounder drill by stepping on third, second and first (in that order), [taking] two steps in the first base coaching box and loping to the dugout in four steps, preferably hitting the same four spots every evening; get a drink of water and jog to centerfield for meditation" (pp. 205–6).

The third category of rituals are the *activity-specific* rituals. Womack (1992) describes the actions of Al Hrabosky when he was a pitcher for the Kansas City Royals:

> Before an important pitch, Hrabosky turns his back on the better and stalks toward second base. He stares into center field . . . Hrabosky then goosesteps back to the mound and glares at the batter. He swings his left foot back and forth across the pitching rubber, takes off his hat with his left hand and wipes across his head with his right forearm. He jerks his head up and down, and from side to side. Finally he pitches. (p. 191)

And finally there are the *rites of protection*. These are actions and rituals performed in order to control "vague, undefined, and potentially threatening events or situations" (Womack, 1992, p. 198). Such situations in sport range from those that are potentially injury-causing to those that may cause the team or the individual to lose the game. Players hide talismans—such as medallions, crosses, lucky charms—in their uniforms or even in their shoes. Other players wear the same equipment that they've worn since their college or junior days—Wayne Gretzky, for example, was renowned for the "old" style of hockey helmet he always wore. And some players prefer to work with particular teammates; Steve Carleton, when he pitched for the St. Louis Cardinals, always insisted that Tim McCarver play as his catcher—no one else.

But why do athletes use these rituals, and how do they believe they work? Anthropologist Bronislaw Malinowski (1927) offered a classic explanation: ritual is used to allay anxiety and to inspire confidence. Another anthropologist, Mary Douglas (1966), had a similar approach: that since ambiguity and uncertainty is threatening, it is dealt with via elaborate rituals that are believed to provide some degree of control over the situation or circumstance. Malcolm B. Hamilton (1995) suggested that superstition is always related to some definite outcome the individual wishes to achieve, and that the practitioners see them as a set of behaviours that are merely the means to an expected end. That is, ritual behaviours are, in essence, attempts to explain, understand, and control reality. Jack McCallum (1992) says simply that such rituals are ways of getting through the tough situations—a crutch, a secret weapon, a way to get a little edge. And, of course, as long as they keep winning, the rituals are clearly "working," and so they go on using them. Once their efficacy has worn off, however, and the team or athlete starts to lose, then another, different ritual is sought out in order to again control the uncertainty in the athlete's life.

Professing Christians and the Dilemma of the Ethic of Competition

Christianity and the Sport Ethic

It is common these days to have elite athletes openly and enthusiastically profess their Christian faith. But many scholars and theologians have argued that there is a serious contradiction between the value system (the ethic) of elite sport and that of Christianity. Shirl Hoffman (1992) points out that Christianity promotes "an ethic that places a premium on the Christian distinctives of submitting ends to means, product to process, quantity to quality, caring for self to caring for others" (p. 122). The ethos of sport, on the other hand, he says, emphasizes "the use of strength, speed, and power to push human limits and aggressively dominate opponents in the quest of victories and championships" (Coakley 2001, p. 94). According to Canadian professor of religious studies Brian Aitken (1992), competitive sport involves "an inordinate desire to win in an absolute sense, a desire to dominate, to obliterate, to wipe out the opponent . . . a desire to achieve a vindictive triumph over the opposition" (p. 239). Hoffmann, therefore, asks the question: "Can the mind of Christ co-exist with the killer instinct?"

> Sport, which celebrates the myth of success, is harnessed to a theology that consistently stresses the importance of losing. Sport, which symbolizes the morality of self-reliance and teaches the just rewards of hard work, is used to propagate a theology dominated by the radicalism of grace ("The first shall be last and the last first"). Sport, a microcosm of meritocracy, is used to celebrate a religion which says all are unworthy and undeserving. (Hoffman, 1992, p. 122)

Stevenson (1991, 1997) investigated these issues by means of in-depth, biographical interviews with a number of Canadian elite athletes; all professing Christians, associated with the Athletes in Action Christian organization at Canadian universities, and who were or recently had been members of a Canadian national team, a professional team, or a college team. These athletes were committed to their sport and clearly valued the experiences and rewards associated with it. But they had also experienced significant problems in trying to live by the normative values of the competitive sport culture. They saw these normative values as being:

1. **The importance of winning:** As athletes they knew that they were expected to strive to win at all costs, to be willing to do anything to achieve success—even to put up with playing with pain and injury if it meant they or their team might win. However, they struggled with this—was winning *really* this important? Was it *really* worth all this stress and the significant possibility of serious, even permanent, injuries?

2. **The importance of social status:** They understood and appreciated that success in sport brings popularity and status, and they had enjoyed these. Yet at the same time, they questioned the continual need to be re-affirming their statuses—they questioned an ethic that continually asked: What have you done for us today? They questioned the need to be continually "paying the price" in dedication, obedience, loyalty, and sacrifice of self in a sport system that jettisoned the worn-out and unworthy without a moment's thought or regret.

3. **Relationships with coach and team:** They realized that contemporary sports were predicated on a hierarchical authority structure—with the coach at the pinnacle of power and obedience as the proper response of all those under him or her. But they struggled with some of the consequences of this power hierarchy, and struggled with the expectations of blind obedience—especially in situations when their own self-interest conflicted with that of the team. They realized that they were supposed to be pleased when a teammate scored a last-minute goal or made a fantastic save, but what if that player was playing in their position?

4. **Relationships with opponents:** They understood the need to get "psyched up" to play another team or to compete in an event. But they struggled with the apparent need to see their opponents as "the enemy." According to Coakley (2001), the competitive sport ethic sees competition as "battles in which the opposition should be intimidated, punished and defeated" (p. 490)—and they had some difficulties with this approach.

5. **Expectations of others:** They appreciated the attention that being an elite athlete brought with it, but they had some difficulties with the expectations that others had of them as "athletes"—the expectations of how they were supposed to behave, the possibilities of now being thought "stuck-up" or "too good for old friends," and so on. They struggled with trying to juggle all of these conflicting expectations.

As a consequence of these difficulties with the ethic of competitive sport, some athletes experienced crises—they spoke of the stress they felt, the injuries they suffered, the strained relationships with other non-athletic friends, the difficulties with their school work, and so on.

Some of these problems became so severe that the athletes were sometimes led to withdraw from their sports for a while. And some were able to return only into a less competitive environment. Others spoke of their need to search for some deeper meaning in their sports involvements. The sport experience was supposed to make them feel good, successful, and fulfilled—yet they reported feeling only emptiness, unhappiness, and struggle. Was this all there was?

Living as a Christian and as an Athlete

If these are the consequences of the clash between the ethic of elite, competitive sport and the values of Christianity, how do professing Christian athletes survive? How do those athletes, who explicitly proclaim their faith by pointing to the sky, or grouping together in public prayer after the game, reconcile the contradictions sufficiently to allow them to continue to compete and yet also feel that they are living out their faith? Stevenson (1991, 1997) examined these questions by asking probing questions of the same Canadian elite athletes; in addition, Dunn and Stevenson (1998) also asked similar questions of a number of non-elite hockey players in a church hockey league in an Eastern Canadian city, once more by means of in-depth interviews (see Box 14.5).

Among both the elite and non-elite athletes, there were those individuals who dealt with the contraction between value systems of their faith and of their sports by simply either ignoring it, or by compartmentalizing their sport and their faith. Some athletes said that when they were at church they were "Christian," but in hockey, they were hockey players and "left their Christianity in the locker room." They said, "When you're in Rome, you do as the Romans do!"

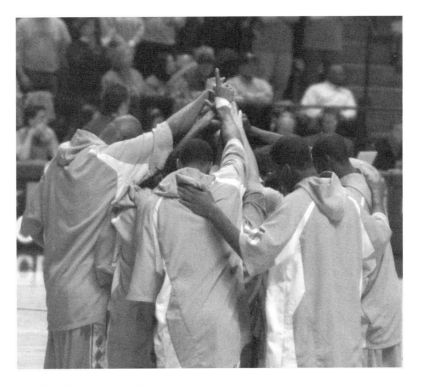

Prayer huddle after a basketball game.

Michelle Donahue Hillison/Shutterstock

Box 14.5   The Three Approaches Used by Christian Athletes in Playing Elite Sport

Stevenson's (1991, 1997) and Dunn and Stevenson's (1998) three groups of Canadian elite and non-elite athletes who were also professing Christians seemed to approach their sports in different ways. One group compartmentalized, or kept separate, their faith and their sport; as Harry said: "I had problems after I became a Christian trying to integrate my faith and my sport. I didn't know how to do that . . . It's still hard because it's like a habit that's been developed where, this is your spiritual life [and] this is your athletic life." Brad agreed: "It just says 'Thou shall not kill', it doesn't say you can't beat someone up . . . I've never had a problem with it because I've never related it. Like I've played sport all my life and I was a Christian all my life, but I never really related it."

A second group of Christian athletes accepted the values of the sport ethic but tried to play in as "Christian" a manner as possible; as Mike said: "You can play a game full-out, that's full contact [where] you hit people, and still have a Christian attitude, because that's part of the game. The other team knows that that's what's happening to them, and they know they're going to get hit." But others, like Alex, worried that in trying to live out his Christianity he had lost his tenacity to win or his willingness to hurt others if necessary. "It's a constant battle" said Alex, "because to really excel [in soccer], [you] use many different methods of achieving things that are not right. There's so many things you do that are against the rules, that you do when the ref's not looking to better your advantage in a situation. . . . I feel awful afterwards but there's things that you do that are very acceptable in the soccer community. And it's like, where do I draw the line?"

The third group of Christian athletes experienced considerable difficulty in continuing their careers as elite athletes because they were constantly conscious of conflicts between their faith and their sporting practices. What this meant for Ken was putting sport "into perspective": "Being a Christian—you have to put your sports into perspective, because it is just part of your life and it's not the main focus of your life anymore." These athletes spoke of their need now to "refocus on their priorities," and to determine which goals were worth pursuing and which were not. Julie remembered: "I said to God many times, Oh Lord, if you don't want me playing, it's fine. You know, I can accept that." But, this withdrawal process was not easy. For some athletes there was a sense of loss; as Hobie said, "I couldn't even look at basketball for a year. I couldn't go to the games. I couldn't do anything." But for others, such as Joe, there was some contentment in following his faith: "All I can do is try my best, and if it works out, great! If not, I really trust the Lord to give me something different. So it really gives you such a peace."

Other athletes admitted that since they really did not know how to integrate their faith into the rest of their lives, it really was not much of a problem. Then there were other elite and non-elite athletes who were more pragmatic: they accepted the dominance of the sport ethic when they were playing their sport—aggression, dominance, "it's all part of the game," they said—but within that context, they tried to play the games as "Christianly" as possible. That is, they tried as much as possible to obey the rules of the game, not to foul unnecessarily, not to deliberately hurt an opponent, and so on. Some took on an approach to their game in which they played "for Christ" and tried to give Him 100 percent of their effort, strength, and will. Ironically, this meant that they now tried to win even more avidly—only this time, "for Christ"! One of their rationales was that with success came the chance to evangelize—people will listen to winners, so winning would give them a chance to speak to others about their faith.

The final group of elite and non-elite athletes were those who were seriously committed to living out their Christian faith in all aspects of their lives—including in their sports. These athletes had considerable difficulties in accommodating their Christian values with the expectations of their sports, whether elite or non-elite. So they tried to put their sports "into perspective," and tried not to let their athletic goals and priorities take over their lives. Most of these athletes reported that they eventually had to withdraw from their sports—at least at the elite levels. They struggled with these decisions, but felt that it was the only way that they could remain true to their beliefs.

Critiques of Evangelical Christianity's Use of Sport

One of the more obvious, contemporary examples of the relationship between sport and Christianity is the highly visible use of sport and sport figures by Evangelical Christian organizations (such as Athletes in Action, Sports Ambassadors, Sports Outreach America) as a means of attracting audiences to their cause and their message. It is the marketing of Evangelical Christianity through the medium of sport—Brian Aitken (1993) calls it "the selling of Jesus." As Oral Roberts once commented, "Sports are becoming the Number One interest of people in America. For us to be relevant we had to gain the attention of millions of people in a way they would understand" (Coakley, 2001, p. 470). Such organizations often use high-profile, professional sports "stars" as the headliners in their campaigns, the honey to attract the clientele that the organizers desire. These sports figures are introduced with great fanfare, and often give a short talk about their own journeys as sports heroes and as Christians, after which the event is then given over to the evangelists-proper, and the sports stars stay around to autograph baseballs or photographs or even Bibles.

Ladd and Mathisen (1999) have argued that this use of sport heroes in evangelism corresponds to American Evangelical Christianity's discovery of marketing techniques as means of reaching the non-evangelical masses. They (and others; for example, Flake, 1992) have characterized this use of sport as a return to, or a revitalization of, muscular Christianity. But if one looks at this phenomenon more closely, it seems clear that there is little about this contemporary use of sport as a marketing tool that is reminiscent of the original tenets of muscular Christianity and its desire to build an exemplary Christian character.

In fact, there has been some substantial criticism of this use of sport and sport heroes as tools of evangelism by such Christian organizations. Aitken (1993) and Hoffman (1992), for example, have each offered a number of such criticisms. Aitken first speaks of the tendency (as he sees it) of such organizations to be opportunistic toward their "star" recruits from the world of sport—he is critical of the way they use them during their periods of popularity but seem to discard them once their public profile becomes diminished. There is, he argues, little in the way of pastoral care in the mission of such organizations, and this is his second criticism. Although people, including athletes, often come to the evangelistic events seeking practical help with life problems, the sports organizations, in Aitken's view, offer them very limited resources— and these tend to be almost exclusively religious remedies, based on a deep-seated belief that faith heals all ills. His third criticism has to do with the inordinate emphasis such organizations place on their statistics—the number of attendees on a given night, the number who "came to Christ," and so on—numbers that, Aitken argues, tend often to be falsely inflated. Obviously, as products of a marketing emphasis, these are the important outcomes, the organization's "return on investment"—appropriate terms and emphasis in the business world, but how appropriate in the "spiritual" world?

Both Hoffman and Aitken are concerned about the sometimes implicit, sometimes explicit ideological messages conveyed in the Evangelical Christian literature and preaching. Aitken is critical of the fundamentalist ideology the organizations tend to embrace—an acceptance of Old Testament morality, conservative politics, and a belief in the "traditional family"—which tends to glorify the "American way of life" and its emphasis on success, conspicuous consumption, obedience to authority, the nuclear family, and right-wing politics. At the same time, Hoffman is concerned about evangelical organizations' deliberate ignoring of social issues, such as racism, gender discrimination, violence and brutality, and especially these social issues in the sport context. There are a number of moral and ethical issues that arise in elite, competitive sport that need to be faced, and about which judgments need to be reached. But Evangelical Christian organizations seem to prefer to concentrate on the evangelistic potential of sport and either whitewash or do not deign to face some of its moral complexities. Indeed, Hoffman says, "when sport is harnessed to the evangelistic enterprise, evangelicals become as much endorsers of the myths reinforced by popular sport as they do of the Christian gospel" (1992, p. 121)—and thus have as much a stake in confirming the "goodness" of sport, and ignoring the "problems," as do the sports promoters themselves.

Aitken, Hoffman, and other writers have also been critical of an approach to competition endorsed by evangelicals called, variously, "Total Release Performance" or "Praise Performance." The idea is that your performance is an act of love toward God, and so you should always put everything you have into it—your effort, attention, strength, determination—everything, 100 percent! In this way, so the Evangelical Christian argument goes, you are expressing to God your gratitude for everything He has done for you. As one of the Canadian athletes in Stevenson's (1991) research explained,

> Because my purpose was to glorify God by using my body, I found that as I began to practise that I was a freer person in my gymnastics. No longer was I competing to make my place on the team or for my scholarship or for my coach or even for myself, but I was competing for Christ, and Christ was the only one in the stands . . . . And so the only way I could fail in Christ was if I didn't try my best . . . . So from that perspective it helped because I knew that I was giving my best, and that was 100% of what I had, and so that was good enough. And even if I didn't then I could just ask for forgiveness and just move on and try to do better next time. (p. 251)

This all sounds rather positive and laudable, but as Aitken points out, one of the implications of such an approach is that any instance of losing must mean that the athlete was in fact *not* giving 100 percent, not trying as hard as they could, not obeying the coach as they should. Another implication is that in this way almost anything can become sanctified—if you are using your talents to the best of your ability, "for God," then that's all you have to be concerned about. Even hitting an opponent as hard as you can becomes an act of worship and so is approved. "I'm going to hit you guys with all the love I have in me," said Rich Saul, a professional football player (Hoffman, 1992, p. 118). Taken to its logical conclusion, one could make a similar argument for robbery, or murder, or even prostitution—if you are doing it to the very best of your ability, then that's all you have to be concerned about. Be the best possible murderer or prostitute that you can be—"for God." Clearly, this makes little sense. There must be some prior, moral, Christian evaluation of the appropriate fit of the activity itself. But, it seems that Evangelical Christian organizations that use sport and sport figures would rather turn a blind eye to the problems and contradictions inherent in elite, competitive sport—where, as Hoffman (1992) points out, "aggression is vented, old scores are settled, number one taken care of, [and] where the discourteous act looms" (p. 114).

CONCLUSIONS

So, what have we learned? We now have an appreciation of just how complex the relationship has been between religion, on the one hand, and sport, games, and physical recreations, on the other hand. We can see how the close integration of religion and games in earlier cultures gave way in early Christianity to a fundamental distrust of anything to do with the physical body—a distrust that could be modified only by reference to an argument of the "usefulness" of certain forms of physical activity; an approach we see in the case of the Puritans and their attitudes toward sports, games, and physical pastimes. This rationale of "usefulness" was seen as particularly appropriate for the application of the ideas of muscular Christianity to the playing of sport. Sport, it was argued, is an excellent arena in which a desirable Christian and manly character could be both demonstrated *and* developed. Sport, then, was justified as a superb means of "building character," and so was able to thrive and develop in late-nineteenth and early twentieth-century society. As Bishop William T. Manning declared in 1925, "Clean, wholesome, well-regulated sport is a most powerful agency for true and upright living. . . . True sport and true religion should be in the closest touch and sympathy. . . . A well played game of polo or of football is in its own way as pleasing to God as a beautiful service of worship in the Cathedral" (Willis & Wettan, 1977, p. 196).

The contemporary relationship between sport and Christianity also appears to be predicated on the theme of "usefulness." The present use of sport and sports heroes by Evangelical Christian organizations is based upon the attractiveness of both to those segments of the population that the organizations are trying to draw to their meetings and rallies—primarily young men. However, as we have seen, this relationship is fraught with problems—of contradictory values, of the lack of pastoral care toward these athletes, and of the turning-of-a-blind-eye by these organizations to some of the ongoing problematic practices in elite, competitive sport.

So, what holds in the future for this relationship? Will Evangelical Christianity continue to find it "useful" to use sport and sports heroes in its campaigns, or will the excesses of high-profile, mass-spectator, commercialized sport eventually prove too much even for these most pragmatic of organizations? Will elite athletes continue to find such apparent succour and comfort in their faiths that they will continue to express it publicly, or will the realities of the inherent contradictions between the values and beliefs of Christianity and those of elite sport eventually prove too much for even the most committed of athletes? And will the value of "usefulness" continue to be the supreme justification in Evangelical Christianity that it currently appears to be, or will some other rationale supplant it—say, the rationale of "grace"; that is, "the fundamental Christian doctrine which teaches that humankind was secured by God in an act of unmerited favour" (Hoffman, 1992, p. 122), or possibly a rationale of "the divine spark called play . . . [the] celebration of humanity's status in the divine order" (Hoffman, 1992, p. 122)? Only time will tell.

CRITICAL THINKING QUESTIONS

1. Religion was at the core of the Olympic Games in Ancient Greece; discuss the role that religion plays in the modern Olympic Games, considering all aspects of the games from the opening ceremonies to the closing ceremonies.
2. Discuss the extent to which the attitudes of the Puritans (in all their complexity) toward games and physical recreations are still represented in the attitudes toward sports and games of contemporary leaders in church, school, and city.
3. Can sport itself be a "religion"? Discuss the issues surrounding this controversy and identify the set of arguments that makes most sense to you.
4. Describe examples of the use of talismans and ritual behaviours in church ceremonies and in sports. Discuss the similarities and the differences between these uses of talismans and ritual behaviours, and compare their purposes in each social setting.
5. How easy is it to live up to your beliefs and ideals in highly stressful and competitive situations? Discuss this issue and provide examples from your own experiences in such social situations, in particular those involving competitive sport.

6. Choose a sport (such as golf, football, swimming, hockey) or choose a level of sport (such as intra-murals, high school, local recreational league, national championships) and try to identify which ideas from muscular Christianity are still present or identifiable in this sport or level of sport.
7. Some writers have offered criticisms of the use of sport and high-profile sports stars by Evangelical Christian organizations. Choose a Christian sports organization and discuss its use of sport and sports stars in its evangelical missions and events.

SUGGESTED READINGS

Dunn, R., & Stevenson, C. L. (1998). The paradox of the church hockey league. *International Review for the Sociology of Sport, 33*, 131–41.

Guttmann, A. (1978). *From ritual to record: The nature of modern sports*. New York: Columbia University Press.

Higgs, R. J. (1995). *God in the stadium: Sports and religion in America*. Lexington, KY: University of Kentucky Press.

Hoffman, S. J. (1992). *Sport and religion*. Champaign, IL: Human Kinetics.

Ladd, T., & Mathisen, J. A. (1999). *Muscular Christianity: Evangelical Protestants and the development of American sport*. Grand Rapids, MI: Baker Books.

Stevenson, C. L. (1991). The Christian-athlete: An interactionist-developmental analysis. *Sociology of Sport Journal, 8*, 362–79.

Stevenson, C. L. (1997). Christian athletes and the culture of elite sport: Dilemmas and solutions. *Sociology of Sport Journal, 14*, 241–62.

WEB LINKS

The National Christian College Athletic Association
http://www.thenccaa.org
General information about NCCAA events, mission and outreach, and member institutions.

The Fellowship of Christian Athletes
http://www.fca.org
Information about the FCA organization, resources that are available, and information specific to students and to adults.

Athletes in Action
http://www.athletesinaction.org
Information about the mission of AIA, the events they host, and their programs.

The Young Men's Christian Association
http://www.ymca.net
The history of the YMCA, its mission, its programs, and its local offices.

Hockey Ministries International
http://www.hockeyministries.org
General information about HMI and a list of the camps it offers.

Motor Racing Outreach
http://www.go2mro.com
Provides a variety of links, gift ideas, as well as the teams and drivers involved in this ministry.

Superstitions Among Hockey Players
http://www.mcq.org/societe/hockey/pages/aasuperstitions_1.html
Provides examples of the superstitions of NHL players.

CHAPTER 15

PERSPECTIVES ON CANADIAN SPORT FUTURES: WAYS TO THINK AHEAD

Dwight Zakus

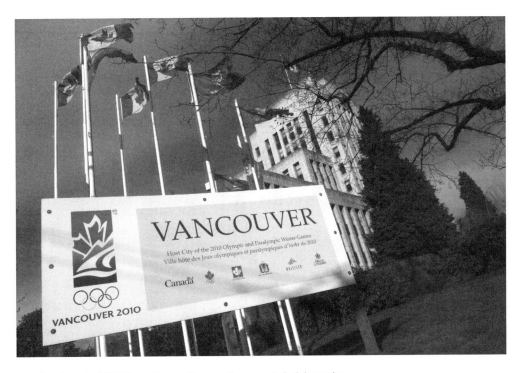

Canadians have the 2010 Winter Olympic Games in Vancouver to look forward to.

Adam Brown/CP Images

Time present and time past
Are both perhaps present in time future,
And time future contained in time past.

T. S. Eliot, "Burnt Norton," *Four Quartets*

We drive into the future using only our rear view mirror.

Marshall McLuhan, Canadian media scholar

What does the future mean to you, a student in your twenties with most of your life ahead of you? Tomorrow is a near enough future to contemplate and deal with, but what will 5, 10, or more years bring? What will life be like when you are 30 years old, or 50 years old? Will you have a family? What careers will you have? What technology will be part of your future life? And how will new inventions, whatever they might be, affect that life? These are a few of the many questions that arise when considering the future.

Remembering back to my undergraduate student days, the future was the next weekend when I would play hockey and party. I now live in a future that I could not imagine back then. I have completed three university degrees, two certificates, taught high school for five years in Canada, and now live and work in Australia. My children are adults, one a university graduate. Back then, I saw my parents as "old" and unable to communicate. In some ways I can understand now how they felt, as there are current trends and music to which I do not relate. I am looking at how my retirement will unfold and whether I will have the health and money to enjoy it. The future concerns many other people and groups in the world, and not only me as an individual.

A number of social actors, soothsayers, fortune-tellers, statisticians, economists, and futurologists, some of whom work for formal organizations, have a role in studying and predicting the future. "Think tanks" exist in government departments and non-governmental organizations (NGOs) for this purpose. In many ways we want to know about the future to have control over our own lives. We all want happiness, prosperity, and wealth, and this is why we build pension funds and make investments. Or, maybe this action toward the future is foreign to you, because you have not yet embarked on a career. To a wide degree we want the future to be a better place and we want assurances that this will be the case. In many ways poet Robert Browning's saying "If a man's grasp cannot exceed his reach, what is a heaven for?" has salience.

Perhaps I sound like your parents, who have encouraged you to think about and plan for the future. Perhaps years ago they set aside money to ensure you could receive a university education. My parents' generation saw a university education as the way to a better life than they had lived. To have a child graduate from university was a status symbol. Your future was determined in the past.

So, why does the future matter? As a species, humans have a proclivity for long-term planning in the modern period. We plan to obtain the things we think will bring us happiness, prosperity, and wealth. I imagine that some of you have planned for the future. Formal organizations complete long-term planning by necessity; part of this planning comes out as policy. An example is the most recent Canadian Sport Policy, published in 2002. This policy declared that

> The Vision of the *Canadian Sport Policy* is to have, by 2012 a dynamic and leading edge sport environment that enables all Canadians to experience and enjoy involvement in sport to the extent of their abilities and interests and, for increasing numbers, to perform consistently and successfully at the highest competitive levels. (Sport Canada, 2006)

In all of this, it is human activity directed to the future conditions that is important. The scholars whose work you have studied in previous chapters are not predicting the future through the materials they present. Yet one might see much to make sense of today and tomorrow in what they write. Remember that today's events (social processes) are part of history once they occur. And history is the record of change in human social activities and structures.

Many would argue that the past is important to understanding the future. An old adage claims that to ignore the past can leave us doomed to repeating it. Canadian history does not provide the complete picture; however, based on current trends, and with some historical understanding, we can make some sense of the possible futures for Canadian sport.

This chapter will begin with a discussion of different conceptual approaches to understanding and predicting the future. Remember that these predictions relate to specific social changes, social actions, and particular value perspectives. An example follows each perspective. Following this, a discussion of general and specific sport futures is made. Here, data are presented that provide indications of potential future directions. In the third section, several structural changes are discussed in terms of the changes they hold for the future of sport.

PREDICTIONS AND ACTIONS ON AND IN THE FUTURE

There are different ways that people think about and predict the future. Each one includes ways of identifying future goals and ways of acting to achieve those goals. Each one also includes particular assumptions and values, and to some degree ideological positions. Three perspectives on the future are discussed in this section. Each perspective should be understood on its own while realizing that it has its own strengths and weaknesses.

Regardless of which perspective of the future you identify with most, I urge you to consider your own assumptions and values in thinking through all three (Malloy, Ross, & Zakus, 2004). By challenging your assumptions and values you engage in critical thinking—thinking that is fundamental to being educated and to making reasoned sense of current and future events. Further, the perspective that makes the most sense for you should also relate to your future goals and actions. For through the value framework basic to your mature thinking processes, you will come to hold a critical perspective on the world and on human action in that world. Often you have not been challenged to think about this perspective, what it means, or why you think and act in particular ways. A key goal of this chapter—and, indeed, this book—is to enhance your thinking, and ultimately your human action, about the world around you and your role in that world.

An Evolutionary View of Change

Many people understand change as an evolutionary process. That is, change occurs across time in some pattern of increasing size and complexity. By studying contemporary and past trends, we can foresee the future. Patterns are discovered cognitively or, more often, through elaborate statistical patterns that identify possible future trends so that estimates and prognoses can be made. In other words, change occurs within the context of the current situation in some iterative process. This perspective embraces a linear model of progress where future trends and events extend from past and present conditions. On the surface the future is positive and the scenarios identified will advance society. From this perspective, the future holds unlimited potential for all humankind; humans need only work hard and follow the dictates of those who are able to identify the appropriate trends to be able to achieve that potential.

Those embracing this pattern of understanding hold a conservative perspective. What is considered appropriate *should be* maintained in the future. Sport as it is currently structured, performed, organized, managed, and operated is the model to continue. Even with a number of tested indicators of the future, when change is necessary it is often a reactive rather than a proactive process. This seems a contradiction, but it is most often the case. To deal with change, "more" is needed. More money, more people, more or larger organizations, more marketing, more effectiveness, or more state intervention are seen as necessary. The issue is not with the current context and operation of sport, but with greater demands on and through sport.

People operating from this perspective will actually resist change. They wish to *conserve* what is (the status quo) and will do so actively. This is a central way in which change is dealt with. For example, Helen Lenskyj's discussion of the gender logic in sport in Chapter 6 overviews the way males have traditionally defined and operated sport, and how they seek to retain this position. Here the values, roles, and traditions in sport are espoused and the historical power enjoyed by men in sport is promoted as the way in which sport *should* or *must* continue.

From this perspective, change is often made in response to legislation, political correctness, or tokenism rather than something more meaningful. The expression "If it ain't broke, don't fix it" is espoused and indicates a gradual change within the context of the current structure, pattern, or operation of sport. The use of rational techniques such as statistical extrapolation is also employed in this context of change.

Information on sport in Canada presented in the second section of this chapter, from Statistics Canada and other research, indicates a decline in participation rates. Further discussion on this aspect of Canadian sport occurs later in the chapter. What can be said here is that a trend is evident; one that overall is not good for Canadian sport.

A Reformist View of Change

In Western history, many changes have been a response to the need for reform. Reformist approaches seek to improve the current state of human life, most often within existing social and power structures. Two long-standing social institutions led many reformist changes while actively retaining their power: the church, and the state. In both cases, some problematic or structural issues arose. As the structure and power relations within the church and state were challenged, those within these institutions responded to challenges to bring the situation back into line, albeit with different outcomes. We witness elements of the conservative approach in these changes, only with a distinction that some major or structural change was required.

One of these was the Protestant Reformation within the Christian church. Dissatisfaction with the power, economic, and social elements of the Catholic Church led Martin Luther in 1517 to challenge the Catholic Church's position by establishing the Protestant Church as a separate structural form to follow Christianity. Christianity was conserved, but within a new religious institutional framework. In this case, a new organization arose, one that reformed elements of the current religious structure in Europe—a major reformation of a key social institution.

In a second major reformation, the Canadian state, following Canada's poor results in the 1976 Montreal Olympics, finally recognized that Canada's sport structure needed reforming. Policy developed focusing on a new approach not only to funding athletes to prepare for major international competitions, but also to how sport was governed and managed (see Macintosh & Whitson, 1990). Canadian sport policy developed over time to deal with varying roles of sport in society. Initial policies sought to support and improve high-performance international sport outcomes, while a parallel recreation policy dealt with general sport participation. The current Canadian Sport Policy (2002) seeks to balance the social-capital aspects of sport with elite athlete achievements.

In other words, Canadian sport policy was reformed over time, not radically changed from one policy to the next. The nature of sport was not questioned. However, the nature of the circumstances in which sport operated was questioned. What resulted was more of a reformation of the current sport-governing model and not of the traditional model of sport governance. However, as reform was instituted, many further major structural and operational changes followed.

A major example of this type of change resulted from the disqualification of Ben Johnson during the 1988 Seoul Olympic Games. The resultant Dubin Inquiry led to many reforms within the current sport structure, but not to a wholesale change in that structure. As a result of this inquiry, global issues pertaining to doping in sport received greater attention. This led to many institutional changes within the structure of Canadian sport. Canada set in place organizations to test for and control the use of banned substances in sport. Educational programs were also developed. These changes led to Canada being acknowledged as a leader in this area and were partially responsible for the World Anti-Doping Agency (WADA) choosing Montreal as its world headquarters.

In these examples, the principles of equality and democracy were affronted. The playing field was not level and it was believed that it must somehow be made more equal. It did not matter that athletes of the former Eastern Bloc nations were state employees and therefore were funded, or that they were systematically using banned performance-enhancing substances and practices to improve their performance. As Jennings (1998) noted, under the surveillance practices of certain socialist state governments and the benign attitudes of many sport leaders at that time, these practices were indifferently controlled and therefore implicitly condoned. Those struggling to remain amateurs (unpaid labour) and those choosing not to use banned substances or practices were competing in an unequal context. Reforms were seen as the appropriate response.

A Radical View of Change

The most strident approach to change is identified as the radical approach. Here, the fundamental understanding of sport—its structure, power relations, and operations—is questioned. Not only questioned, but also seen as being in need of wide-ranging fundamental change. That is, current definitions and structures of sport are problematic and are not fulfilling the values and goals they purport, so change is demanded.

At the heart of this approach is action directed at rectifying the inequalities. Most often these inequalities relate to capitalism and the resultant class-based society. The social matters identified in all of the preceding chapters of this book indicate this focus. Issues of power differences, market operations, and tacit inequality are central within this type of social structure. Change proposed within this approach demands a fundamental change of society, a breaking down of the inequalities inherent in capitalism. There are examples where this change followed a revolutionary pattern—Russia in 1917, China in the 1950s—however, in most Western societies this approach was not followed.

A number of activist groups have worked to push for positive social change and a better future for Canadians. One group was the "Bread, Not Circuses" coalition of Toronto-based community groups (Lenskyj, 2000). Their focus was on a number of social issues (housing, poverty, social programs) and action directed against the City of Toronto's bids for the 1996 and 2008 Olympic Games. This coalition felt that funds directed to hosting the Olympics were immoral and misdirected, because so many social issues remained unresolved. In the end, the bids went ahead but were not successful. Other activist groups such as "Creative Resistance" and "Impact on Community Coalition" carry on organized resistance to Canadian bidding/ hosting of Olympic Games.

To fundamentally change the social and economic basis of Canadian society is an unlikely scenario. What, then, is possible? A first response has been made by the state to attempt to rectify the inequalities. Welfare-state programs (see Chapters 7, 8, 11, and 12) are one response, but not a radical one. Second, individual social action through protest and lobbying is indicated. In Canada, women's groups pushed change through in both general and sport-specific legislation by more radical means such as pressure groups (lobbying government) and open protest activities (large public demonstrations and marches).

In the end, however, both of these actions led to reformist change, not the radical change behind political protest. A widely used social concept to explain why this lesser type of change occurs is "hegemony." The concept of hegemony is indicated when particular groups in society are able to maintain a wider status quo. Hegemony is used to understand how dominant coalitions of social groups, including dominant members of the economic, political, social, religious, and sport groups and organizations, actively seek to impose their ideas as the key ones in a society. Through this imposition of dominant ideas other ideas are reduced and marginalized. The dominant groups are also able to co-opt the ideas of subordinate groups in society. In fact, they actively seek to change the thinking of people toward the dominant ideas. This reduces the opposition to radical changes in society, and the world. Throughout this book you have read about power relations and the social action used to maintain the status quo. In fact, all change is difficult, as humans seek constancy and stability in life. To actively seek change is the domain of the few, rather than the majority. Having said this, there are indicators that we employ to identify possible futures. The following section describes these indicators.

CURRENT TRENDS

Examining historical data is one way in which we use the past to foresee what might happen in the future. Different social actors (politicians, economists, academics) and institutions (governments, privately funded think tanks, NGOs—for example the United Nations) extrapolate from historical data to identify possible future trends. For example, stock markets and government departments use techniques based on past statistical information to evaluate what prices, economic activity, or other social conditions might be and how they might be addressed. In this we caution that American author Mark Twain's comment of there being "lies, damned lies, and statistics" could be operational. While such information is helpful and reasonably accurate, human lives are not predictable. Under neo-liberalism, however, the numbers guide legislation, policy development and analysis, and program outcomes. They cannot be avoided, only understood within their limits to inform.

Another way in which the past is used is to look for patterns. Often in human history, patterns have repeated themselves (with some obvious inherent differences). For example, labour disputes in Major League Baseball (MLB) have a long history, one that has been repeated in other major professional sports (as in the most recent NHL lockout season of 2004–05). Again, this is not to say that history *will* repeat itself, but certainly similar circumstances might lead to similar future events. What does this indicate for sport?

Several demographic characteristics can provide information on what the future of Canadian sport *might* be. This includes population growth and aging; immigration as a percentage of population; degree of urbanization; and sport participation rates. Each of these is discussed in the following sections.

Population Growth and Aging

Canada is an aging country with a low birth rate, and consequently seeks immigrants to continue to grow. Population growth was approximately 1 percent per annum between 1996 and 2001, and the population was projected to increase by less than 1 percent to 2006 (Statistics Canada, 2002).

The "baby-boomer" post–World War II age group (those born between 1946 and 1965) is seen as a key social indicator for several issues into the early twenty-first century. As this cohort ages and the size of the population to support their retirement, health needs, and workforce inputs becomes disproportionately smaller, several economic and social issues will accrue. In 2001 the baby boomers were aged 36 to 55 years. According to 2001 population projections, this age group totals approximately 32 percent of the total population and will remain around that level until 2006, when the first part of the cohort reaches retirement age. The proportion of seniors (65+ years of age) is projected to rise to 23 percent of the population by 2041, up from 12 percent in 1995 (compare with Foot, 1989).

With regard to sport, we ask which sports will continue to have participants and will produce national- and international-calibre athletes. Likewise, how much will certain sport spectator markets grow or be maintained? Sport Canada (1998) reported that 38.3 percent of the 55-plus age group felt that age was a factor in their non-participation in sport. A further 23.6 percent reported that health and injury kept them from sport (these figures for females are 40 percent and 24 percent, respectively). With female life expectancy higher than that of males, who currently represent the majority of participants in sport, the overall figure for the age-55+ female participation rate might further decline. The above two factors, added to general social and economic pressures such as lower household disposable income; increasing costs of sport equipment, registration, and membership fees; limited leisure time; and the availability of numerous other competing leisure activities (e.g., home computers, Internet access, and increased grandchild care) point to significant economic impacts on sport, sport participation, and the management of sport in the future (Sport Canada, 1998, pp. 60–2).

Immigration

Immigration to Canada will remain a significant factor in the makeup of the country in the future. Immigration was a significant factor in the settling of Canada, and it remains a key to Canada's population growth. Since 1986, immigration to Canada contributed to 48 to 51 percent of Canada's population growth. In the 1996 census, immigrants made up 17 percent of the population (Boyd & Vickers, 2000). Throughout the 1980s, immigrants increasingly came from places other than the United States, the United Kingdom, and Europe, and in 1996 people from places such as Asia, the subcontinent, Africa, and the Caribbean made up 48 percent of all immigrants (Boyd & Vickers, 2000).

With an increasing proportion of the population being not of Anglo-American, European, or Canadian origins, what will be the effect on sport in Canada? Will these new people follow Canada's traditional sports? What sports do they bring with them? What are the implications on sport facilities and state subsidies as a result of this shift? Are the newcomers sport spectators? For which sports? Will they become socialized as Canadians and support Western sport as participants and spectators? For example, at the World Basketball Championships in Toronto in 1994, the Greek and Italian teams received huge ovations when they played, but the Canadian team did not. This prompted Canadian coach Ken Shields to ask, "Where are the Canadians?"

These questions point to changes that will influence the future of Canadian sport. Many immigrants will come to live more as Canadians and will participate actively and as spectators in Canadian sport, rather than holding on to the identity of their or their ancestors' country of origin. It is difficult to determine how many immigrants will come to cheer for Canadian athletes in major international competitions, or who and how many will be representative athletes for Canada. Further, their influences in the social construction of sport indicate that change will occur as they bring with them their backgrounds in the structure and operation of sport, providing a rich mosaic of new sport interests. For example, Indian, Pakistani, and Caribbean cricket players and a multitude of citizens who follow the "world game" of football (soccer) point to a future for these sports in Canada, not to mention the folk games and sports of new immigrants. Also, as they come from nations with different or non-existent volunteering backgrounds, will they become part of this important feature of Canadian life and sport? This also points to the notion that Canada's cultural pluralism, enshrined in the federal constitution and national policy, and indicated in the concept of Canada being a cultural mosaic, will accommodate a wider panoply of sports.

Urbanization

In 1931, 54 percent of the population lived in urban centres; that percentage rose to 70 per-cent in 1961 and 78 percent in 1996 (Statistics Canada, 2002). Most of this population is located along the United States border. These statistics have implications for sport in the pro-vision of teams, leagues, and facilities in both urban and rural settings. In rural settings there are fewer children, youths, and adults to populate teams or leagues for competition. It is increasingly difficult to have separate teams and leagues for boys and girls. The contraction of the hinterland has a considerable effect on sport. Many villages and towns have disappeared, and as they disappear so too do the school playing fields, the local arena, and other recreational facilities (although the disappearance of schools and sport facilities might also be a cause). This then becomes a "catch-22" situation as there are few or no facilities available to allow sport participation, too few participants to warrant demand, and too few taxpayers to fund the facil-ities, and further decline occurs (see Gruneau & Whitson, 1993, pp. 205–10).

Conversely, growing urban populations and the effects of urban sprawl increase the pressures on the provision of teams, leagues, coaches, and managers for sport. Rising population also puts greater demands on parks, pools, arenas, stadiums, tracks, and other sport facilities in urban set-tings. Increasingly, green, public open space for recreation and sport is reduced or limits are placed on this space by urban sprawl and reduced state budgets. Both aspects, the human and the matériel, put pressure on local and provincial state provision of sport. Add to this the demands for large, publicly funded stadiums and arena facilities for professional or elite sport, and the result is further pressure on the state (at all levels, in this case). An interesting paradox is evident here as this claim is not supported by a 1998 Sport Canada document, which indicates that "the unavailability of sport facilities and programs ranked last among the reasons for non-participation" in sport (Sport Canada, 1998, p. 57)—suggesting that current provision is not a problem.

Nonetheless, urbanization is a double-edged sword, for the state has to balance financial and political pressures to ensure that Canadians are continually able to access sport. Local, provincial, and national sport organizations also are under pressure to find and train athletes, coaches, managers, and administrators for both rural and urban sport. These factors provide major challenges for those in government and sport.

Sport Demographics

To understand the statistical trends in sport, two documents must be examined. The first is the above-mentioned 1998 Sport Canada document (and its earlier 1994 Highlights), which iden-tifies trends for the 15-plus age groups. The second is Kremarik's (2000) summary of sport trends for 5- to 14-year-olds derived from the 1998 General Social Survey (GSS). Between the two, observations can be made about the total Canadian population.

Both documents define sport participation to include those who engage in a particular sport at least once a week, but do not include activities for recreation that might be defined as sport by some people (e.g., walking, aquafitness, bicycling, body building, hiking, jogging, skateboarding). The data presented here are therefore limited as the separation between sport as recreation (schoolyard softball) and sport in an organized league (a formal community softball league) is questionable. It does, however, raise the question of whether sport participation can be studied and understood only in the context of formal (usually adult-organized) teams and leagues.

Kremarik (2000) noted that 2.2 million children aged 5 to 14 (54 percent of this age range) participated in some form of sport in 1998. Further, nearly half of this total participated in more than one sport. He also indicated that soccer (31 percent), swimming (24 percent), hockey (24 percent), baseball (22 percent), and basketball (13 percent) were the top five of ten sports this age group actively participated in (Kremarik, 2000, p. 21). While this article does not have as many data as the Sport Canada publication, it does provide insight as to why 5- to 14-year-olds are involved in sport.

Kremarik (2000) did further statistical analysis of the GSS data to understand the degree to which parental involvement in sport and family income affect sport participation among this group. His findings confirm that children from families where at least one parent is active in a sport or is a volunteer (coach, manager, administrator) are more likely to participate. There is some evidence here to support socialization theory. This is important for the future of sport as it indicates that participants, support for particular sports, and volunteers to support the whole sport system are being generated.

As noted in Chapter 1, socialization in and via sport is significant. Think back on your own involvement and history in sport, reflecting particularly on the socialization aspect. This also raises a number of interesting questions. What will new immigrants bring to Canadian sport? Will their children be socialized in and through sport—and if so, how? Will traditional Canadian sports continue or will new sports rise to prominence? How well will volunteerism work under these conditions? More simply stated, how will future generations of Canadian children and youth become participants and future volunteers in sport?

Another key variable affecting sport participation in the 5 to 14 age group was family income. Offord, Lipman, and Duku (1998) suggested that income is a barrier for children from lower-income households. Analysis by Kremarik (2000, pp. 22–23) found participation rates were influenced by household income. For example, those in households with incomes of $80,000 and over had a 72.9-percent participation rate; $40,000 to $80,000 a 62.5-percent rate; and household incomes of less than $40,000 a 49.4-percent rate. Further, children and youths from two-parent households where both parents were active in sport and with family incomes of $80,000 were 12 times more likely to be in sport than those in a home with an inactive parent and family income of less than $20,000 (Kremarik, 2000, p. 23). Again, the current class structure of Canadian society and of sport in our society contains inequalities that are detrimental to wider participation and the overall development of individuals and society.

Sport Canada data for those aged 15 and older indicate that participation rates have fallen and the participation rates of each gender are widening (see Table 15.1). Similar results were found in each GSS for the influence of income on sport participation, level of education attainment, labour force participation, and mother tongue. An interesting difference between

Table 15.1   Active Sport Participation of Canadians, 15+ Years Old

	1992		1998		
	000s	%	000s	%	Net Change
Total	9,594	45.1	8,309	34.2	−10.9
Males	5,454	52.3	5,140	43.1	−9.2
Females	4,141	38.1	3,169	25.7	−12.4
15–18	1,185	76.8	1,121	68.2	−8.6
19–24	1,375	61.3	1,235	51.1	−10.2
25–34	2,483	52.8	1,781	38.6	−14.2
35–54	3,196	43.0	2,937	31.4	−11.6
55 and over	1,355	25.3	1,234	19.8	−5.5

Source: Sport participation in Canada. CH24-1/200-1E-IN. The Department of Canadian Heritage. Reproduced with the permission of the Minister of Public Works and Government Services Canada, 2006.

the two surveys was seen in the most popular sports. In the 1992 summary, the sports with most participants were hockey, baseball, volleyball, golf, and bowling. By 1998 the order had changed to golf, hockey, baseball, swimming, and basketball. The fact that participation rates for hockey were not the highest is interesting. Whether this is a shift in interest or a result of age demographics posits an interesting topic for further research.

By comparison, a Conference Board of Canada (2005) study provides interesting data on participation rates, although the age categories are slightly different. Table 15.2 provides additional information on active and volunteer participants and gender-related data. It is evident that active participation falls as age increases, which would be expected, while volunteering increases inversely until the late-50+ age groupings. It seems odd that the knowledge, interest, and involvement of older Canadians are not used more widely in the delivery of sport.

Another variable of interest for the future of sport noted in the Sport Canada report concerns participation rates in volunteer positions in coaching, administration, and officiating (see Table 15.3 and Table 15.4; see also Hall, Lasby, Gumulla, & Tryon, 2006). First, the number of female coaches has risen by 300 percent since the early 1990s, while the number of 15- to 18-year-olds who coach has doubled. These are strong positive signs for the future of sport in Canada. Levels of education and income held constant over the two surveys, with the number of indirect contributions rising with higher education and income levels.

Table 15.2   Active Sport Participation of Canadians, 16+ Years Old (percentage of total population in 2004)

	Active Participants	**Volunteers**	**Attendees**
By Gender			
Males	39.0	20.8	47.2
Females	23.4	15.9	43.8
By Age Group			
Under 20	67.2	27.6	63.8
20–29	53.7	23.3	56.0
30–39	42.5	27.1	62.7
40–49	33.3	28.9	58.7
50–59	29.6	18.8	50.0
60+ Years	26.1	7.2	41.1

Source: Strengthening Canada: The socio-economic benefits of sport participation in Canada. Conference Board of Canada. (2005). Downloaded from <www.conferenceboard.ca> on 16 September 2006.

Table 15.3   Indirect Involvement in Sport, Comparison of 1992 and 1998 (as a percentage of the total population)

	1992	**1998**	**Change**
Administration/helper	9.2	7.0	−2.2%
Referee	2.6	3.9	+1.3
Coach	3.9	7.1	+3.2
Spectator	23.9	31.5	+7.6

Source: Sport participation in Canada. (1998). CH24-1/2000-1. The Department of Canadian Heritage. Reproduced with the permission of the Minister of Public Works and Government Services Canada, 2006.

Spectatorship at amateur sport events is an interesting variable. The change through the 1990s was 8 percent. Of this, 55 percent of spectators were 15 to 18 years old, and a further 36 percent were 19 to 24 years old. What one can surmise from these figures is that the cohorts of late teens and young adults (who may also be parents) are more highly involved than those in the older age categories. As nearly 31 percent of the total population is involved in amateur sport, one can argue that socialization is occurring and future sport participants and spectators are being developed. This rate must be juxtaposed with that for elite professional and entertainment sport. Clearly there will be overlap between the two, but a comparison of live audience participation would be interesting.

We can compare this to data of the above-mentioned Conference Board of Canada study. That study found that nearly 13.7 million adult Canadians (defined as those 16 years and older), or 55 percent of all adults, took part in sport as active participants, volunteers, attendees, or some combination of these roles in 2004. Table 15.5 provides comparative data to

Table 15.4   Direct and Indirect Involvement in Sport (1998 figures)

	Thousands	%	Thousands	%	Thousands	%
Population aged 15 and over	24,260		11,937		12,323	
Regularly participate in sport	8,309	34.2	5,140	43.1	3,169	25.7
Through a club or organization	4,599	19.0	2,238	19.6	2,261	18.3
Competition and/or tournament	2,992	12.3	2,076	17.4	916	7.4
Coach	1,729	7.1	962	8.1	766	6.2
Referee/official/umpire	937	3.9	537	4.5	399	3.2
Administrator/helper	1,706	7.0	842	7.1	864	7.0
Spectator at amateur sport competition	7,651	31.5	4,040	33.8	3,611	29.3

Source: Based on data from the Statistics Canada General Social Survey, 1998.

Table 15.5   Activity of Canadian Adults in Sport, by Type of Participation (adult population)

	Number (percentage of total population)
Active participants only	1.821 million (7.3)
Volunteers only	249 thousand (1.0)
Attendees only	4.240 million (17)
Active participants and volunteers	299 thousand (1.2)
Active participants and attendees	3.068 million (12.3)
Volunteers and attendees	1.472 million (5.9)
Total for all three categories	2.569 million (10.3)
Total active participants	31%
Total volunteers	18.3%
Total attendees	45.5%
Total all types	54.9%

Source: Strengthening Canada: The socio-economic benefits of sport participation in Canada. Conference Board of Canada. (2005). Downloaded from <www.conferenceboard.ca> on 16 September 2006.

Table 15.4. However, those actively participating comprise only 7.3 percent of the adult population, evidence that we are more a nation of spectators than participants.

STRUCTURAL CHANGES AND THE FUTURE OF CANADIAN SPORT

This section looks at the larger or macro level of social structure to point to future issues in Canadian sport—there are many, as previous chapters have exhibited. In this chapter, only a few structural topics are addressed, but not necessarily the key ones. Sport is seen as a central feature of modern society and also as a cultural component of Canadian society. While it embraces a set of socially constructed activities and structures, sport must be understood in relation to the cultural elements that complete its place in those social activities and structures. Sport is a system of symbols and signs that define it beyond the definitions usually employed. Following the discussion on sport as a cultural component of Canadian society, we will focus on a few aspects of the underlying capitalist nature and operation of our society. Much that was presented in previous chapters makes note of this fact.

The nature of capitalism and the future of sport are inextricably intertwined, for the market base of our society is in a dialectical relationship with the cultural structures arising from that base. Capitalism as the economic engine of global society has been resilient and has adapted to pressures that might lead to its decline. Several scholars at different historical moments have predicted the end of capitalism, but this has not happened for several centuries. In predicting the future we encourage you to think of what sport might be like under such conditions (an economic system other than capitalism), even though this is not a likely scenario.

Sport in Canadian Culture

Most often sport is seen as a subcultural element of the general (that is, Canadian, regional) culture that embraces a series of its own subcultural elements (that is, within each type of sport, within sport teams and clubs, and within different sport organizations). With the implementation of the 1995 North American Free Trade Agreement (NAFTA), the question of Canadian sovereignty took on greater importance. Canada has always struggled to maintain a separate identity both culturally and economically in its relationship first with Britain and now the United States. As a colonial or dependent state, Canada had to define and protect its identity as a unique and separate nation. What, then, is this identity? Are we what former Prime Minister Brian Mulroney claimed: a nation that is culturally defined by hockey?

As noted in Chapter 12, Sport, Politics, and Policy, the state claimed sport to be a central, important feature of how Canadians see and understand themselves. To further emphasize this, in 1994 the federal government passed an act to recognize ice hockey (winter) and lacrosse (summer) as Canada's national sports (National Sports of Canada Act, Chapter N-16.7). These, of course, are symbolic elements of what partially defines Canada's cultural identity.

Culture has many definitions; however, language, common understandings, identifiable ways of living, symbols that point to a common identity (e.g., flag, anthem, currency, buildings, historic sites), and ways of thinking are seen as the key elements (see Chapter 1 in Gruneau & Whitson, 1993, for a discussion of this concept). If one thinks about what it is that makes being Canadian unique, one begins to make sense of culture. Culture is an important element of any society and comes to be protected by legislation and government bureaus.

In a previous section we noted that hockey no longer has the largest participant base, pointing out a unique cultural contradiction. Many arguments would arise over the place of hockey in defining "Canadianness" (see Kidd, 1970, and Metcalfe, 1987, for a wider discussion of this topic). For example, the 1972 Canada–USSR hockey series illustrates an absolute high of Canadian sport achievement. The dramatic late goal by Canada's Paul Henderson gave Canadians cause to celebrate both being Canadian and being the world power in hockey. Many of your parents and grandparents will remember fondly the pride and excitement in this moment.

For some time, Canada enjoyed supremacy in a series of Canada Cup victories. This position, however, has declined. Recent inconsistent outcomes in world, junior, and women's competitions, and pre-2002 Olympic Winter Games (OWG), have eroded Canada's position in world hockey and now threaten part of Canadian cultural identity. This naturally leads to the question of how relevant hockey is to all Canadians and how culturally reduced Canadians feel when defeated in various world hockey competitions (cf. Jackson, 1994) or, conversely, ecstatic when a Canadian athlete wins a gold medal in half-pipe snowboarding.

The most recent medal standings at the OWG for Canada were as follows: 1992 = ninth, 1994 = seventh, 1998 and 2002 = fourth, and 2006 = fifth. Yet the national mood appeared low as the men's hockey team finished second in 1992, fourth in 1994, and second in 1998. In Canada, the "home of hockey," anything less than a gold medal in men's ice hockey adversely affects the national mood. The gold-medal win by the men's team in the 2002 OWG led to euphoric celebrations throughout Canada, seemingly overriding achievements by other Canadian athletes (and especially of the women's ice hockey team). February 24, 2002, might become as revered to current youth and children as did the day Paul Henderson scored the series-winning goal in 1972. Both events reclaimed Canada's position as the best nation in world ice hockey, however suspect that claim might be in reality. It also seriously downplays the outstanding record of Canada's women's hockey teams as more focus is given to the men's teams in the media.

The Canadian women's team followed its 2002 gold medal in the Salt Lake City Games with an impressive run through the Torino OWG in 2006. They won the Olympic gold medal in the women's ice hockey tournament, outscoring their opponents by 46 goals to one. This restores them to the top of women's international hockey as they have won every world championship since this competition's inception in 1990 (with the exception of a silver medal in 2005). Because the women's national team has been superlative, the number of females playing hockey has increased significantly. In 1990, just over 8,100 girls and women played hockey. This number grew to 50,000 in 2001–02 and is now over 70,000 players. The number of girls' and women's teams has grown from 517 in 1990 to more than 2,600 during this same time period (Canadian Hockey Association, 2006).

Exactly how much sport contributes to Canadian identity is open to debate. There does seem to be some degree to which this correlation makes intuitive sense. For example, the success for Donovan Bailey and the men's 4 × 100m relay team gold medals in the 1996 Olympic Games, Sandra Schmirler's many curling victories, the Blue Jays 1992 World Series win, and, at the regional level, Grey Cup victories and parties add much to this identity. On the other hand, just as many Canadians can remember where they were when Canada defeated the former USSR in 1972, many also remember Ben Johnson's 100-metre race in the 1988 Seoul Olympics as an identifying moment. This later moment had less of the euphoria, and the sad outcome has had a long-term effect on the Canadian psyche. For good or bad, sport has come to occupy a central position in Canadian identity.

Canada's national and international teams have come to represent more than their own performances. Their successes and failures influence Canadians to different degrees. One does not have to be a fan or sport aficionado to revel in outcomes of local, regional, national, or international teams. Spontaneous crowd outbursts, flag waving, and euphoric cheering by the general population are expressions of nationalistic joy that is easily witnessed. As both fans and non-fans exhibit this behaviour, they are saying something important about being Canadian.

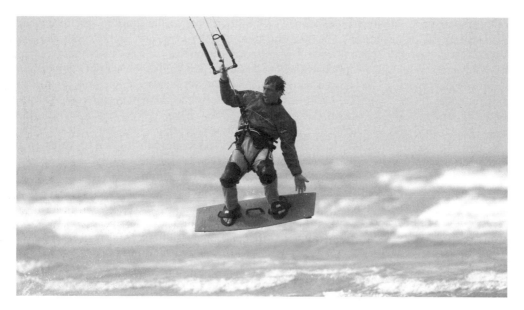

Are extreme sports the future of sport?

CP Images

While Canadian identity might not be linked with hockey as profoundly as in the past, sport continues to be a key element of our culture. Today we can observe the tensions between traditional sports and newer sport forms. Will future generations of Canadians cheer only for our mogul and aerial skiers, half-pipe and slalom snowboarders, or eXtreme-games athletes? Or will they continue to show support for our curlers, gymnasts, fencers, and wrestlers? Will the Canadian state and the IOC continue with traditional sports, or focus on those sports that are more commercially viable? It is likely that if Canadian athletes show strongly in the newer sports, attention, funding, and inclusion of the newer sport forms will follow.

Government Involvement in Sport

The Canadian state, at all levels, provides economic and structural support for what are identified as merit goods and public goods in the sport sector (Berrett, Slack, & Whitson, 1993). A *merit good* results when citizens feel great pride over an athlete's Olympic or World gold-medal win, where the basis for that athlete's success results from a state-developed and -funded sport program. A *public good* in sport occurs when a major sport facility or games festival is funded in part by the state, for example, the facilities for and the holding of the 1988 Calgary OWG and now the 2010 Vancouver OWG. Under current economic circumstances, the question arises of how much longer this funding will continue.

The complexities of the funding structure and the rise of managerialism and economic rationalism in the 1980s indicate that the state is struggling to be all things to all sports. With diminishing funds and more sports seeking recognition and support, those achieving international success and large participant bases will likely continue to receive government funding.

Perhaps a larger issue for state sport-governing bodies is their success in international competitions and the number of participants competing at the lower levels of the total sport structure who develop into elite athletes. Canada's success at the Olympic Games has been varied

Table 15.6   Olympic Results—Summer and Winter Games

	Gold Medals	Silver Medals	Bronze Medals
Pre 1969 Task Force			
1908	3	3	9
1912	3	2	3
1920 (OSG/OWG totals)*	2/1	3/0	3/0
1924	0/1	3/0	1/0
1928	4/1	4/0	7/0
1932	2/1	5/1	8/5
1936	1/1	3/0	5/0
1948	0/2	1/0	2/1
1952	1/1	2/0	0/1
1956	2/0	1/1	3/2
1960	0/2	1/1	0/1
1964	1/1	2/0	0/0
1968	1/1	3/1	1/1
Post 1969 Task Force			
1972	0/0	2/1	3/0
1976	0/1	2/1	3/0
1980**	0/0	0/1	0/1
1984**	10/2	18/1	16/1
1988 (19 & 13 on medal table)***	3/0	2/2	5/3
1992 (11 & 9 on medal table)	7/2	4/3	7/2
1994 (OWG only) (3rd)	3	6	4
1996 (OSG only) (21st)	3	11	8
1998 (OWG only) (4th)	6	5	4
2000 (OSG only) (27th)	3	3	8
2002 (OWG only) (4th)	6	3	8
2004 (OSG only) (21st)	3	6	3
2006 (OWG only) (5th)	7	10	7

* OSG-Summer Olympic Games; OWG-Winter Olympic Games.
** Boycotts occurred in each of these Olympic Games.
*** Numbers in parentheses indicate Canada's position in the overall medal table for the OSG and OWG.

Source: Zakus, 1988, p. 150 and IOC Web page.

(see Table 15.6 for the medal counts). While an Olympic medal count does not indicate the overall effectiveness of a sport system, it is widely used as a way of measuring the value of a country's viability in the world of sport. The question is whether a medal count is sufficiently impressive to continue the current level of funding.

An analysis of the talent identification and development programs at the national, provincial, and territory levels, as well as their overall coherence, would be necessary to substantiate this claim. However, the results from major competitions indicate these systems are problematic (see also Chapters 7, 8, and 12). On the other hand, the question of how the sport governing bodies can attract more participants and develop successful world-class athletes (future outputs) becomes central. For example, with Vancouver to host the 2010 OWG, the federal government initiated an *Own the Podium* funding program strategy. The concern, however, with many of these types of programs is what happens when the games are over. How will future athletes and programs be funded?

New Technologies and Sport

Improved sport science and sport medicine knowledge result in better performances by elite athletes. The advance in knowledge of training programs, including better nutrition, strength and conditioning, recovery, psychological and tactical preparation, and skills elements, are basic to this improvement. This raises an interesting point: how far can "normal" applications of new research-based science advance elite sport performance? This question raises interesting moral and ethical issues as many elite athletes or their support staff seek alternate substances and practices to ensure success.

Among these, issues concerning drug use in sport are well known. Clearly, more must be done to rid sport of performance-enhancing substances and practices. Sport history is replete with doping issues, as John Hoberman (1992) and Terry Todd (1987) note. Doping in sport has a long history and will likely be with us for some time. It appears that recent attempts to catch drug cheats and ongoing doping scandals do not surprise many people. The dilemma is that the Montreal-based World Anti-Doping Agency—chaired by a Canadian, Richard Pound—struggles to keep up with the cheaters and with the changing technologies for cheating.

An issue in sport that will have more dramatic consequences is related to new genetic knowledge and future practices. The Human Genome Project, which maps the human DNA sequence, is leading to a number of medical advances. The ability to generate, implant, and ultimately enhance body tissues (heart, muscle, tendon, bone) might lead to a type of "cyber-athlete." Other genetic research has led to cloning; it will not be long before "designer babies" are born via in vitro fertilization. The genetic factors sought in these babies could potentially be those necessary to produce top sport performers (Cole, 1994). Cole (as cited in Featherstone) elaborated on this when she noted:

> the potential consequences here for, to take an example, sport are tremendous. Not only is there the capacity to enhance performance and repair, or replace body parts to produce cyber-bodies. There is also the potential to genetically design optimum types of bodies best suited for particular sports. (p. 22)

The debate over the potential impact of gene therapy, stem cell technology, alternate medicines, electro-pharmaceutical enhancement of brain function, and, at the atomic level, nanotechnological enhancements is well underway. While these technologies and their potential use in health care—let alone sport—are in the early stages, researchers in these fields already receive correspondence from athletes willing to be "guinea pigs." Clearly, debates over this type of human performance manipulation will continue in the world of sport. It is more a question of when rather than if we will see genetically altered and otherwise doped athletes, or cyborgs (human-like robots with digitally controlled prostheses) in sport.

The above focuses directly on the human body. New knowledge about the science and techniques of training are enhancing athletic ability. Since the end of the Cold War the application of military technology has led to incredible improvements in sport equipment, apparel, and facilities. High-technology metals, synthetic polymers, and computer chip applications now make sport equipment and facilities stronger, lighter—and more expensive.

For example, golf club and ball development has reached a point where the length of the course, or the ability to extend the length of the course, is outstripped by golfers' ability to hit the ball greater distances. Top professional golfers now drive their tee-shots more than 300 yards on average. Many use only three clubs on most par 4 holes—driver, wedge, and putter. A question raised here is whether it is the equipment or the athlete creating these results.

The same comments could be made on racing bicycles, tennis racquets, protective equipment for collision sports, and suits worn by swimmers, track athletes, and skiers, among others. Although standards are set and testing of new equipment occurs through governing bodies for sport, new twists to old equipment can add unseen benefits. For example, recently Australian cricketer Ricky Ponting's cricket bat was ruled illegal due to a graphite strip along the back of the bat. This harkens back to Major League Baseball banning "corked" bats and the initial introduction of graphite hockey sticks.

Sport vocabulary now contains statements about "fast" swimming pools, luge/bobsleigh runs, and athletics tracks. The materials and construction techniques used in these facilities permit athletes to swim, slide, run, or jump to greater records. Again, is it better athletic performance, or is it these new modalities creating the improvements? The need to host major national (Canada Games) or international (Olympics, world championships) sport competitions to build or improve existing facilities is widely held as the reason for holding such events. Major league sport franchise owners also push for new facilities at taxpayers' expense. Expensive ballparks, stadiums, and arenas are quickly outdated or do not have the facilities necessary to generate more revenues (club seating, corporate boxes) as new building materials, techniques, and designs evolve. Many new sport facilities have short lives, costing governments considerable amounts in public infrastructure investment.

Both human and matériel technological developments will give rise to numerous future debates. The question of what this means to the average person on the street must be raised. Does it matter that some people seek out and pay huge amounts for designer drugs, genetic materials, or babies? Will the contest be between genetic or pharmaceutical corporations to decide which has the best product to replace the competition of sport? Will humans enjoy watching these genetically constructed "athletes" and cyborgs over normal humans? How much of this is science fiction and how much the future of sport?

This debate raises fundamental issues about the human and social nature of sport. Clearly this will be an important issue at the top end of sport production, but is not likely to be as significant for the average active athlete. Other than being consumers of new clothes, shoes, and other sporting goods, most of us will continue in sport the same way people have for years. Here again much of the debate focuses on elite and professional sport. For many of us this discussion is fascinating, but not the reality of sport as we encounter it throughout life other than in the equipment, footwear, and apparel we purchase to improve our ability in sport and extend the consumer culture of current times.

Another key development has been in virtual spectating and involvement in sport. Massive changes in Internet technology and the integration of telephony with cable and satellite digital broadcasting results in many different ways that people can "consume" sport (as passive participants and spectators). Sport fans are now able to watch multiple sports programs, often during the same time slot as the television industry expands. This includes watching sport on their fridges, watches, and cell phones. With WiFi, Bluetooth, and other forms of electronic connectivity, sport programs and news sites are available 24/7.

From these new forms of interaction, albeit non-social ones, people are able to enter into fantasy leagues in a wide number of sports, often with others they do not—and never will—directly know. Sport gambling also expands with interactive digital technology. Seemingly beyond governments to control, people can gamble and place bets from anywhere to anywhere in the world. Real-time scores and interactivity expand the way people obtain information on sport, the way they can participate in sport, and the way they gamble. With increasing telephony and digital media this aspect of sport indicates an interesting future.

THE FUTURE OF CANADIAN SPORT IN THE GLOBAL CONTEXT

Attempting to predict the future of Canadian sport is fraught with difficulty. The predictions will likely be based on incorrect assumptions and perhaps poor value judgments, leaving the prognosis faulty. Should this, however, deter us from trying to make sense of that future? Canadian society is generally based on a liberal-democratic, capitalist structure and is part of the global capitalist structure. Sport, which is a central feature of Canadian society, therefore has to be understood within this context.

As Canada's economy is part of the wider global economy, sport in Canada is part of the broader, global structure of sport. This position must also be understood in terms of Ralston Saul's (2005) discussion of globalism. Globalism, a neo-conservative ideology, claims free markets and free trade are the primary forces for the future of world development. The implications for the movement of athletes globally are significant. One need only look at the NBA and NHL to see these patterns or to the Bosman Ruling (European football) and the Curt Flood case in MLB to show the implications of player movements and the new legal frameworks constituted to deal with player "migrations." To understand Canadian sport, we must look at and make sense of sport in the larger social context. Maguire (1999) provides an extensive analysis of this context and a wider understanding of the global movement of athletes. Much has been written lately about globalization and the place of sport in this expanded world. In this section we will look at some of these assumptions and attempt to indicate what might happen to Canadian sport.

Sport, as with any other area of society, is affected by the changes inherent in capitalism, and more recently globalism. As discussed in previous chapters, sport has to generate products and services through production and build markets for consumption to sell those goods and services to realize the extra value they contain. Capital must expand by realizing the extra value through favourable market exchange if the economic system is to remain viable. Sport and its nexus with several other industries (e.g., tourism, events, and especially the media) point to the ways in which capital investment has grown.

For example, professional sport franchises continue to be part of larger media and entertainment complexes. As Harvey, Law, and Cantelon (2001) note, more than 31 percent of the total professional sport franchises in North America are part of media and entertainment corporations. Here, vertical and horizontal integration of different forms of capital (corporations) are merged. Each element of the new, larger integrated organization contributes value to that overall corporate operation.

What does this mean for Canada and Canadians? What does this mean for Canadian cities attempting to become "world class" (see Whitson & Macintosh, 1993)? With the move of the Québec Nordiques to Denver in 1995 and the Winnipeg Jets to Phoenix in 1996, we witnessed the move of Canadian teams to larger population centres in the United States—that is, to larger markets, both for live and television audiences and for commercial opportunities.

Will this be a scenario to be repeated with, for example, the Calgary Flames and Edmonton Oilers? With salaries escalating and being set in U.S. dollars, with small market reaches and with other limitations on their operations, Canadian teams face this question constantly. This assumes that hockey teams in Vancouver, Montreal (already owned by U.S. interests), and Toronto will retain their NHL franchises because they operate in larger markets. This assumption, however, might not save these franchises. Vancouver lost its NBA team, the Grizzlies, to Memphis in 2001 and Montreal's MLB team, the Expos, moved to Washington, D.C. in 2005.

The four most recent NHL expansion franchises were located in U.S. cities. Finally, not since the 1992–93 season has a Canadian NHL franchise won the Stanley Cup.

Canadian top-level professional sport is on the edge of chaos. *Globe and Mail* columnist James Christie's 2001 top sport losses included "Joe Fan" in the number one position (Christie, 2001). Christie was commenting on how sport fans have suffered the greatest losses within the changing milieu of sport. From this, the question "Will Canadians have only U.S.–based major league teams to cheer for in the future?" holds saliency.

With the CFL continuing to experience variable support and ongoing crises, lacrosse and soccer failing to maintain professional leagues, and market conditions unable to support major league franchises, it is likely that Canada will continue as a hinterland or dependent source of athletes and fans. Certainly a large number of Canadian towns and cities are capable of supporting professional, semi-professional, and development-level franchises.

Perhaps a key example of this is major junior hockey. The Canadian Hockey League (CHL) and its three divisions (Western, Ontario, Quebec) continue to provide the majority of new players for the NHL and its farm teams, although this is at a falling rate. There are 59 CHL franchises with 50 teams in 10 Canadian provinces and nine teams in four American states (although the league will expand again in 2006–08). This trio of leagues is seen globally as a key pathway to being drafted into the NHL. Not only are Canadian youths seeking places on these teams, but European and United States players also migrate to compete in the CHL.

Because of the strength of the CHL, and with viable minor-league farm teams in other Canadian cities (e.g., Winnipeg, Saint John, St. John's, Halifax, Hamilton), professional hockey will continue to exist. Curling continues to attract spectators and media attention; however, this might be age-related. The CFL will continue as a culturally unique sport in localized markets. Baseball will continue to locate development-level franchises in Canadian cities both large and small. Figure skating will continue to enjoy a following, although it is clearly within the media and entertainment complex (e.g., International Management Group's Ice Capades). The Canadian Professional Golf Association will continue to hold its tournament season; however, it will struggle for recognition of the Canadian Open, part of the U.S. Professional Golfers' Association annual tour.

Canada is part of the North American market economy, but it cannot compete with the major U.S. media and entertainment corporations for audiences and revenues. Its population continues to be roughly a tenth that of the United States and its dollar remains at less than par with the U.S. dollar. As Canada remains a dependent state within the North American system, it will remain in a secondary position in sport production and consumption. However, this is not a negative situation. Bigger is not necessarily better. Whether Canada will retain all or some of its remaining major professional sport leagues is open to debate. If we look back to the 1950s we see that Canada had only two major professional sport franchises, the Toronto Maple Leafs and the Montreal Canadiens. For the moment, Canada has eight major league franchises—six in hockey, one in baseball, and one in basketball. Are Canadians and Canadian sport any better or worse off at this time? It can be argued there is considerable currency in smaller, localized professional sport franchises and leagues.

Smaller franchises and leagues compete in markets comparable to their size. That is, to exist they do not have to compete globally for markets, revenues, and media exposure. In identity building, smaller localized franchises have many positive impacts: the first points to local community identity building; the second is in rivalry with other local, similar franchises; the third is in the effect on local production and consumption patterns. Sport can continue to fulfil its social and cultural role within the local environment. For example, two Canadian universities (Laval in football and Lakehead in men's hockey) are funded through the private sector; others are investigating this possibility.

This notion of local leagues holds importance with regard to spectatorship in another way. Major league sport demands faculties that permit more differentiated, expensive, and value-added revenues. More and more franchises want club and corporate boxes where they can charge for the space and for the services provided (food and beverage). The cost of tickets is therefore beyond the reach of most of the middle and working classes to afford.

Furthermore, television will allow sport fans to actively participate in "live" events through interactive digital technology and through "narrowcasting" of televised sport. Even this form of participation is being segmented into packages of channels for sport fans. For example, hockey fans are able to buy a package of games, much as they would have bought a package of games in the arena. Again, this is not necessarily a bad thing. Further, this might add to the number of fans for live local amateur sport and local leagues.

CONCLUSIONS

As radical change is not likely on the broader level, can radical change occur in smaller ways? Even this is not likely, as conservative forces are able to control the sport agenda through economic, media, and ideological means (especially with many neo-conservative governments in power). Although sport is touted to be a social practice that has emancipating and egalitarian potential, those pushing for radical change are not able to mount the necessary resistance and resources. The Olympic movement, with Olympism as its guiding philosophy, is regarded as the epitome of sport. Its games support and promote elite sport, which draws the agenda and resources away from a truly egalitarian structure for sport. Radical sport movements linked historically to workers' movements illustrate this radical type of sport structure; then again, this restructuring remains unrealized (remember that many of these movements were based in societies attempting to operate on socialist principles).

Within most liberal-democratic capitalist states, the future of change is firmly in the control of conservatives and reformists. With sport linked to many values and higher ideals, it seems both ironic and sad that the current situation does not permit these values full expression in the way sport is understood, structured, and provided.

Because change is a constant in life, we must expect and be ready to deal with it. Clearly, a proactive stance is better than a reactive one. Nor can we hope that serendipity will operate. For we wish, as humans, to make changes that are seen as better and not simply to react to situations that are often imposed on us. We have, in other words, the ability to be volitional. We can work within the current structure of sport or we can become involved in oppositional groups (such as the Bread not Circuses coalition in Toronto). Or we can create new futures for sport, through new sport types (e.g., snowboarding, eXtreme sports) or new structures for sport (e.g., eXtreme Games, Gay Games) (Rinehart, 1998).

While for many people sport is a central feature of their lives, it is not a necessary condition, merely a sufficient one. Those studying sport and how sport operates at all levels of society (i.e., from the local to the global levels) must realize that the individual problems we encounter will not necessarily be resolved at the structural level or become a structural issue. However, using our imaginations and implementing ideas can make new futures for sport.

Hall, Slack, Smith, and Whitson (1992) followed the premise of sociologist C. Wright Mills in their book. Mills wrote that it is

> necessary for anyone who wishes to understand the changing nature of sport or any other significant feature of social life to relate the personal troubles of individuals' lived experience to the public issues of social structure. (p. 236)

For some, sport is a given fact of their life. It is part of their family life and is an ongoing activity through family generations. For others it is a socially, economically, or otherwise unobtainable desire. Canada has a vast sport system, but it does not provide opportunities for all or wider success through athletic achievement or simply through opportunities to participate (e.g., the disabled, economically disadvantaged). Why this situation exists must not be seen as appropriate or acceptable. If sport is seen as a basic social right, then we must challenge these disparities and push for change so that all Canadians have the opportunities to pursue the sport(s) of their choice.

Challenging one's own assumptions of what sport is, how it is structured, its cultural position, the social opportunities it might or should provide, and how it should operate are key to the future of Canadian sport. As indicated in several places throughout this text, each individual has the volition and the ability to identify and work toward change.

It is possible to understand this type of change by examining available statistics and making estimations of the future (toward a conservative change). Some might look at social structures and seek to change the power relations in and resultant from those structures (toward a reform in the structure). Others might take a more active role and seek to break down the structures that inhibit, exclude, or operate unequally (through a more radical action). While we collectively struggle to identify who we are as individuals and also collectively as a nation, sport provides unique and important ideas and outcomes for this activity.

Sport provides a basis of social discourse and a daily activity for many of us. While we might not all be directly active in sport, we will likely connect through the mediation of sport. Whatever our involvement, we must critically reflect and morally act to improve our own and others' involvement and enjoyment of sport. That is, we must use critical thinking to follow Mills's (1959) promise by seeking to resolve personal troubles of those who cannot access sport in some way or by actively lobbying for better sport facilities, resources, and public and private organizations for the delivery and governance of sport. Through human volition we are capable of creating a better future—if we follow McLuhan's suggestion, by looking in the rear-view mirror we can create a better future with knowledge of the past and its shortcomings.

CRITICAL THINKING QUESTIONS

1. In May 2006 a census of Canada was completed. This new information and reports emanating from this data were not available when this edition was written. Students are encouraged to look up the latest data from the StatsCan website and the Conference Board of Canada (2005) report on involvement in sport, and suggest what trends are evident. How have sport and sport activity changed? What are the reasons, in your estimation, for these changes? What might happen between the current date and the next data collection?
2. What features of Canadian sport could contribute to maintaining a unique and separate country and culture? Which sports can accomplish this identity?
3. How do the figures in Table 15.1 indicate ways the local, provincial, and federal levels of government might ensure the continuation of sport? What special features of sport would be part of that future?
4. Would cyborg sport be marketable? Why? How?
5. In the discussion of structural issues and the future of sport, certain aspects of sport provision were not included (e.g., for disabled people, First Nations people, economically disadvantaged people). Identify the current state of sport for these groups and how we might address the structural issues you have noted. Find statistics and other arguments for this discussion.

6. (a) On a piece of paper draw a line down the middle of the page. On the left side list the arguments for bids by Canadian cities to host future Olympic Games. On the right side list the negative aspects of such a bid. (b) What action(s) might be taken to decide whether to bid for these games?

7. Debate the idea that hockey is Canada's unique cultural characteristic (you may have to identify the cultural characteristics of Canada to enter this debate). Back up your position with substantive information and data.

8. In the future, will current new sport forms (e.g., skateboarding, snowboarding, aerial and mogul skiing, mountain-bike trick riding) be attractive to participants, consumers, the media, and the organizers of major games (although several are already in the Olympics)? Or will more traditional sports continue to be attractive?

9. Complete a poll of 20 to 30 students asking them what sports they participate in, what sports they watch live or on television, and what sports they want to see in the Olympics. Compare the figures you obtain with those presented in the second section of this chapter, those found on television, and those in the Olympic Games and Winter Olympic Games programs. What do the results of this informal poll indicate?

10. Will movements such as anti-globalization and the "slow movement" influence the commercialization of sport, the levels of participation in sport, and the future of sport generally? Look up information on these movements and prepare arguments for and against their possible influence.

11. In terms of the three perspectives on the future, identify which one makes the most sense to you, and why this is so.

SUGGESTED READINGS

Coakley, J., & Dunning, E. (2000). *Handbook of sport studies*. London: Sage.

Gruneau, R., & Whitson, D. (1993). *Hockey night in Canada: Sport, identities and cultural politics*. Toronto: Garamond Press.

Macintosh, D., & Whitson, D. (1990). *The game planners: Transforming Canada's sport system*. Montreal & Kingston: McGill–Queen's University Press.

Maguire, J. (1999). *Global sport: Identities, societies, civilizations*. Cambridge: Polity Press.

Malloy, D. C., Ross, S., & Zakus, D. H. (2004). *Sport ethics: Concepts and cases in sport and recreation*. Toronto: Thompson Educational Publishing.

Wright Mills, C. (1959). *The sociological imagination*. New York: Free Press.

WEB LINKS

The Amateur Athletic Foundation of Los Angeles
http://www.aafla.org
Funded by some of the 1984 Los Angeles Olympic Games windfall. A major library and electronic collection of Olympic and sport materials.

Canadian Olympic Committee
http://www.olympic.ca
Current and historical information on Canada at the Olympics. Links to other sport and Olympic sites.

International Olympic Committee
http://www.olympic.org

The "grandparent" of all sport organizations. Several internal links to different parts of the IOC, and links to other elements of the Olympic family. Future Games sites are also linked through this site.

The Conference Board of Canada

http://www.conferenceboard.ca

A non-governmental, not-for-profit research organization: "specialists in economic trends, as well as organizational performance and public policy issues" (from their website). Another of their reports provided background reading for this chapter and students are encouraged to access this site for future statistical information. The document is *The World and Canada: Trends Reshaping Our Future.*

Sport Canada

http://www.pch.gc.ca/sportcanada/

Covers the development of sport nationally. Includes links to all national sport governing bodies and other national and international sport sites.

Statistics Canada Website

http://www.statscan.ca

Contains a number of pages and links with recent studies on the nature of Canada, Canadians, and how they live their lives.

References

Aboriginal Sports/Recreation Association of B.C. (1995, October). Media release on the 1997 North American Indigenous Games planned for Victoria, B.C.

Adams, M. L. (2006). A game of whose lives? Notes on gender and identity in a hockey mad culture. In D. Whitson & R. Gruneau (Eds.), *Artificial ice: Hockey, commerce, and cultural identity* (pp. 71–84). Peterborough, ON: Broadview Press.

Adler, P., & Adler, P. (1991). *Backboards and blackboards: College athletes and role engulfment.* New York: Columbia University Press.

Aitken, B. W. W. (1993). The emergence of born-again sport. In C. Prebish (Ed.), *Religion and sport.* Westport, CT: Greenwood Press.

Albom, M. (2000, July 16). Parents often drop ball in youth sports. *Detroit Free Press.*

Alfermann, D., Stambulova, N., & Zemaityte, A. (2004). Reactions to sport career termination: A cross-national comparison of German, Lithuanian, and Russian athletes. *Psychology of Sport and Exercise, 5,* 61–75.

American Academy of Pediatrics. (2000). Intensive training and sports specialization in young athletes. *Pediatrics, 106,* 154–157.

Ammirante, J. (2006). Globalization in professional sport: Comparisons and contrasts between hockey and European football. In D. Whitson & R. Gruneau (Eds.), *Artificial ice: Hockey, culture, and commerce* (pp. 237–261). Peterborough, ON: Broadview Press.

Anderson, D., Broom, E., Pooley, J., Rhodes, E., Robertson, D., & Schrodt, B. (1989). *Foundations of Canadian physical education, recreation, and sport studies.* Dubuque, IA: Wm. C. Brown.

Andrews, D. (1996). The fact(s) of Michael Jordan's blackness: Excavating a floating racial signifier. *Sociology of Sport Journal, 13,* 125–158.

Andrews, D. (2004). Sport in the late capitalist moment. In T. Slack (Ed.), *The commercialization of sport* (pp. 1–28). London: Routledge.

Andrews, D. (Ed.). (2001). *Michael Jordan, Inc.: Corporate sport, media culture, and late modern America.* Albany: SUNY Press.

Anshel, M. H. (1997). *Sport psychology: From theory to practice.* Scottsdale, AZ: Gorsuch Scarisbrick.

Armstrong-Doherty, A. (1995). Athletic directors' perceptions of environmental control over interuniversity athletics. *Sociology of Sport Journal, 12,* 75–95.

Association of Universities and Colleges of Canada. (1966). *Physical education and athletics in Canadian universities and colleges.* Ottawa: Canadian Association of Health, Physical Education, and Recreation.

Athens 2004 Olympics Broadcast Report. (2004). Retrieved September 6, 2006 from http://www.olympic.org/uk/utilities/reports.

Atkinson, M. (2002). Fifty million viewers can't be wrong: Professional wrestling, sports entertainment, and mimesis. *Sociology of Sport Journal, 19*, 47–66.

Atkinson, M. (2007). It's still part of the game: Violence and masculinity in Canadian ice hockey. In L. Fuller, *Sport, rhetoric, gender and violence: Historical perspectives and media representations*. New York: Palgrave MacMillan.

Augustine, St. (1961). *Confessions*. Harmondsworth, UK: Penguin Books.

Baillie, P. H. F., & Danish, S. J. (1992). Understanding the career transition of athletes. *The Sport Psychologist, 6*, 77–98.

Bairner, A. (2001). *Sport, nationalism and globalization*. New York, NY: SUNY Press.

Bakardjieva, M. (2005). *Internet society: The internet in everyday life*. London: Sage.

Baker, J. (2003). Early specialization in youth sport: A requirement for adult expertise? *High Abilities Studies, 14*, 85–94.

Bandura, A., & Walters, R. (1963). *Social learning and personality development*. New York: Holt, Rinehart & Winston.

Bannerji, H. (2000). *The dark side of the nation: Essays on multiculturalism, nationalism and gender*. Toronto: Canadian Scholars Press.

Barnes, J. (1996). *Sports and the law in Canada*, 3rd edition. Toronto and Vancouver: Butterworths.

Barney, R. K. (1993). Golden egg or fools' gold? American Olympic Commercialism and the IOC. In *International Olympic Academy, Proceedings: Thirty-third session of the International Olympic Academy* (p. 17). Olympia, Greece.

Barney, R. K. (1996). Prologue: The Ancient Games. In *Historical dictionary of the modern Olympic Movement* (pp. xxi–xxxxi). Westport, CT: Greenwood Press.

Barney, R. K., Wenn, S., & Martyn, S. (2002). *Selling the five rings: The International Olympic Committee and the rise of Olympic commercialism*. Salt Lake City: University of Utah Press.

Bausell, R., Bausell C., & Siegel, D. (1991). *The links among alcohol, drugs and crime on American college campuses: A national followup study*. Towson, MD: Towson State University.

Beal, B. (2002). Symbolic interactionism and cultural studies: Doing critical ethnography. In J. Maguire & K. Young (Eds.), *Theory, sport & society* (pp. 353–373). Amsterdam: JAI.

Beamish, R. (1990). The persistence of inequality: an analysis of participation among Canada's high performance athletes. *International Review for the Sociology of Sport, 25*, 143–55.

Beamish, R. (2002). Karl Marx's enduring legacy for the sociology of sport. In J. Maguire & K. Young (Eds.), *Theory, sport & society* (pp. 25–39). Amsterdam: JAI.

Beamish, R., & Borowy, J. (1988). *Q. What do you do for a living? A. I'm an athlete*. Kingston, ON: The Sport Research Group.

Becket, H. W. (1882). *The Montreal snow shoe club: Its history and record*. Montreal: Becket Brothers.

Bellamy, R., (1998). The evolving television sports marketplace. In L. Wenner (Ed.), *MediaSport* (pp. 73–87). New York: Routledge.

Bellamy, R., & Shultz, K. (2006). Hockey Night in the United States? The NHL, major league sports, and the evolving television/media marketplace. In D. Whitson & R. Gruneau (Eds.), *Artificial ice: Hockey, culture, and commerce* (pp. 163–180). Toronto: Broadview Press.

Benedict, J. (1998). *Athletes and acquaintance rape*. Thousand Oaks, CA: Sage.

Berrett, T., Slack, T., & Whitson, D. (1993). Economics and the pricing of sport and leisure. *Journal of Sport Management, 7*, 199–215.

Bhabha, H. K. (1994). *The location of culture*. London: Routledge.

Birrell, S., & Richter, D. (1987). Is a diamond forever? Feminist transformations of sport. *Women's Studies International Forum, 10*, 395–410.

Blanchard, M. (2004, October 15). Le Canadien déficitaire: des chiffres confirmés. *La Presse* (Montreal), p. S5.

Blinde, E. (1989). Unequal exchange and exploitation in college sport: The case of the female athlete. *Arena Review, 13*, 110–123.

Blumer, H. (1995). Society as symbolic interaction. In D. McQuarie (Ed.), *Readings in contemporary sociological theory: From modernity to post-modernity* (pp. 206–213). Englewood Cliffs, NJ: Prentice Hall.

Bompa, T. (1995). *From childhood to champion athlete*. Toronto: Veritas.

Booth, D., & Loy, J. (1999). Sport, status, and style. *Sport History Review, 30*, 1–26.

Borowy, J., & Little, M. (1991). *A time and space just for us*. Toronto: Central Neighbourhood House.

Bottomore, T. (1964). *Elites and society*. New York: Basic Books.

Bourdieu, P. (1984). *Distinction: A social critique of the judgment of taste*. Cambridge: Harvard University Press.

Bourdieu, P. (1998). *Practical reason: On the theory of action*. Stanford, CA: Stanford University Press.

Bowler, G. (2005, December 10). Yule be sorry. *The Globe and Mail*, p. D55.

Boyd, M., & Vickers, M. (2000, Autumn). 100 years of immigration to Canada. *Canadian Social Trends*, 2–12.

Boyle, R., & Haynes, R. (2000). *Power play: Sport, the media and popular culture*. Harlow, UK: Pearson Education Limited.

Boyle, R., & Haynes, R. (2003). New media sport. In A. Bernstein and N. Blain (Eds.), *Sport, media, culture: Global and local dimensions* (pp. 95–114). London: Frank Cass.

Brackenbridge, C. H. (2001). *Spoilsports: Understanding and preventing sexual exploitation in sport*. London: Routledge.

Brailsford, D. (1969). *Sport and society: Elizabeth to Anne*. London: Routledge and Kegan Paul.

Breton, R. (1964). Institutional completeness of ethnic communities and personal relations of immigrants. *American Journal of Sociology, 70*, 193–205.

Brewer, B. W. (1993). Self-identity and specific vulnerability to depressed mood. *Journal of Personality, 61*, 343–364.

Brohm, J. M. (1978). *Sport: A prison of measured time*. London: Ink Links.

Brookes, R. (2002). *Representing sport*. New York: Oxford University Press.

Brown, A. (1980). Edward Hanlan: The world sculling champion visits Australia. *Canadian Journal of History of Sport and Physical Education, 11*, 1–44.

Brown, D. (1986). Militarism and Canadian private education: Ideal and practise, 1861–1918. *Canadian Journal of History of Sport and Physical Education, 17*, 46–59.

Bryant, J. E., & McElroy, M. (1997). *Sociological dynamics of sport and exercise*. Englewood, CO: Morton.

Burnet, J. R., & Palmer, H. (1988). *"Coming Canadians": An introduction to a history of Canada's people*. Toronto: McClelland & Stewart in Association with the

Multiculturalism Program, Department of the Secretary of State and the Canadian Government Publishing Centre, Supply and Services, Canada.

Burstyn, V. (1999). *The rites of men*. Toronto: University of Toronto Press.

Butcher, J., Linder, K. L., & Johns, D. P. (2002). Withdrawal from competitive youth sport: A retrospective ten-year study. *Journal of Sport Behavior, 25*, 145–163.

Butsch, R. (Ed.). (1990). *For fun and profit: The transformation of leisure into consumption*. Philadelphia: Temple University Press.

Caillois, R. (1961). *Man, play and games*. New York: The Free Press.

Canada. (1970). *A proposed sports policy for Canadians*. Ottawa: Ministry of Health and Welfare.

Canada. (1992). Sport, the way ahead: The report of the Minister's Task Force on Federal Sport Policy. Ottawa, Minister of State, Fitness and Amateur Sport, p. 187.

Canadian Association for Health Physical Education Recreation and Dance. (1989). *Quality daily physical education rationale handbook*. Ottawa: Government of Canada Fitness and Amateur Sport.

Canadian Broadcasting Corporation. (2004). *Fair game: Pioneering Canadian women in sports*. Retrieved from http://archives.radio-canada.ca/IDCC-1-41-714-4219/sports/women_sports/; and http://archives.radio-canada.ca/IDCC-1-41-714-4246/sports/women_sports/.

Canadian Centre for Ethics in Sport (CCES). (2002, July). *Public opinion survey on youth and sport: Final report*.

Canadian Charter of Rights and Freedoms. (1982). Retrieved from http://www.laurentia.com/ccrf/ccrf-prnt.html.

Canadian Fitness and Lifestyle Research Institute (CFLRI). (1999). *1999 physical activity monitor*. Retrieved from http://www.cflri.ca.

Canadian Fitness and Lifestyle Research Institute (CFLRI). (2000). *2000 physical activity monitor*. Ottawa: Canadian Fitness and Lifestyle Research Institute.

Canadian Fitness and Lifestyle Research Institute (CFLRI). (2004). *2004 capacity study*. Retrieved from http://www.cflri.ca/eng/statistics/surveys/capacity2004.php.

Canadian Heritage. (2005a). *A Canada for all: Canada's action plan against racism—An overview*. Retrieved November 16, 2005 from http://www.canadianheritage.gc.ca/multi/plan_action_plan/index_e.cfm.

Canadian Heritage. (2005b). *Sport Canada's policy on Aboriginal peoples' participation in sport*. Retrieved from http://www.pch.gc.ca/progs/sc/pol/aboriginal/index_e.cfm.

Canadian Institute for Health Information. (2004). *Improving the health of Canadians*. Ottawa: Canadian Institute for Health Information.

Canadian Interuniversity Sport (CIS). (2000a). *CIS guideline on athletic awards*. Retrieved from http://www.cisport.ca/awards/awards_criteria.htm.

Canadian Interuniversity Sport (CIS). (2000b). *2000–2001 awards data collection*. Retrieved from http://www.cisport.ca/awards/2000_data.htm.

Canadian Interuniversity Sport (CIS). (2002). *Historical snapshot*. Retrieved from http://www.cisport.ca/about/history/htm.

Canadian Interuniversity Sport (CIS). (2005a). *2005 equity practices questionnaire final report*. Retrieved from http://www.cisport.ca/e/research/index.cfm.

Canadian Interuniversity Sport (CIS). (2005b). *Analysis of male and female coaches in CIS sports*. Retrieved from http://www.cisport.ca/e/research/index.cfm.

Canadian Intramural Recreation Association. (2002). *Organizational profile and overview*. Retrieved from www.intramurals.ca/cira/overview.html.

Canadian Olympic Committee (COC). (2004). *Annual report, 2004*. Retrieved from https://www.olympic.ca/EN/organization/publications/reports/2004report.pdf.

Canadian Teachers' Federation. (1990). *A capella: A report on the realities, concerns, expectations and barriers experienced by adolescent women in Canada*. Ottawa: Canadian Teachers' Federation.

Cantelon, H. (2006). Have skates, will travel: Canada, international hockey, and the changing hockey labour market. In D. Whitson & R. Gruneau (Eds.), *Artificial ice: Hockey, culture, and commerce* (pp. 215–235). Peterborough, ON: Broadview Press.

Chad, K. E., Humbert, M. L., & Jackson, P. L. (1999). The effectiveness of the Canadian Quality Daily Physical Education Program on school physical education. *Research Quarterly for Exercise and Sport, 70*, 55–64.

Chandler, J. M. (1992). Sport is not a religion. In S. J. Hoffman (Ed.), *Sport and religion* (pp. 55–61). Champaign, IL: Human Kinetics.

Charbonneau, L. (2002, February). Universities give $2.4 million in student athlete awards. *University Affairs, 32*.

Chartrand, J. M., & Lent, R. W. (1987). Sports counseling: Enhancing the development of the student-athlete. *Journal of Counseling and Development, 66*, 164–167.

Chelladurai, P., & Danylchuk, K. E. (1984). Operative goals of intercollegiate athletics: Perceptions of athletic administrators. *Canadian Journal of Applied Sports Sciences, 9*, 33–41.

Chiswick, B. R., & Miller, P. W. (2002, March). Do enclaves matter in immigrant adjustment? Discussion paper 449. Bonn, Germany: Institute for the Study of Labor.

Christie, J. (2001). Past year saw its share of losers. *Globe and Mail* [online]. Retrieved from www.globeandmail.com.

Clarkson, S. (2002). *Uncle Sam and us: Globalization, neoconservatism, and the Canadian state*. Toronto: University of Toronto Press.

Coakley, J. (2001). *Sport in society: Issues and controversies*, 7th ed. New York: McGraw-Hill.

Coakley, J. (2004). *Sport in society: Issues and controversies*, 8th ed. New York: McGraw Hill.

Coakley, J., & Donnelly, P. (2004a). *Sport in society: Issues and controversies*, 1st Canadian ed. Toronto: McGraw-Hill Ryerson.

Coakley, J., & Donnelly, P. (2004b). Sports and children: Are organized programs worth the effort? In *Sport in society: Issues and controversies*, 1st Canadian ed. Toronto: McGraw-Hill Ryerson.

Cole, C. (1994). Resisting the canon: Feminist cultural studies, sport, and technologies of the body. In C. Cole & S. Birrell (Eds.), *Women, sport, and culture* (pp. 5–29). Champaign-Urbana, IL: Human Kinetics.

Conference Board of Canada. (2004, December). *National household survey on participation in sport*. Ottawa: Conference Board of Canada.

Conference Board of Canada. (2005). *Strengthening Canada: The socio-economic benefits of sport participation in Canada*. Retrieved from http://www.conferenceboard.ca.

Conley, C. (1999). The agreeable recreation of fighting. *Journal of Social History, 33*, 57–72.

Connell, R. W. (1995). *Masculinities*. Los Angeles: University of California Press.

Connell, R. (2005). *Masculinities*, 2nd ed. Berkeley: University of California Press.

Cosentino, F. (1974). Ned Hanlan—Canada's premier oarsman: A case study of nineteenth century professionalism. *Ontario History, 66*, 241–250.

Cosentino, F. (1975). A history of the concept of professionalism in Canadian sport. *Canadian Journal of History of Sport and Physical Education, 6*, 75–81.

Cosentino, F. (1998). *Afros, Aboriginals and amateur sport in pre World War One Canada*. Canada's Ethnic Group Series, Booklet No. 26. Ottawa: The Canadian Historical Society.

Costas, B. (2000). *Fair ball: A fan's case for baseball*. New York: Broadway Books.

Cragg, S., Cameron, C., Craig, C. L., & Russell, S. (1999, November). *Canada's children and youth: A physical activity profile*. Ottawa: Canadian Fitness and Lifestyle Research Institute Publication.

Crompton, J. (2004). Beyond economic impact: An alternative rationale for the public subsidy of major league sports facilities. *Journal of Sport Management, 18*, 40–58.

Crossman, J., Hyslop, P., & Guthrie, B. (1994). A content analysis of the sports section of Canada's national newspaper with respect to gender and professional/amateur status. *International Review for the Sociology of Sport, 29*, 123–134.

Crossman, J., Vincent, J., & Speed, H. (forthcoming). The times they are a-changin': Gender comparisons in three national newspapers of the 2004 Wimbledon Championships.

CTV.ca. (2006, May 29). Edmonton police, mayor plan for hockey hooligans. CTV.ca Retrieved from http://www.ctv.ca/servlet/ArticlesNews/story/CTVNews/20060529/edmonton_security_060529/20060529?hub=TopStories.

Curtis, J., & McTeer, W. (1990). Sport involvement and academic attainment in university: Two studies in the Canadian case. In L. Vander Velden & J. H. Humprey (Eds.), *Psychology and sociology of sport: Current selected research 2* (pp. 177–192). New York: AMS Press.

Curtis, J., McTeer, W., & White, P. (1999). Exploring effects of school sport experiences on sport participation in later life. *Sociology of Sport Journal, 16*, 348–365.

Curtis, J. E., & Birch, J. S. (1987). Size of community of origin and recruitment to professional and Olympic hockey in North America. *Sociology of Sport Journal, 4*, 229–244.

Dagg, A., & Thompson, P. (1987). *MisEducation*. Toronto: Ontario Institute for Studies in Education Press.

Dahrendorf, R. (1995). Toward a theory of social conflict. In D. McQuarie (Ed.), *Readings in contemporary sociological theory: From modernity to post-modernity* (pp. 74–82). Englewood Cliffs, NJ: Prentice Hall.

Dalla Costa, M. (2005, December 23). Road to Turin: We want a medal—at any cost. *The London Free Press*. Retrieved from http://www.lfpress.com/cgi-bin/publish.cgi?p=117235&x=articles&s=olympics.

Dallaire, C., & Denis, C. (2005). Asymmetric hybridities: Youths at Francophone games in Canada. *Canadian Journal of Sociology, 30*, 143–169.

Danish, S. J., & Nellen, V. C. (1997). New roles for sport psychologists: Teaching life skills through sport to at-risk youth. *Quest, 49*, 100–113.

Danish, S. J., Owens, S. S., Green, S. L., & Brunelle, J. P. (1997). Building bridges for disengagement: The transition process for individuals and teams. *Journal of Applied Sport Psychology, 9*, 154–167.

Danylchuk, K. E. (1995). Academic performance of intercollegiate athletes at a Canadian university: Comparisons by gender, type of sport and affiliated faculty. *Avante, 1*, 78–93.

Darnell, S., & Sparks, B. (2005). Inside the promotional vortex: Canadian media construction of Sydney Olympic triathlete Simon Whitfield. *International Review for the Sociology of Sport, 40*, 357–376.

Davis, C. (1999). Eating disorders, physical activity, and sport: Biological, psychological, and sociological factors. In P. White & K. Young (Eds.), *Sport and gender in Canada* (pp. 85–106). Don MIlls, ON: Oxford University Press.

Davis, K., & Moore, W. E. (1945). Some principles of stratification. *American Sociological Review, 10,* 242–249.

Deacon, B. (2001, November). *Physical education curriculum review report.* British Columbia Ministry of Education, Curriculum Branch. Retrieved from http://www.bced.gov.bc.ca/irp/reports/pereport.pdf.

Deacon, J. (1997, January 20). Darkening the hockey dream. *Maclean's,* p. 54.

Deacon, J. (2001, March 26). Rink rage. *Maclean's,* pp. 21–24.

Debord, G. (1967). *Society of the spectacle.* Detroit: Black and Red.

de Coubertin, P. (2000). Why I revived the Olympic Games. In N. Müller (Ed.), *Pierre de Coubertin, Olympism: Selected writings* (pp. 542–546). Lausanne: International Olympic Committee.

Deford, F. (1980, March 3). A heavenly game? *Sports Illustrated,* pp. 59–70.

Denis, C. (1997). *We are not you: First Nations & Canadian modernity.* Peterborough, ON: Broadview Press.

Department of National Health and Welfare. (1969). *Report of the task force on sports for Canadians.* Ottawa: The Queen's Printer for Ontario.

Desrosiers, E. (2005, December 28). Noël à longueur d'année. *Le Devoir* (Montreal), p. B5.

Dodd, M. (2006, April 30). Sport or not a sport? Pot is split on poker. *USA Today,* p. 13C.

Dollard, J., Doob, L., Miller, N., Mowrer, O., & Sears, R. (1939). *Frustration and aggression.* New Haven, CT: Yale University Press.

Donnelly, P. (1996). The local and the global: Globalization in the sociology of sport. *Journal of Sport & Social Issues, 20,* 239–257.

Donnelly, P. (1999). Who's fair game? Sport, sexual harassment, and abuse. In P. White & K. Young, *Sport and gender in Canada* (pp. 107–128). Don Mills, ON: Oxford University Press.

Donnelly, P. (2000). *Taking sport seriously: Social issues in Canadian sport.* Toronto: Thompson Publishing.

Donnelly, P. (2002). George Herbert Mead and an interpretive sociology of sport. In J. Maguire & K. Young (Eds.), *Theory, sport & society* (pp. 83–102). Amsterdam: JAI.

Donnelly, P. (2004). Sport and risk culture. In K. Young (Ed.), *Sporting bodies, damaged selves: Sociological studies of sports-related injury* (pp. 29–58). Amsterdam: Elsevier.

Donnelly, P., & Kidd, B. (2003). Realizing the expectations: Youth, character, and community in Canadian sport. In Canadian Centre for Ethics in Sport, *The sport we want: Essays on current issues in community sport in Canada* (pp. 25–44). Ottawa: Canadian Centre for Ethics in Sport.

Douglas, M. (1966). *Purity and danger.* London: Routledge and Kegan Paul.

Drummond, M. (2002). Masculinity and self-identity in elite triathlon, bodybuilding and surf lifesaving. In D. Hemphill & C. Symons (Eds.), *Gender, sexuality and sport: A dangerous mix* (pp. 39–48). Sydney: Walla Walla Press.

Dubin, C. L. (1990). *Commission of inquiry into the use of drugs and banned substances intended to increase athletic performance.* Ottawa: Supply and Services Canada.

Duncan, M. C., & Hasbrook, C. (1988). Denial of power in televised women's sports. *Sociology of Sport Journal, 5,* 1–21.

Duncan, M., & Messner, M. (1998). The media image of sport and gender. In L. Wenner (Ed.), *MediaSport* (pp. 170–185). London: Routledge.

Dunn, R., & Stevenson, C. L. (1998). The paradox of the church hockey league. *International Review for the Sociology of Sport, 33,* 131–141.

Dunning, E. (1999). *Sport matters: Sociological studies of sport, violence and civilization.* London: Routledge.

Dunning, E., & Sheard, K. (1979). *Barbarians, gentlemen, and players: A sociological study of the development of rugby football.* Oxford: Martin Robertson.

Durant, W. (1926). *The story of philosophy.* New York: Simon & Schuster.

Durkheim, E. (1951). *Suicide: A study in sociology.* New York: The Free Press.

Dworkin, S., & Messner, M. (2002). Introduction: Gender relations and sport. *Sociological Perspectives, 45,* 347–52.

Eitzen, D. S. (2005). *Sport in contemporary society: An anthology.* Boulder: Paradigm.

Eitzen, D. S., & Sage, G. H. (2003). *Sociology of North American sport,* 7th ed. New York: McGraw-Hill.

Ekos Research Associates. (1992, September). *The status of the high performance athlete in Canada: Final report.* Submitted to Sport Canada Directorate, Fitness and Amateur Sport.

Elias, N., & Dunning, E. (1986). *Quest for excitement: Sport and leisure in the civilizing process.* Oxford: Basil Blackwell.

Eliot, T. S. (1943). Little Gidding. *Four quartets,* pp. 31–39. New York: Harcourt, Brace & World.

Engh, F. (1999). *Why Johnny hates sports.* Garden City Park, NY: Avery.

Epp, R., & Whitson, D. (Eds.). (2001). *Writing off the rural West: Globalization, governments, and the transformation of rural communities.* Edmonton: University of Alberta Press.

Ericsson, K. A., Krampe, R. T., & Tesch-Romer, C. (1993). The role of deliberate practice in the acquisition of expert performance. *Psychological Review, 100,* 363–406.

Ewing, M. E., & Seefeldt, V. (1990). *American youth and sports participation.* Youth Sports Institute of Michigan State University. Sponsored by the Athletic Footwear Association, Palm Beach, Florida.

Fawcett, B. (1992). The trouble with globalism. In M. Wyman (Ed.), *Vancouver forum* (pp. 183–201). Vancouver: Douglas & McIntyre.

Fejgin, N. (1994). Participation in high-school competitive sports: A subversion of school mission or contribution to academic goals? *Sociology of Sport Journal, 11,* 211–230.

Figler, S. K., & Whitaker, G. (1991). *Sport and play in American life.* Dubuque, IA: Wm. C. Brown.

Firth, C. E. (1968). *Macaulay's History of England,* Volume 1. New York: AMS Press.

Flake, C. (1992). The spirit of winning: Sport and the total man. In Shirl J. Hoffman (Ed.), *Sport and religion* (pp. 161–176). Champaign, IL: Human Kinetics.

Foer, F. (2004). *How soccer explains the world: An (unlikely) theory of globalization.* New York: Harper Perennial.

Foot, D. (1989). Public expenditures, population aging, and economic dependency in Canada: 1920–2021. *Population Research and Policy Review, 8,* 97–117.

Fort, R. D. (2003). *Sports economics.* Upper Saddle River, NJ: Pearson Education.

Fougère, M., & Mérette, M. (1999). *Population ageing, intergenerational equity, and growth: Analysis with an endogenous growth overlapping generations model.* Ottawa: Department of Finance. Retrieved from http://www.carleton.ca/economics/seminar percent20papers/ Merette-14Jan2000.pdf.

Freidman, T. (1999). *The Lexus and the olive tree.* New York: Farrar, Strauss & Giroux.

Frideres, J. S. (1988). Racism. In *The Canadian encyclopedia,* 2nd ed., Vol. III. Edmonton: Hurtig Publishers, 1816.

Frisby, W., Alexander, T., Taylor, J., Tirone, S., Watson, C., Harvey, J., & Laplante, D. (2005). *Bridging the recreation divide: Listening to youth and parents from low income families across Canada*. Ottawa: Report for the Canadian Parks and Recreation Association.

Fromm, Z. (2005). *Economic issues of Vancouver–Whistler 2010 Olympics*. Toronto: Pearson Prentice-Hall.

Galeano, E. (1998). *Soccer in the sun and shadow* (Trans. M. Fried). London: Verso.

Ganley, T., & Sherman, C. (2000, February). Exercise and children's health. *Physician and Sports Medicine, 28*(2). Retrieved from http://www.physicianandsportsmedicine.com.

Gibbons, S. L., & Van Gyn, G. H. (1996). It's more complex than coed vs. non coed: The British Columbia project on gender equitable coed physical education. *CAHPER Journal, 62*, 4–10.

Gibbons, S. L., Van Gyn, G. H., Wharf-Higgins, J., & Gaul, C. A. (2000). Girls' participation in physical education. *CAHPERD Journal, 66*, 26–32.

Gibbons, S. L., Wharf-Higgins, J., Gaul, C. A., & Van Gyn, G. H. (1999). Listening to female students in high school physical education. *Avante, 5*, 1–20.

Giddens, A. (1989). *Sociology*. Oxford: Polity Press.

Gillespie, G. (2001). The imperial embrace: British sportsmen and the appropriation of landscape in nineteenth century Canada. Doctoral dissertation, University of Western Ontario.

Glazer, N. (1970). Ethnic groups in America: From national culture to ideology. In M. Kurokawa (Ed.), *Minority responses* (pp. 74–86). New York: Random House.

Goldlust, J. (1987). *Playing for keeps: Sport, the media and society*. Melbourne: Longman Cheshire.

Gould, D. (1984). Psychosocial development and children's sport. In J. R. Thomas (Ed.), *Motor development during childhood and adolescence* (pp. 212–236). Minneapolis, MN: Burgess.

Grant, C., & Darley, F. (1993). Reaffirming the coach-athlete relationship: A response from intercollegiate athletics. *The Counseling Psychologist, 21*, 441–444.

Grant, P., & Wood, C. (2004). *Blockbusters and trade wars: Popular culture in a globalized world*. Vancouver: Douglas & McIntyre.

Greendorfer, S. L., & Blinde, E. M. (1985). Retirement from intercollegiate sport: Theoretical and empirical considerations. *Sociology of Sport Journal, 2*, 101–110.

Greendorfer, S. L., & Lewko, J. (1978). The role of family members in sport socialization of children. *Research Quarterly, 49*, 146–152.

Griffin, P. (1998). *Strong women, deep closets: Lesbians and homophobia in sport*. Champaign, IL: Human Kinetics.

Grossberg, L., Wartella, E., Whitney, D., & Wise, J. (Eds.). (2006). *MediaMaking: Mass media in a popular culture*. Thousand Oaks, CA: Sage.

Grossman, D. (2006, February). Students flocking to fringe sports. *Toronto Star*.

Grove, J. R., Lavallee, D., & Gordon, S. (1997). Coping with retirement from sport: The influence of athletic identity. *Journal of Applied Sport Psychology, 9*, 191–203.

Grover, R. (1998, June 1). Online sports: Cyber fans are roaring. *Business Week*, p. 155.

Gruneau, R. (1972). An analysis of Canada Games' Athletes, 1971. Unpublished master's thesis, University of Calgary, Calgary.

Gruneau, R. (1983). *Class, sports and social development*. Amherst: University of Massachusetts Press.

Gruneau, R. (1988). Modernization or hegemony: Two views on sport and social development. In J. Harvey & H. Cantelon (Eds.), *Not just a game: Essays in Canadian sport sociology* (pp. 9–32). Ottawa: University of Ottawa Press.

Gruneau, R. (1989). Making spectacle: A case study in television sports production. In L. Wenner (Ed.), *Media, sports and society* (pp. 134–154). Newbury Park, CA: Sage.

Gruneau, R., & Whitson, D. (1993). *Hockey night in Canada: Sport, identities and cultural politics.* Toronto: Garamond Press.

Guttmann, A. (1978). *From ritual to record: The nature of modern sports.* New York: Columbia University Press.

Guttmann, A. (1988). *A whole new ball game: An interpretation of American sports.* Chapel Hill, NC: University of North Carolina Press.

Hackett, R., & Gruneau, R. (2000). *The missing news: Filters and blind spots in Canada's press.* Toronto: Garamond Press.

Haley, B. (1978). *The healthy body and Victorian culture.* Cambridge, MA: Harvard University Press.

Halifax Herald. (2005, 20 December). Sagueneens apologize to Nolan for fans' conduct, p. C1.

Hall, A., Slack, T., Smith, G., & Whitson, D. (1991). *Sport in Canadian society.* Toronto: McClelland & Stewart Inc.

Hall, M. A. (2002). *The girl and the game: A history of women's sport in Canada.* Peterborough, ON: Broadview Press.

Hall, M., Lasby, D., Gumulla, G., & Tryon, C. (2006). *Caring Canadians, involved Canadians: Highlights of the 2004 Canada survey of giving, volunteering and participating.* Ottawa: Minister of Industry.

Hamilton, M. B. (1995). *The sociology of religion: Theoretical and comparative perspectives.* London and NY: Routledge.

Hannerz, U. (1996). *Transnational connections: Culture, people, places.* London: Routledge.

Hardman, K., & Marshall, J. (2000). The state and status of physical education in schools in international context. *European Physical Education Review, 6,* 203–229.

Hargreaves, J., & McDonald, I. (2000). Cultural studies and the sociology of sport. In J. Coakley & E. Dunning (Eds.), *Handbook of sport studies* (pp. 48–60). London: Sage.

Harris, H. A. (1972). *Sport in Greece and Rome.* London: The Camelot Press.

Hartman-Stein, P., & Potkanowicz, E. (2003). Behavioral determinants of healthy aging: Good news for the Baby Boomer generation. *Online Journal of Issues in Nursing, 48.* Retrieved from https://www.nursingworld.org/ojin/topic21/tpc21_5.htm.

Harvey, J. (1988). Sport policy and the welfare state: An outline of the Canadian state. *Sociology of Sport Journal, 5,* 315–329.

Harvey. J. (2000). What's in a game? In P. Donnelly (Ed.), *Taking sport seriously.* Toronto: Thompson Educational Publishing.

Harvey, J. (2006). Whose sweater is this? The changing meanings of hockey in Quebec. In D. Whitson & R. Gruneau (Eds.), *Artificial ice: Hockey, commerce, and cultural identity* (pp. 29–52). Peterborough, ON: Broadview Press.

Harvey, J., & Houle, F. (1994). World economy, global culture and new social movements. *Sociology of Sport Journal, 11,* 337–355.

Harvey, J., & Law, A. (2005). Resisting the global media oligopoly? The Canada Inc. response. In M. Silk, D. Andrews, & C. Cole (Eds.), *Sport and corporate nationalisms* (pp. 187–225). New York: Berg.

Harvey, J., & Proulx, R. (1988). Sport and the state in Canada. In J. Harvey & H. Cantelon, *Not just a game: Essays in Canadian sport sociology* (pp. 93–112). Ottawa: University of Ottawa Press.

Harvey, J., Law, A., & Cantelon, H. (2001). North American professional team sport franchises ownership patterns and global entertainment conglomerates. *Sociology of Sport Journal, 18,* 435–57.

Harvey, J., Rail, G., & Thibault, L. (1996). Globalization and sport: Sketching a theoretical model for empirical analyses. *Journal of Sport & Social Issues, 20,* 258–277.

Hayden, P. (1996). *The summer Paralympic Games: A history of the Paralympic Games and the 1996 Canadian Paralympic team.* Retrieved from http://www.cwba.ca/program/parahsty.html.

Healthy weights, healthy lives. (2004). Toronto: Report of Ontario's Chief Medical Officer of Health.

Hecimovich, M. (2004, April). Sport specialization in youth: A literature review. *Journal of the American Chiropractic Association.*

Heritage Canada. (2002). Evaluation of the 2001 IAAF World Championships in athletics (WCA) in Edmonton, Alberta, Final report. Retrieved September 6, 2006 from http:// www.canadianheritage.gc.ca/progs/em-cr/eval/2002/2002_pdf/WCA_eval2002_e.pdf.

Hildebrand, K., Johnson, D., & Bogle, K. (2001). Comparison of patterns of alcohol use between high school and college athletes and non-athletes. *College Student Journal, 35,* 358–370.

Hoberman, J. (1992). *Mortal engines: The science of performance and the dehumanization of sport.* New York: The Free Press.

Hoberman, J. (2005). *Testosterone dreams: Rejuvenation, aphrodisiac, doping.* Berkeley and Los Angeles: University of California Press.

Hoffman, S. J. (1992). *Sport and religion.* Champaign, IL: Human Kinetics.

Holland, A., & Andre, T. (1994). Athletic participation and the social status of adolescent males and females. *Youth & Society, 25,* 388–407.

Hollingshead, K. (1998). Tourism, hybridity, and ambiguity: The relevance of Bhabha's "third space" cultures. *Journal of Leisure Research, 30,* 121–156.

Holmes, J., & Silverman, E. (1992). *We're here, listen to us.* Ottawa: Canadian Advisory Council on the Status of Women.

Homans, G. (1964). Bringing men back in. *American Sociological Review, 29,* 809–818.

Homer. (1973). *The Iliad.* Edited by E. V. Rieu. London: Lane.

Homer. (2001). *The Odyssey.* Edited by R. L. Reickhoff. New York: Forge.

Hoover, N. C. (1999). *National survey: Initiation rites and athletics for NCAA sports teams.* Retrieved from http://www.alfred.edu/news/html/hazing_study_99.html.

Hoover, N. C., & Pollard, N. J. (2000). *Initiation rites in American high schools: A national survey.* Retrieved from http://www.alfred.edu/new/html/hazing_study.html.

Horin, A. (2005, August 7). Boys who are too uncool for school. *Sydney Morning Herald.* Retrieved from http://www.smh.com.au.

Horne, J. (2006). *Sport in consumer culture.* London: Palgrave Macmillan.

Howell, C. (2001). *Blood, sweat and cheers: Sport and the making of modern Canada.* Toronto: University of Toronto Press.

Hughes, C. (2005, October 6). Don't impose phys ed (Letter to the editor). *Toronto Star,* A25.

Hughes, T. (1857). *Tom Brown's school days by an old boy.* New York: Hurst and Company. 1904.

Hughes, T. (1861). *Tom Brown at Oxford.* London: Macmillan.

Hughes, T. (1994). *Tom Brown's schooldays.* London: Penguin Books.

Humbert, M. L. (1995). On the sidelines: The experiences of young women in physical education classes. *Avante, 1,* 58–77.

Humbert, M. L., & Chad, K. E. (1998). Determining barriers to implementing quality daily physical education. *Journal of the International Council for Health, Physical Education, Recreation, Sport, and Dance, 34*, 12–17.

Hums, M. A., MacLean, J., Richman, J. M., & Pastore, D. L. (1994). Influences on women's intercollegiate sport in the United States and Canada. *Journal of the International Council for Health, Physical Education, Recreation, Sport, and Dance, 31*, 34–37.

Hurtig, M. (2002). *The vanishing country: Is it too late to save Canada?* Toronto: McClelland & Stewart.

Hutchison, R. (1988). A critique of race, ethnicity, and social class in recent leisure-related research. *Journal of Leisure Research, 20*, 10–30.

Ingham, A., Howell, J., & Schilperoort, T. (1988). Sport and community: A review and exegesis. *Exercise and Sport Science Review, 15*, 427–465.

Inglis, S. (1991). Influence in and around interuniversity athletics. *Journal of Sport Management, 5*, 18–33.

Iyer, P. (2000). *The global soul.* New York: Vintage Books.

Jackson, R. (1986). The effect of international sport on Canadian interuniversity athletics. In A. W. Taylor (Ed.), *The role of interuniversity athletics: A Canadian perspective* (pp. 39–42). Ottawa: Sports Dynamic.

Jackson, S. J. (1994). Gretzky, crisis & Canadian identity in 1988: Rearticulating the Americanization of culture debate. *Sociology of Sport Journal, 11*, 428–446.

Jackson, S. J. (1998a). A twist of race: Ben Johnson & the Canadian crisis of racial and national identity. *Sociology of Sport Journal, 15*, 21–40.

Jackson, S. J. (1998b). Life in the (mediated) Faust Lane: Ben Johnson, national affect and the 1988 crisis of Canadian identity. *International Review for the Sociology of Sport, 33*, 227–238.

Jackson, S. J. (1998c). The 49th paradox: The 1988 Calgary Winter Olympic Games and Canadian identity as contested terrain. In M. Duncan, G. Chick, & A. Aycock (Eds.), *Diversions and divergences in the fields of play* (pp. 191–208). Greenwich, CT: Ablex.

James, C. E. (1995). Negotiating school through sports: African Canadian youth strive for academic success. *Avante, 1*, 20–36.

James, C. E. (2005). *Race in play: Understanding the socio-cultural worlds of student-athletes.* Toronto: Canadian Scholars' Press Inc.

James, C. L. R. (1963). *Beyond a boundary.* London: Hutchinson.

Jennings, A. (1998). Sport lies, and . . . . Presentation to the Danish Gymnastics and Sports Association. Retrieved June 13, 2006 from http://www.playthegame.org/Knolwege%20/Articles/Sport_lies.asp.

Jhally, S. (1989). Cultural studies and the sports/media complex. In L. Wenner (Ed.), *Media, sports and society* (pp. 70–93). Newbury Park, CA: Sage.

Jobling, I. (1970). Sport in nineteenth century Canada: The effects of technological changes on its development. Doctoral dissertation, the University of Alberta.

Johns, D. P. (2004). Weight management as sport injury: Deconstructing disciplinary power in the sport ethic. In K. Young (Ed.), *Sporting bodies, damaged selves: Sociological studies of sports-related injury* (pp. 117–136). Amsterdam: Elsevier.

Johnson, J. (2000). *Sport hazing experiences in the context of anti-hazing policies: The case of two southern Ontario universities.* Unpublished master's thesis, University of Toronto.

Johnson, J., & Miller, P. S. (2004). Changing the initiation ceremony. In J. Johnson & M. Holman (Eds.), *Making the team: Inside the world of sport initiations and hazing.* Toronto: Canadian Scholars' Press Inc.

Jones, J. C. H., & Ferguson, D. G. (1988). Location and survival in the National Hockey League. *Journal of Industrial Economics, 36,* 443–57.

Jones, R., & LeBlanc, R. (2005). Sport, sexuality and representation in advertising: The political economy of the pink dollar. In S. J. Jackson & D. L. Andrews (Eds.), *Sport, culture and advertising: Identities, commodities and the politics of representation* (pp. 119–135). London: Routledge.

Kazemipur, A., & Halli, S. S. (2001). The changing color of poverty in Canada. *Canadian Review of Sociology and Anthropology, 38,* 217–238.

Kellner, D. (1995). *Media culture.* London: Routledge.

Kenyon, G. (1977). Factors influencing the attainment of elite track status in track and field. *Post Olympic conference proceedings.* Ottawa: Coaching Association of Canada.

Kenyon, G., & McPherson, B. (1973). Becoming involved in physical activity and sport: A process of socialization. In G. L. Rarick (Ed.), *Physical activity: Human growth and development.* New York: Academic Press.

Kenyon, G. S. (1969). Sport involvement: A conceptual go and some consequences thereof. In G. S. Kenyon (Ed.), *Aspects of contemporary sport sociology.* Chicago: The Athletic Institute.

Kerr, D., & Beaujot, R. (2003). Child poverty and family structure in Canada, 1981–1997. *Journal of Comparative Family Studies, 34,* 321–35.

Kerr, G. (1996). The role of sport in preparing youth for adulthood. In B. Galway & J. Hudson (Eds.), *Youth in transition: Perspectives on research and policy.* Toronto: Thompson Educational Publishing.

Kerr, G., & Dacyshyn, A. (2000). The retirement experiences of elite, female gymnasts. *Journal of Applied Sport Psychology, 12,* 115–133.

Kidd, B. (1970). Canada's "national" sport. In I. Lumsden (Ed.), *Close the 49th Parallel etc.: The Americanization of Canada* (pp. 257–74). Toronto: University of Toronto Press.

Kidd, B. (1983). In defense of Tom Longboat. *Canadian Journal of History of Sport, 14,* 34–65.

Kidd, B. (1984). The myth of the ancient Games. In A. Tomlinson & G. Whannel (Eds.), *Five ring circus: Money, power and politics at the Olympic Games* (pp. 71–83). London and Sydney: Pluto Press.

Kidd, B. (1996a). Chapter nine: Worker sport in the new world: The Canadian story. In A. Kuger & J. Riordan (Eds.), *The story of worker sport* (pp. 143–156). Champaign, IL: Human Kinetics.

Kidd, B. (1996b). *The struggle for Canadian sport.* Toronto: University of Toronto Press.

Kidd, B. (1999). The economic case for physical education. *CAHPERD Journal, 65,* 4–10.

Kidd, B., & Eberts, M. (1982). *Athlete's rights in Canada.* Toronto: Queen's Printer.

Kilmarten, M. (1994). *The masculine self.* Toronto: Maxwell Macmillan.

King, C. R., & Springwood, C. F. (2001). *Team spirits: Essays on the history and significance of Native American mascots.* Lincoln: University of Nebraska Press.

Kirkwood, K. (2004). Out of the Olympic closet: Abandoning prohibitions on doping in favour of a harm reduction approach. Unpublished Dissertation. London, ON: The University of Western Ontario.

Klein, A. (1991). *Sugarball: The American game, the Dominican dream.* New Haven, CT: Yale University Press.

Klein, A. (1997). *The Owls of the two Laredos: Baseball and nationalism on the Texas-Mexican border.* Princeton, NJ: Princeton University Press.

Knickman, J., & Snell, E. (2002). The 2030 problem: Caring for aging baby boomers. *Health Services Research, 37,* 849–884.

Knowles, V. (2000). Forging our legacy: Canadian citizenship and immigration 1900–1977. Ottawa: Citizenship and Immigration Canada. Retrieved November 17, 2005 from http://www.cic.gc.ca/english/department/legacy/acknowledge.html.

Koukouris, K. (1994). Constructed case studies: Athletes' perspectives of disengaging from organized competitive sport. *Sociology of Sport Journal, 11,* 114–39.

Kremarik, F. (2000, Autumn). A family affair: Children's participation in sport. *Canadian Social Trends,* 20–24.

Labbé, R. (2004, February 22). Dollar favorable ou pas, le Canadien va perdre de l'argent, *La Presse* (Montreal), p. S3.

Ladd, T., & Mathisen J. A. (1999). *Muscular Christianity: Evangelical Protestants and the development of American sport.* Grand Rapids, MI: Baker Books.

Landers, D., & Landers, D. (1978). Socialization via interscholastic athletics: Its effects on delinquency. *Sociology of Education, 51,* 299–303.

Langford, I. (2004, February 10). Cherry's comments: Racially insensitive and nonsensical. *torontObserver.* Retrieved July 5, 2006 from http://observer.thecentre.centennialcollege.ca/opinion/cherry_ian021004.htm.

Lathrop, A. H., & Murray, N. (1998). A discipline under siege: Who took the physical out of education? *Avante, 4,* 92–100.

Lavallee, D. (2005). The effect of a life development intervention on sports career transition adjustment. *The Sport Psychologist, 19,* 193–202.

Lavoie, M. (1989). Stacking, performance differentials, and salary discrimination in professional ice hockey: A survey of evidence. *Sociology of Sport Journal, 6,* 17–35.

Lavoie, M. (1997). *Avantage numérique: L'argent et la Ligue nationale de hockey.* Hull: Vents d'Ouest.

Lavoie, M. (2003). The entry draft in the National Hockey League: Discrimination, style of play, and team location. *American Journal of Economics and Sociology, 62,* 383–406.

Lavoie, M., & Whitson, D. (2003). The economics of sport. In J. Crossman (Ed.), *Canadian sport sociology* (pp. 139–155). Toronto: Thomson Nelson.

LeBeau, S. (2006). (No title). In Mad about hockey—Superstitions. Retrieved from http://www.mcq.org/societe/hockey/pages/aasuperstitions_3.html.

LeClair, J. (1992). *Winners and losers: Sport and physical activity in the '90s.* Toronto: Thompson Educational Publishing.

Leger Marketing. (2002, February). Leger Marketing poll of Canadian spectator preferences. Montreal: Leger Marketing.

Leichliter, J., Meilman, P., Presley, C., & Cashin, J. (1998). Alcohol use and related consequences among college students with varying levels of involvement in college athletics. *Journal of College Health, 46,* 257–262.

Lenskyj, H. (1986). *Out of bounds: Women, sport and sexuality.* Toronto: Women's Press.

Lenskyj, H. (1990). Power and play: Gender and sexuality issues in sport and physical activity. *International Review for the Sociology of Sport, 25,* 235–245.

Lenskyj, H. (1993). Running risks: Compulsive exercise and eating disorders. In C. Brown & K. Jasper (Eds.), *Consuming passions: Feminist counselling approaches to weight preoccupation and eating disorders* (pp. 91–108). Toronto: Second Story Press.

Lenskyj, H. (1994). *Women, sport and physical activity: Selected research themes.* Ottawa: Sport Information Resource Centre.

Lenskyj, H. (2000). *Inside the Olympic industry: Power, politics and activism.* Albany NY: SUNY Press.

Lenskyj, H. (2003). *Out on the field: Gender, sport and sexualities.* Toronto: Women's Press.

Leonard II, W. M. (1998). *A sociological perspective of sport,* 3rd ed. Boston: Allyn and Bacon.

Levin, R. C., Mitchell, G. J., Volcker, P. A., & Will, G. F. (2000, July). *The report of the independent members of the Commissioner's Blue Ribbon Panel on baseball economics.*

Levitt, A. (2004, February 5). *Independent review of the combined financial results of the National Hockey League 2002–2003 season.* Retrieved from http://www.nhlcbanews.com/levittreport.html.

Lewi, D. (2006, January 31). Canada's first multicultural hockey league. *torontObserver.* Retrieved February 28, 2006 from http://tobserver.thecentre.centennialcollege.ca/read_articles.asp?article_id=681.

Li, P. S. (1990). Race and ethnicity. In Peter S. Li (Ed.), *Race and ethnic relations in Canada* (pp. 3–17). Toronto: Oxford University Press.

Limbert, J., Crawford, S. M., & McCargar, L. J. (1994). Estimates of the prevalence of obesity in Canadian children. *Obesity Research, 2,* 321–327.

Lindsay, P. L. (1969). A History of Sport in Canada, 1807–1867. Doctoral dissertation, University of Alberta.

Lindsay, P. L. (1970). The impact of military garrisons on the development of sport in British North America. *Canadian Journal of History of Sport and Physical Education, 1,* 33–44.

Lindsay, P. L. (1972). George Beers and the national game concept: A behavioural approach. Proceedings of the Second Canadian Symposium on the History of Sport and Physical Education, 27–44.

Longley, N. (2000). The underrepresentation of French Canadians on English Canadian NHL teams. *Journal of Sports Economics, 1,* 236–256.

Longley, N. (2004). The professional football industry in Canada: Economic and policy issues. In R. Fort & J. Fizel (Eds.), *International sports economics* (pp. 209–21). Westport, CT: Praeger.

Lorenz, K. (1966). *On aggression.* New York: Harcourt, Brace, & Jovanovich.

Lorimer, R., & McNulty, J. (1996). *Mass communication in Canada,* 3rd ed. Toronto: Oxford University Press.

Lowes, M. D. (1999). *Inside the sports pages.* Toronto: University of Toronto Press.

Loy, J., & Booth, D. (2002). Émile Durkheim, structural functionalism and the sociology of sport. In J. Maguire & K. Young (Eds.), *Theory, sport & society* (pp. 41–62). Amsterdam: JAI.

Loy, W. J., & Booth, D. (2000). Functionalism, sport and society. In J. Coakley & E. Dunning (Eds.), *Handbook of sport studies* (pp. 8–27). London: Sage.

Lull, J. (2000). *Media, commerce, culture: A global approach.* NY: Columbia University Press.

Lumpkin, A. (2005). *Physical education, exercise science, and sport studies,* 5th ed. Boston: McGraw-Hill.

MacAloon, J. (1990). Steroids and the State: Dubin, melodrama and the accomplishment of innocence. *Public Culture, 2,* 41–64.

Macdonald, C. (1976). The Edmonton Grads, Canada's most successful team: A history and analysis of their success. Master's thesis, University of Windsor.

MacIntosh, D. (1990). Interschool sport programs in Canada. *CAHPER Journal, 56,* 36–40.

MacIntosh, D., & Whitson, D. (1990). *The game planners.* Montreal: McGill–Queen's University Press.

MacIntosh, D., Bedecki, T., & Franks, C. E. S. (1987). *Sport and politics in Canada: Federal government involvement since 1961.* Kingston & Montreal: McGill–Queen's University Press.

MacLachlan, I., & Sawada, R. (1997). Measures of income inequality and social polarization in Canadian metropolitan areas. *Canadian Geographer, 41*, 377–97.

MacNeill, M. (1996). Networks: Producing Olympic ice hockey for a national television audience. *Sociology of Sport Journal, 13*, 103–124.

Macpherson, A., Rothman, L., & Howard, A. (2006). Body-checking rules and childhood injuries in ice hockey. *Pediatrics, 117*, 143–147.

Maguire, J. (1999). *Global sport: Identities, societies, civilizations.* Cambridge: Polity Press.

Maguire, J. A. (1993). Globalization, sport development and the media/sport production complex. *Sport Science Review, 2*(1), 29–47.

Maitland, F. W. (1906). *The life and letters of Leslie Stephen.* London: Duckworth and Co.

Majors, R. (1990). Cool pose: Black masculinity and sports. In M. Messner & D. Sabo (Eds.), *Sport, men, and the gender order: Critical feminist perspectives* (pp. 109–114). Champaign, IL: Human Kinetics Press.

Malinowski, B. (1927). *Coral gardens and their magic.* London: Routledge and Kegan Paul.

Malloy, D. C., Ross, S., & Zakus, D. H. (2000). *Sport ethics: Concepts and cases in sport and recreation.* Toronto: Thompson Educational.

Malloy, D. C., Ross, S., & Zakus, D. H. (2004). *Sport ethics: Concepts and cases in sport and recreation,* 2nd ed. Toronto: Thompson Educational Publishing.

Mannix, D. P. (1958). *Those about to die.* New York: Ballantine Books.

Marchie, A., & Cusimano, M. (2003). Bodychecking and concussions in ice hockey: Should our youth pay the price? *Canadian Medical Association Journal, 169*, 124–128.

Marcia, J. E. (1993). The ego identity status approach to ego identity. In J. E. Marcia, A. S. Waterman, D. R. Matteson, S. L. Archer, & J. L. Orlofsky (Eds.), *Ego identity: A handbook for psychosocial research* (pp. 3–21). New York: Springer-Verlag.

Martens, F. L. (1985). Academic achievement of intercollegiate athletes in physical education at the University of Victoria. *CAHPER Journal, 51*, 14–22.

Martens, M., Dams-O'Connor, K., & Beck, N. (2006). A systematic review of college student-athlete drinking: Prevalence rates, sport-related factors, and interventions. *Journal of Substance Abuse Treatment, 31*, 305–316.

Martens, M., Watson, J., & Beck, N. (2006). Sport-type differences in alcohol use among intercollegiate athletes. *Journal of Applied Sport Psychology, 18*, 136–150.

Marx, K. (1844). Economic and philosophical manuscripts. In *Karl Marx: Early writings.* Markham, ON: Penguin Books. 1975.

Marx, K. (1963). Economic and philosophical manuscripts. In T. B. Bottomore (Ed.), *Karl Marx: Early writings* (pp. 61–220). New York: McGraw-Hill.

Marx, K. (1972). Thesis on Feuerbach. In R. C. Tucker (Ed.), *The Marx-Engels reader* (pp. 107–109). New York: W.W. Norton & Company.

Marx, K. (1977). *Capital, vol. I.* New York: Vintage Books.

Marx, K., & Engels, F. (1948). *Manifesto of the communist party.* New York: International Publishers.

Mason, D. (2002). Get the puck outta here: Media transnationalism and corporate identity. *Journal of Sport and Social Issues, 26*(2), 140–167.

Mason, D. (2006). "Expanding the footprint"? Questioning the NHL's expansion and relocation strategy. In D. Whitson & R. Gruneau (Eds.), *Artificial ice: Hockey, culture, and commerce* (pp. 181–199). Peterborough, ON: Broadview Press.

Mathews, A. W. (1974). *Athletics in Canadian universities.* Ottawa: The Association of Universities and Colleges in Canada.

McBride, P. (1975). *Culture clash: Immigrants and reformers, 1880–1920*. Boston: R & E Associates.

McCallum, J. (1992). Green cars, black cats and lady luck. In S. J. Hoffman (Ed.), *Sport and religion* (pp. 203–211). Champaign, IL: Human Kinetics.

McChesney, R. (1999). *Rich media, poor democracy*. New York: The New York Press.

McElroy, M. (1983). Parent-child relations and orientations toward sport. *Sex Roles: A Journal of Research, 9,* 997–1004.

McGowan, E., & Rail, G. (1996). Up the creek without a paddle: Canadian women sprint racing canoeists' retirement from international sport. *Avante, 2,* 118–136.

McNeal, R. (1995). Extracurricular activities and high-school dropouts. *Sociology of Education, 68,* 62–81.

McPherson, B. (1977). Factors influencing the attainment of elite hockey status. *Post Olympic conference proceedings*. Ottawa: Coaching Association of Canada.

McQuarie, D. (Ed.). (1995). *Readings in contemporary sociological theory: From modernity to post-modernity*. Englewood Cliffs, NJ: Prentice Hall.

McTeer, W., & Curtis, J. (1999). Intercollegiate sport involvement and academic achievement: A follow-up study. *Avante, 5,* 39–55.

Mead, G. H. (1962). *Mind, self, & society from the standpoint of a behaviourist*. Chicago and London: The University of Chicago Press.

Melnick, M., Sabo, D., & Vanfossen, B. (1992a). Educational effects of interscholastic athletic participation on African-American and Hispanic youth. *Adolescence, 27,* 295–308.

Melnick, M., Sabo, D., & Vanfossen, B. (1992b). Educational effects of interscholastic athletic participation on social, educational, and career mobility of Hispanic girls and boys. *International Review for Sociology of Sport, 27,* 57–75.

Merrigan, P., & Trudel, P. (2004). *Dernière minute de jeu: Les millions du hockey*. Montreal: Hurtubise HMH.

Messner, M. (1990). When bodies are weapons: Masculinity and violence in sport. *International Review for the Sociology of Sport, 25,* 203–218.

Messner, M. (1992). *Power at play: Sports and the problem of masculinity*. Boston: Beacon.

Metcalfe, A. (1970). The form and function of physical activity in New France, 1534–1759. *Canadian Journal of History of Sport and Physical Education, 1,* 45–64.

Metcalfe, A. (1987). *Canada learns to play: The emergence of organized sport, 1807–1914*. Toronto: McClelland & Stewart.

Meynaud, J. (1966). *Sport et politique*. Paris: Payot.

Miliband, R. (1969). *The state in capitalist society*. London: Quartet Books. Thousand Oaks, CA: Sage.

Miller, P. S., & Johnson, J. (1998). *Handbook on orientation and transition for students at the University of Toronto*. Toronto: Faculty of Physical Education and Health, University of Toronto.

Miller, P. S., & Kerr, G. (2002). The athletic, academic, and social experiences of intercollegiate student-athletes. *Journal of Sport Behavior, 25,* 346–367.

Miller, P. S., & Kerr, G. (2003). The role experimentation of intercollegiate student-athletes. *The Sport Psychologist, 17,* 197–220.

Miller, S. (1989, April). Sport sections responding to audience interest and needs. *Scripps-Howard Editors' Newsletter, 13.*

Mills, C. W. (1959). *The sociological imagination*. London: Oxford University Press.

Mills, D. (1998). *Sport in Canada: Everybody's business*. Ottawa: Standing Committee on Canadian Heritage, Subcommittee on the Study of Sport in Canada.

Ministry of Education. (2001). *Report of the Minister's Advisory Group on the provision of co-instructional activities*. Ottawa: The Queen's Printer for Ontario.

Morgan, C. (1995). In search of the phantom misnamed honour: Duelling in Upper Canada. *The Canadian Historical Review, 76*, 529–562.

Moriarty, D., & Holman-Prpich, M. (1987). Canadian interuniversity athletics: A model and method for analyzing conflict and change. *Journal of Sport Management, 1*, 57–73.

Morissette, R., & Bérubé, C. (1996). *Longitudinal aspects of earnings inequality in Canada*. Ottawa: Analytical Studies Branch, Statistics Canada.

Morissette, R., Zhang, X., & Drolet, M. (2002). The evolution of wealth inequality in Canada, 1984–1999. Ottawa: Statistics Canada, p. 187.

Morley, D. (2005). Media. In T. Bennett, L. Grossberg, & M. Morris (Eds.), *New keywords: A revised vocabulary of culture and society* (pp. 211–214). Malden, MA: Blackwell Publishing.

Morrow, D. (1979). Lionel Pretoria Conacher. *Journal of sport History, 6, 1*, 5–37.

Morrow, D. (1981). The powerhouse of Canadian sport: The Montreal Amateur Athletic Association, inception to 1909. *Journal of Sport History, 8*, 20–39.

Morrow, D. (1986). A case study in amateur conflict: The athletic war in Canada, 1906–1908. *British Journal of Sports History, 3*, 183–190.

Morrow, D. (1987). Sweetheart sport: Barbara Ann Scott and the Post World War Two image of the female athlete in Canada. *Canadian Journal of History of Sport and Physical Education, 18*, 36–54.

Morrow, D., & Leyshon, G. (1987). George Goulding: A case study in sporting excellence. *Canadian Journal of History of Sport and Physical Education, 18*, 26–51.

Morrow, D., & Wamsley, K. B. (2005). *Sport in Canada: A history*. Toronto: Oxford University Press.

Morrow, D., Keyes, M., Simpson, W., Cosentino, F., & Lappage, R. (1989). *A concise history of sport in Canada*. Toronto: Oxford University Press.

Mott, M., & Allardyce, J. (1989). *Curling capital: Winnipeg and the roarin' game, 1876–1988*. Winnipeg: University of Manitoba Press.

Mullick, R. (2002, February). Warren Moon. *CFL legends*. The Official Site of the Canadian Football League. Retrieved from http://www.cfl.ca/CFLLegends/moon.html.

Murphy, G. M., Petitpas, A. J., & Brewer, B. W. (1996). Identity foreclosure, athletic identity, and career maturity in intercollegiate athletes. *The Sport Psychologist, 10*, 239–246.

Murphy, P., Williams, J., & Dunning, E. (1990). *Football on trial: Spectator violence and development in the world of football*. London: Routledge.

Nack, W., & Yaeger, D. (1999, September 13). Who's coaching your kid? The frightening truth about child molestation in youth sports. *Sports Illustrated*, 39–53.

National Coaching Certification Program (NCCP). (1988). *Coaching theory I manual*. Gloucester, ON: Coaching Association of Canada.

Naylor, D. (2004, February 21). Poor boys no more. *The Globe and Mail*, p. S1.

Nelson, E. & Robinson, B. (1999). *Gender in Canada*. Scarborough: Prentice Hall Allyn & Bacon.

Nelson, M. B. (1991). *Are we winning yet? How women are changing sports and sports are changing women*. New York: Random House.

Nelson, M. B. (1994). *The stronger women get, the more men love football: Sexism and the American culture of sports*. New York: Harcourt Brace.

NHL. (2004a). *NHL collective bargaining agreement background*, Press release, NHL.

NHL. (2004b). *What fans say: 2003–2004 season study*. Retrieved from http://www.nhlcbanews.com/fansurvey.html.

Nissenbaum, S. (1996). *The battle for Christmas*. New York: Knopf.

Nixon, H. (1996). Explaining pain and injury attitudes and experiences in sport in terms of gender, race, and sports status factors. *Journal of Sport and Social Issues, 20*, 33–44.

Nixon, H. L., & Frey, J. H. (1996). *A sociology of sport*. Belmont: Wadsworth.

Norfolk Capital and Triax. (2001). *Executive summary: OSHC 2001 limited partnership class A units*. (The document was officially released on January 8, 2002.)

North, J., & Lavallee, D. (2004). An investigation of potential users of career transition services in the United Kingdom. *Journal of Sport and Exercise, 5*, 77–84.

Novak, M. (1976). *The joy of sport*. New York: Basic Books.

O'Brien, S. (2004). *The Canadian Football League: The phoenix of professional sports leagues*. Morrisville, NC: Lulu Press.

Offord, D., Lipman, E., & Duku, E. (1998). *Sports, the arts, and community programs: Rates and correlates of participation*. Ottawa: Human Resources Development.

Okihiro, N. R. (1984). Extracurricular participation, educational destinies and early job outcomes. In N. Theberge & P. Donnelly (Eds.), *Sport and the sociological imagination* (pp. 334–349). Fort Worth, TX: Texas Christian University Press.

Ontario University Athletics (OUA). (2001). The constitution and by-laws. Ontario University Athletics in the Canadian Interuniversity Athletic Union.

Owram, D. (1996). *Born at the right time: A history of the baby boom generation*. Toronto: University of Toronto Press.

Pal, L. (2006). *Beyond policy analysis: Public issue management in turbulent times*. Toronto: Nelson.

Paraschak, V. (1997). Variations in race relations: Sporting events for Native Peoples in Canada. *Sociology of Sport Journal, 14*, 1–21.

Parkin, F. (1978). Social stratification. In T. Bottomore & R. Nisbet (Eds.), *A history of sociological analysis* (pp. 599–632). London: Heinemann Educational Books.

Parsons, T. (1961). An outline of the social system. In T. Parsons, E. Shils, K. D. Naegele, & J. R. Pitts (Eds.), *Theories of society: Foundations of modern sociological theory*, Vol. I (pp. 30–79). New York: The Free Press of Glencoe.

Pearson, R. E., & Petitpas, A. (1990). Transitions of athletes: Developmental and preventive perspectives. *Journal of Counseling and Development, 69*, 7–10.

Pearton, R. (1986). Violence in sport and the special case of soccer hooliganism in the United Kingdom. In R. Rees & A. Miracle (Eds.), *Sport and social theory* (pp. 67–84). Champaign, IL: Human Kinetics.

People for Education. (2001). *The 2001 Tracking Report*. Retrieved from http://www.peopleforeducation.com.

Physical activity promotion and school physical education. (1999, September). *Research Digest, 3*(7). Retrieved from http://www.fitness.gov.

Pitter, R. (2006). Racialization and hockey in Canada: From personal troubles to a Canadian challenge. In D. Whitson & R. Gruneau (Eds.), *Artificial ice: Hockey, culture, and commerce* (pp. 123–139). Peterborough, ON: Broadview Press.

Play Therapy UK. (n.d.). Definition of play. Retrieved December 29, 2006 from http://www.playtherapy.org.uk/AboutPlayTherapy/PlayDefinition1.htm.

Prebish, C. S. (1984). Heavenly father, divine goalie: Sport and religion. *The Antioch Review, 42*, 306–318.

Preuss, H. (2004). *The economics of staging the Olympics*. Cheltenham, UK: Edward Elgar.

Pronger, B. (1990). *The arena of masculinity*. New York: St. Martin's Press.

Pronger, B. (1993, January 25). Push 'em back. *University of Toronto Bulletin*, 20.

Psycho-physiological contributions of physical activity and sports for girls. (1998, March). *Research Digest, 3*(1). Retrieved from http://www.fitness.gov.

Public Broadcasting Service. (2004). *The real Olympics: A history of the ancient and modern Olympics Games*. Alexandria, VA: PBS Home Video.

Rail, G. (2000). Contextualizing the Mills report: Pro sport, corporate welfare and the Canadian state. *Avante, 6*, 1–11.

Ralston Saul, J. (2005). *The collapse of globalism and the reinvention of the world*. Camberwell, Australia: Penguin/Viking.

Rayner, M. (1998, July 16). CIAU faces split over scholarships. *Western News*.

Real, M. (1998). Mediasport: Technology and the commodification of postmodern sport. In L. Wenner (Ed.), *MediaSport* (pp. 14–26). London: Routledge.

Ricardo, D. (1951). *On the principles of political economy and taxation*. Cambridge: Cambridge University Press.

Rice, C., & Russell, V. (1995). EmBodying equity. *Our Schools Our Selves* (September, pp. 14–36; December, pp. 32–54).

Rice, C., & Russell, V. (2002). *Embodying equity*. Toronto: Green Dragon Press. Retrieved from http://www3.sympatico.ca/equity.greendragonpress.

Richardson, D. (2000). Pay, performance, and competitiveness in the National Hockey League. *Eastern Economic Journal, 26*, 393–418.

Rinehart, R. E. (1998). *Players all: Performance in contemporary sport*. Bloomington, IN: Indiana University Press.

Robertson, R. (1992). *Globalization: Social theory and global culture*. New York: Russell Sage.

Robinson, L. (1998). *Crossing the line: Sexual harassment and abuse in Canada's national sport*. Toronto: McClelland & Stewart.

Robinson, L. (2002). *Black tights: Women, sport, and sexuality*. Toronto: HarperCollins.

Rosenberg, D. (2003). Athletics in the Ward and beyond: Neighborhoods, Jews, and sport in Toronto, 1900–1939. In R. C. Wilcox, D. L. Andrews, R. Pitter, & R. L. Irwin (Eds.). *Sporting dystopias: The making and meanings of urban sport cultures* (pp. 137–152). Albany, NY: State University of New York Press.

Rosenstein, J. (1997). *In whose honor? America Indian mascots in sports*. New Jersey: New Day Films.

Rowe, D. (1996). The global love-match: Sport and television. *Media, Culture & Society, 18*, 565–582.

Rowe, D. (1999). *Sport, culture and the media*. Buckingham, UK: Open University Press.

Rowe, D., Lawrence, G., Miller, T., & McKay, J. (1994). Global sport? Core concern and peripheral vision. *Media, Culture & Society, 16*, 661–675.

Sabo, D., Melnick, M., & Vanfossen, B. (1993). High school athletic participation and post-secondary educational and occupational mobility: A focus on race and gender. *Sociology of Sport Journal, 10*, 44–56.

Sage, G. (2004). The sporting goods industry: From struggling entrepreneurs to national business to transnational corporations. In T. Slack (Ed.), *The commercialisation of sport* (pp. 29–51). London: Routledge.

Sage, G. H. (1997). Physical education, sociology, and sociology of sport: Points of intersection. *Sociology of Sport Journal, 14,* 317–339.

Sage, G. H. (1998). *Power and ideology in American sport,* 2nd ed. Champaign, IL: Human Kinetics.

Schaefler, C., & Kaduson, H. (1994). *The quotable play therapist.* Northvale: Jason Aronson.

Scherer, J. (2001). Globalization and the construction of local particularities: A case study of the Winnipeg Jets. *Sociology of Sport Journal, 18,* 205–230.

Scherer, J. (forthcoming). Globalization, promotional culture and the production/consumption of on-line games: Engaging Adidas's beat rugby campaign. *New Media & Society.*

Scherer, J., & Jackson, S. (2004). From corporate welfare to national interest: Newspaper analysis of the public subsidization of NHL hockey debate in Canada. *Sociology of Sport Journal, 21,* 36–60.

Scherer, J., & Jackson, S. (2005). *Globalization, new media technologies and the production/consumption of allblacks.com.* Paper presented at the 2005 Conference of the North American Society for the Sociology of Sport in Winston-Salem, North Carolina.

Schiller, D. (1999). *Digital capitalism.* Cambridge, MA: The MIT Press.

Schlossberg, N. (1981). A model for analyzing human adaptation to transition. *The Counseling Psychologist, 9,* 2–18.

Schneider, A., & Butcher, R. (2000). An ethical analysis of drug testing. In W. Wilson & E. Derse, *Doping in elite sport: The politics of drugs in the Olympic movement* (pp. 129–152). Champaign, IL: Human Kinetics.

Schneider, M. (1988). *Often invisible: Counselling gay and lesbian youth.* Toronto: Central Toronto Youth Services.

Schneider, V. E. (1997). Interuniversity athletics: Separation from physical education. *Avante, 3,* 88–97.

Scott, R. (1987). *Jackie Robinson: Baseball great.* New York: Chelsea House Publishers.

Semotiuk, D. M. (1986). Internal factors affecting elite sport in Canadian universities. In A. W. Taylor (Ed.), *The role of interuniversity athletics: A Canadian perspective* (pp. 59–76). Ottawa: Sports Dynamic.

Sennnett, R., & Cobb, J. (1973). *The hidden injuries of class.* New York: Vintage Books.

Short, J. R., & Kim, Y. H. (1999). *Globalization and the city.* New York: Longman.

Siedentop, D. (2004). *Introduction to physical education, fitness and sport,* 5th ed. Boston: McGraw-Hill.

Silk, M. (2001). Together we're one? The place of the nation in media representations of the 1998 Kuala Lumpur Commonwealth Games. *Sociology of Sport Journal, 18,* 277–301.

Silver, J. (1996). *Thin ice: Money, politics, and the demise of an NHL franchise.* Halifax: Fernwood Books.

Smith, A. (1976). *An inquiry into the nature and causes of the wealth of nations.* Chicago: University of Chicago Press.

Smith, M. (1983). *Violence and sport.* Toronto: Butterworths.

Soroka, L. (2000). Male/female urban income inequality: The soaring nineties. *Canadian Journal of Regional Science/Revue canadienne des sciences régionales, 23,* 489–506.

Sparkes, R. (2000). Child sexual abuse in sport. In P. Donnelly, *Taking sport seriously: Social issues in Canadian sport* (pp. 108–111). Toronto: Thompson Publishing, Inc.

Special Olympics. (2006). *From backyard camp to global movement: The beginnings of Special Olympics*. Retrieved from http://www.specialolympics.org/Special+Olympics+Public+Website/English/About_Us/History/default.htm.

Spector, M. (2004, February 13). Not a pretty picture: Treadmill to obscurity. *National Post*, p. D8.

Spence, C. (1999). *The skin I'm in: Racism, sports and education*. Halifax: Fernwood.

Spence, J., & Gauvin, L. (1996). Drug and alcohol use by Canadian university athletes: A national survey. *Journal of Drug Education, 26*, 275–287.

Spence, J., Mandigo, J., Poon, P., & Mummery, W. (2001). A survey of physical education enrolment at the secondary level in Alberta. *Avante, 7*, 97–106.

Spencer, H. (1961). The nature of society. In T. Parsons, E. Shils, K. D Naegele, & J. R. Pitts (Eds.), *Theories of society: Foundations of modern sociological theory, Vol. I* (pp. 139–143). New York: The Free Press of Glencoe.

Spitzer, G. (2004). A Leninist monster: Compulsory doping and public policy in the G.D.R. and the lessons for today. In J. Hoberman & V. Moller (Eds.), *Doping and public policy* (pp. 133–144). Odense: University Press of Southern Denmark.

Sport Canada. (1998). *Sport participation in Canada*. Report prepared by Statistics Canada for Sport Canada. Ottawa: Minister of Public Works and Government Services Canada.

Sport Canada. (2002). *The Canadian sport policy*. Retrieved August 21, 2006 from http://www.canadianheritage.gc.ca/progs/sc/pol/pcs-csp/index_e.cfm.

Sport Canada. (2004). *Investing in sport participation: A discussion paper*. Ottawa.

Sport Canada. (2005). *Contribution guidelines 2006–2007*. Retrieved August 21, 2006 from http://www.canadianheritage.gc.ca/progs/sc/contributions/2006-2007/2006-2007_e.pdf.

Sport Canada. (2006). The Canadian sport policy (2002). Retrieved February 1, 2006 from http://www.pch.gc.ca/progs/pol/pcs-csp/indexc.efm.

Sport Participation in Canada. (1998). Report prepared by Statistics Canada for Sport Canada. Ottawa: Minister of Public Works and Government Services Canada.

Sporttek Performance Technology. (2006). FIFA World Cup 2006 limited edition watches. Retrieved December 27, 2006 from http://www.sporttek.co.uk/CASIO_FIFA_World_Cup_2006.html.

Spreitzer, E. (1994). Does participation in interscholastic athletics affect adult development? A longitudinal analysis of an 18–24 age cohort. *Youth & Society, 25*, 368–387.

Statistics Canada. (1998). *General Social Survey*. Ottawa: General Social Surveys Division, Statistics Canada.

Statistics Canada. (2001). Census, "Religions in Canada" analytic series, Catalogue 96F0030XIE2001015. Retrieved from http://www.statcan.ca/english/census01/products/analytic/companion/rel/canada.cfm.

Statistics Canada. (2002). Canadian statistics: Population. Retrieved from http://www.statcan.ca/english/Pgdb/popula.htm#pop/.

Statistics Canada. (2003). 2001 Census, Analysis series: Canada's ethnocultural portrait: The changing mosaic. Retrieved November 16, 2005 from http://www12.statcan.ca/english/census01/products/analytic/companion/etoimm/canada.cfm.

Statistics Canada. (2004). *Canadian community health survey*. Special Surveys Division. Retrieved from http://www.statcan.ca/Daily/English/040615/d040615b.htm.

Status of Women Canada. (2000). *Economic gender equality indicators*. Retrieved from http://www.swc-cfc.gc.ca/pubs/egei2000/egei2000_e.pdf.

Staudohar, P. D. (1996). *Playing for dollars: Labor relations and the sports business*. Ithaca: ILR Press & Cornell University Press.

Staudohar, P. D. (2005). The hockey lockout of 2004–05. *Monthly Labor Review, 128*, 23–9.

Stein, G. (1997). *Power play: An inside look at the business of the National Hockey League*. Secaucus, NJ: Birch Lane Press.

Stephan, Y., Bilard, J., Ninot, G., & Delignières, D. (2003a). Bodily transition out of elite sport: A one-year study of physical self and global self-esteem among transitional athletes. *Journal of Sport and Exercise Psychology, 1*, 192–207.

Stephan, Y., Bilard, J., Ninot, G., & Delignières, D. (2003b). Repercussions of transition out of elite sport on subjective well-being: A one-year study. *Journal of Applied Sport Psychology, 15*, 354–371.

Stephens, T., & Craig, C. (1990). *The well-being of Canadians*. Ottawa: CFLRI.

Stevenson, C. (1999). Becoming an international athlete: Making decisions about identity. In J. Coakley & P. Donnelly (Eds.), *Inside sports* (pp. 86–95). London & New York: Routledge.

Stevenson, C. L. (1986). College athletics and "character": The decline and fall of socialization research. In D. Chu & J. Segrave (Eds.), *Sport and higher education* (pp. 249–266). Champaign, IL: Human Kinetics.

Stevenson, C. L. (1991). The Christian-athlete: An interactionist-developmental analysis. *Sociology of Sport Journal, 8*, 362–379.

Stevenson, C. L. (1997). Christian athletes and the culture of elite sport: Dilemmas and solutions. *Sociology of Sport Journal, 14*, 241–262.

Stoddart, B. (1994). Sport, television, interpretation and practice reconsidered: Televised sport and analytical orthodoxies. *Journal of Sport and Social Issues, 18*, 76–88.

Stodolska, M., & Jackson, E. L. (1998). Discrimination in leisure and work experienced by a white ethnic minority group. *Journal of Leisure Research, 30*, 23–46.

Summerfield, L. (1990). Promoting physical activity and exercise among children. (n.p.): ERIC Clearinghouse on Teaching and Teacher Education ED328556.

Taylor, A. W. (1986). *The role of interuniversity athletics: A Canadian perspective*. Ottawa: Sports Dynamic.

Theberge, N. (2000). *Higher goals*. Albany, NY: SUNY Press.

Theberge, N., & Cronk, A. (1986). Work routines in newspaper sports departments and the coverage of women's sports. *Sociology of Sport Journal, 5*, 195–203.

Thelin, J. R. (1994). *Games colleges play: Scandal and reform in intercollegiate athletics*. Baltimore: Johns Hopkins Press.

The Sports Network (TSN). (1991). *Hockey, a white man's game?* Documentary. Toronto: The Sports Network.

Thomas, W. I., & Thomas, D. (1929). *The child in America*. Chicago: Alfred Knopf.

Thompson, S. T. (2002). Sport, gender, feminism. In J. Maguire & K. Young (Eds.), *Theory, sport & society* (pp. 105–127). Amsterdam: JAI.

Tirone, S. (2000). Racism, indifference and the leisure experiences of South Asian Canadian teens. *Leisure/Loisir: The Journal of the Canadian Association of Leisure Studies, 24*, 89–114.

Tirone, S. (2005). The challenges and opportunities faced by migrants and minorities in their leisure: An international perspective. Presented at the 10th International Metropolis Conference, Toronto.

Tirone, S., & Pedlar, A. (2000). Understanding the leisure experience of a minority ethnic group: South Asian teens and young adults in Canada. *Loisir et Societe/Society and Leisure, 23*, 145–169.

Todd, J., & Todd, T. (2000). Significant events in the history of drug testing and the Olympic movement: 1960–1999. In W. Wilson & E. Derse (Eds.), *Doping in elite sport: The politics of drugs in the Olympic movement* (pp. 65–128). Champaign, IL: Human Kinetics.

Todd, T. (1987). Anabolic steroids: The gremlins of sport. *Journal of Sport History, 14,* 87–107.

Torregrosa, M., Boixadós, M.,Valiente, L., & Cruz, J. (2004). Elite athletes' image of retirement: The way to relocation in sport. *Psychology of Sport and Exercise, 5,* 35–43.

Tremblay, M. S., Inman, J. W., & Willms, J. D. (2000). The relationship between physical activity, self-esteem, and academic achievement in 12-year-old children. *Pediatric Exercise Science, 12,* 312–323.

Tremaine Drahota, J. A., & Eitzen, D. S. (1998). The role exit of professional athletes. *Sociology of Sport Journal, 15,* 263–278.

United States Congress. (1972). *Title IX of the education amendments of 1972.* Retrieved from http://www.usdoj.gov/crt/cor/coord/titleixstat.htm.

United Way of Greater Toronto. (April, 2004). Poverty by postal code: The geography of neighbourhood poverty 1981–2001. Prepared jointly by the United Way and Canadian Council on Social Development, Toronto.

University of Toronto. (2004). *UTSC alumna makes history in sports and equality.* Retrieved from http://www.utsc.utoronto.ca/~advancement/alumni/blaney_broker.html.

Vancouver 2010. (2006). *Own the Podium—2010.* Retrieved from http://www.vancouver2010.com/en/WinterGames/OwnPodium.

Vaughan, G. (1996). *The puck stops here.* Fredericton: Goose Lane Editions.

Vertinsky, P., Batth, I., & Naidu, M. (1996). Racism in motion: Physical activity and the Indo-Canadian female. *Avante, 2,* 1–23.

Wagner, P. (1976). Puritan attitudes towards physical recreation in 17th century New England. *Journal of Sport History, 3,* 139–151.

Wakeford, C. (2003). Can small markets compete? Empirics on competitive balance in the NHL, Major paper, MA program, Department of Economics, University of Ottawa.

Wamsley, K. B. (1999). The public importance of men and the importance of public men: Sport and masculinities in nineteenth century Canada. In P. White & K. Young (Eds.), *Sport and gender in Canada* (pp. 24–39). New York: Oxford University Press.

Wamsley, K. B., & Kossuth, R. (2001). Fighting it out in nineteenth century Upper Canada/Canada West: Masculinities and physical challenges in the tavern. *Journal of Sport History, 27,* 405–30.

Wamsley, K. B., & Whitson, D. (1998). Celebrating violent masculinities: The boxing death of Luther McCarty. *Journal of Sport History, 25,* 419–31.

Wanta, W. (2006). The coverage of sports in print media. In A. Raney & J. Bryant (Eds.), *Handbook of sports and media* (pp. 105–115). New Jersey: Lawrence Erlbaum Publishers.

Warshaw, R. (1988). *I never called it rape.* New York: Harper and Row.

Washburne, R. F. (1978). Black underparticipation in wildland recreation: Alternative explanations. *Leisure Sciences, 1,* 175–189.

Weber, M. (1946). Class, status, party. In H. Gerth & C. W. Mills (Eds.), *From Max Weber: Essays in sociology* (pp. 180–195). New York: Oxford University Press.

Weider, B. (1976). The *strongest man in history: Louis Cyr.* Toronto: Mitchell Press.

Weiler, P. (2000). *Leveling the playing field: How the law can make sports better for fans.* Cambridge, MA: Harvard University Press.

Weisz, E., & Kanpol, B. (1990). Classrooms as socialization agents: The three R's and beyond. *Education, 111,* 100–04.

Welk, G. J. (1999). The youth physical activity model: A conceptual bridge between theory and practice. *Quest, 51,* 5–23.

Wells, C. (1996, March). Physical activity and women's health. *Research Digest, 2*(5). Retrieved from http://www.fitness.gov.

Wenner, L. A. (Ed.). (1998). *MediaSport.* London: Routledge.

West, C., & Zimmerman, D. (1991). Doing gender. In J. Lorber & S. Farrell (Eds.), *The social construction of gender* (pp. 13–37). London: Sage Publications.

Whannel, G. (2005). Pregnant with anticipation: The pre-history of television sport and the politics of recycling and preservation. *International Journal of Cultural Studies, 8,* 405–426.

White, G., Katz, J., & Scarborough, K. (1992). The impact of professional football games upon violent assaults on women. *Violence and Victims, 7,* 157–171.

White, P., & Wilson, B. (1999). Distinctions in the stands: An investigation of Bourdieu's "habitus," socio-economic status and sport spectatorship in Canada. *International Review for the Sociology of Sport, 34,* 245–64.

White, P., & Young, K. (1999a). Is sport injury gendered? In P. White & K. Young (Eds.), *Sport and gender in Canada* (pp. 69–84). Don Mills, ON: Oxford University Press.

White, P., & Young, K. (Eds.). (1999b). *Sport and gender in Canada.* Don Mills, ON: Oxford University Press.

White, P. G., & Curtis, J. E. (1990). Participation in competitive sport among anglophones and francophones in Canada: Testing competing hypotheses. *International Review for the Sociology of Sport, 25,* 125–142.

Whitson, D. (1998). Circuits of promotion: Media, marketing and the globalization of sport. In L. A. Wenner (Ed.), *MediaSport* (pp. 57–72). London: Routledge.

Whitson, D. (2001). Hockey and Canadian identities: From frozen rivers to revenue streams. In D. Taras & B. Rasporich (Eds.), *A passion for identity: Canadian studies for the 21st century* (pp. 217–236). Toronto: Nelson.

Whitson, D., & Gruneau, R. (Eds.). (2006). *Artificial ice: Hockey, commerce, and cultural identity.* Peterborough, ON: Broadview Press.

Whitson, D., & Macintosh, D. (1993). Becoming a world class city: Hallmark events and sport franchises in the growth strategies of western Canadian cities. *Sociology of Sport Journal, 10,* 221–40.

Whitson, D., Harvey, J., & Lavoie, M. (2000). The Mills report, the Manley subsidy proposals, and the business of major-league sport. *Canadian Public Administration, 43,* 127–156.

Wickberg, E. B. (1988). Chinese. *The Canadian encyclopedia,* 2nd ed., Vol. I (pp. 415–417). Edmonton: Hurtig Publishers.

Williams, J. (1994). The local and the global in English soccer and the rise of satellite television. *Sociology of Sport Journal, 11,* 376–397.

Willis, J. D., & Wettan, R. G. (1977). Religion in sport in America: The case for the sports bay in the Cathedral Church of St. John the Divine. *Journal of Sports History, 4,* 189–207.

Willis, P. (1990). *Common culture: Symbolic work at play in the everyday cultures of the young.* Philadelphia: Open University Press.

Willis, P., Dolby, N., & Dimitriadis, G. (Eds.). (2004). *Learning to labor in new times*. London: Routledge Falmer.

Wilson, B. (1997). Good blacks and bad blacks: Media constructions of African-American athletes in Canadian basketball. *International Review for the Sociology of Sport, 32,* 177–189.

Wilson, B. (1999). "Cool pose" incorporated: The marketing of black masculinity in Canadian NBA coverage. In P. White & K. Young (Eds.), *Sport and gender in Canada* (pp. 232–253). Don Mills, ON: Oxford University Press.

Wilson, B. (2006). Selective memory in a global culture: Reconsidering links between youth, hockey, and Canadian identity. In D. Whitson & R. Gruneau (Eds.), *Artificial ice: Hockey, culture, and commerce* (pp. 53–70). Peterborough, ON: Broadview Press.

Wilson, B., & White, P. (2002). Revive the pride: Social process, political economy, and a fan-based grassroots movement. *Sociology of Sport Journal, 19,* 119–148.

Wilson, T. C. (2002). The paradox of social class and sports involvement: The roles of cultural and economic capital. *International Review for the Sociology of Sport, 37,* 5–16.

Winter, J. (1997). *Democracy's oxygen: How corporations control the news*. Montreal: Black Rose Books.

Wolff, K. (2004). *The cost of hockey*. Retrieved from http://www.cbc.ca/sports/columns/ forthekids/cost.html.

Womack, M. (1992). Why athletes need ritual: A study of magic among professional athletes. In Shirl J. Hoffman (Ed.), *Sport and religion* (pp. 191–202). Champaign, IL: Human Kinetics.

Woolcock, M. (1998). Social capital and economic development: Toward a theoretical synthesis and policy framework. *Theory and Society, 27,* 151–208.

WordNet. (n.d.). Sport. Retrieved December 29, 2006 from http://wordnet.princeton.edu/ perl/webwn?s=sport.

World Anti-Doping Agency (WADA). (2003). *World anti-doping code* (version 3.0). Retrieved from http://www.wada-ama.org/docs/web/standards_harmonization/code/ code_v3.pdf.

Wright, J., & Clarke, G. (1999). Sport, the media and the construction of compulsory heterosexuality: A case study of women's rugby. *International Review for the Sociology of Sport, 34,* 227–243.

Wuest, D. A., & Bucher, C. A. (2003). *Foundations of physical education and sport*, 42nd ed. St. Louis: McGraw-Hill.

Yesalis, C. E., & Bahrke, M. S. (2002). History of doping in sport. *International Sports Studies, 24,* pp. 32–76.

Young, A. J. (1988). *Beyond heroes: A sport history of Nova Scotia*, Vol. 2. Hantsport, NS: Lancelot Press.

Young, J. (1997). The subterranean world of play. In H. Gerth & S. Thornton (Eds.), *The subcultures reader* (pp. 71–80). New York: Routledge.

Young, K. (1991). Sport and collective violence. *Exercise and Sport Science Review, 19,* 539–87.

Young, K. (1993). Violence, risk, and liability in male sports culture. *Sociology of Sport Journal, 10,* 373–96.

Young, K. (2002). From sports violence to sports crime: Aspects of violence, law, and gender in the sports process. In M. Gatz, M. Messner, & S. Ball-Rokeach (Eds.), *Paradoxes of youth and sport* (pp. 207–24). New York: SUNY Press.

Young, K. (Ed.). (2004). *Sporting bodies, damaged selves: Sociological studies of sports-related injury.* Amsterdam: Elsevier.

Young, K., & Wamsley, K. B. (1996). State complicity in sports assault and the gender order in twentieth century Canada: Preliminary observations. *Avante, 2,* 51–69.

Young, K., & White, P. (1995). Sport, physical danger and injury: The experiences of elite women athletes. *Journal of Sport and Social Issues, 19,* 45–61.

Young, K., White, P., & McTeer, W. (1994). Body talk: Male athletes reflect on sport, injury, and pain. *Sociology of Sport Journal, 11,* 175–94.

Zakus, D. H. (1988). A preliminary examination of the dialectical change in "modern" sport and of the intervention of the Canadian state in sport between 1968 and 1988. Unpublished doctoral dissertation, University of Alberta.

Zirin, D. (2005). *What's my name, fool? Sports and resistance in the United States.* Chicago: Haymarket Books.

CREDITS

This page constitutes an extension of the copyright page. We have made every effort to trace the ownership of all copyrighted material and to secure permission from copyright holders. In the event of any question arising as to the use of any material, we will be pleased to make the necessary corrections in future printings. Thanks are due to the following authors, publishers, and agents for permission to use the material indicated.

Chapter 1. 1: Yellow Dog Productions/The Image Bank/Getty Images 8: Based on data from Statistics Canada General Social Survey, 1998. 12: MATT DUNHAM/AP/CP Images 13: DAVE MARTIN/AP/CP Images

Chapter 2. 21: © CORBIS 29: KEVIN FRAYER/CP Images

Chapter 3. 41: Source: Library and Archives Canada/W. H. Coverdale collection of Canadiana/Accession no. 1970-188-2096/C-040148 57: Courtesy of Dr. Don Morrow

Chapter 4. 61: Photograph by Action Sports International, www.asiphoto.com 65: JACQUES DEMARTHON/AFP/Getty Images

Chapter 5. 79: Reprinted by permission of Harvey Alberta Trophy/Elite Sportwear Awards 79: From "Little Gidding," *Collected Poems* by T. S. Eliot (1943) pp. 31–39. Used with permission. 91: From the Public Archives of Nova Scotia/Tom Connors Collection

Chapter 6. 99: IT Stock Free/Picture Quest/Jupiter Images 106: © Royalty-Free/Corbis 112: Source: Economic Gender Equality Indicators 2000, 2002. Reproduced with the permission of the Minister of Public Works and Government Services, Courtesy of Statistics Canada and Status of Women Canada, 2006. Statistics Canada, "Canadian Social Trends," Catalogue 11-008, Spring 2001, no. 60. 113: Based on data from the Statistics Canada National Population Health Survey, 1996.

Chapter 7. 119: Bigshots/Photodisc Red/Getty Images 123: Based on data from the Statistics Canada General Social Survey, 1998. 124: © Clifford White Photography 133: © BananaStock/SuperStock

Chapter 8. 139: © Dimitri Iundt/TempSport/Corbis 147: KEVIN FRAYER/CP Images 152: Reprinted with permission of CAHPERD.

Chapter 9. 159: Photo by Matt Silver/TRU Athletics 170: ROB LINKE/CP Images

Chapter 10. 177: Bob Thomas/Stone/Getty Images 181: CP PHOTO/STRCOC/J. Gibson 184: Horne, J. and Manzenreiter, W. (2002: 197). The world cup and television football. In J. Horne and W. Manzenreiter (Eds.), *Japan, Korea and the 2002 World Cup*. London: Routledge. ISBN: 9780415275620/ISBN-10: 0415275628 189: CBC Still Photo Collection

Chapter 11. 197: ADRIAN WYLD/CP Images 204: JONATHAN HAYWARD/CP Images 213: Based on data from the Statistics Canada CANSIM database <http://cansim2.statcan.ca>, Table 176-0064, Series V37426.

Chapter 12. 221: CHUCK STOODY/CP Images 222: AP/CP Images 226: From *Beyond Policy Analyis*, Third Edition, by PAL, 2006. Reprinted with permission of Nelson, a division of Thomson Learning: www.thomsonrights.com. Fax 800 730-2215. 233: The Department of Canadian Heritage. Reproduced with the permission of the Minister of Public Works and Government Services Canada, 2006. 233: Sport Canada. (2002). *The Canadian sport policy*. The Department of Canadian Heritage. Reproduced with the permission of the Minister of Public Works and Government Services Canada, 2006.

Chapter 13. 239: © Stephane Reix/For Picture/Corbis **241:** © Comstock/SuperStock

Chapter 14. 257: CP PHOTO/Frank Gunn **264:** © Hulton-Deutsch Collection/CORBIS **266:** Reprinted with permission of Gerry Bowler. **268:** *L'Histoire du Hockey au Quebec.* Donald Guay. (1990). Reprinted with permission of Editions JCL. **268:** *L'Histoire du Hockey au Quebec.* Donald Guay. (1990). Reprinted with permission of Editions JCL. **268:** *L'Histoire du Hockey au Quebec.* Donald Guay. (1990). Reprinted with permission of Editions JCL. **271:** Michelle Donahue Hillison/Shutterstock

Chapter 15. 277: Adrian Brown/CP Images **277:** From "Burnt Norton" from *Collected Poems* by T. S. Eliot (1943). Used with permission. **285:** Sport participation in Canada. CH24-1/2000-1E-IN. The Department of Canadian Heritage. Reproduced with the permission of the Minister of Public Works and Government Services Canada, 2006. **286:** *Strengthening Canada: The socio-economic benefits of sport participation in Canada.* Conference Board of Canada. (2005). Downloaded from <www.conferenceboard.ca> on 16 September 2006. **286:** Sport participation in Canada. (1998). CH24-1/2000-1. The Department of Canadian Heritage. Reproduced with the permission of the Minister of Public Works and Government Services Canada, 2006. **287:** Based on data from the Statistics Canada General Social Survey, 1998. **287:** *Strengthening Canada: The socio-economic benefits of sport participation in Canada.* Conference Board of Canada. (2005). Downloaded from <www.conferenceboard.ca> on 16 September 2006. **290:** CP Images

INDEX